Essentials of Complementary and Alternative Medicine

Essentials of Complementary and Alternative Medicine

Edited by Brendon Gould

SYRAWOOD
PUBLISHING HOUSE

New York

Published by Syrawood Publishing House,
750 Third Avenue, 9th Floor,
New York, NY 10017, USA
www.syrawoodpublishinghouse.com

Essentials of Complementary and Alternative Medicine
Edited by Brendon Gould

International Standard Book Number: 978-1-68286-480-7 (Hardback)

The publisher's policy is to use permanent paper from mills that operate a sustainable forestry policy. Furthermore, the publisher ensures that the text paper and cover boards used have met acceptable environmental accreditation standards.

Trademark Notice: Registered trademark of products or corporate names are used only for explanation and identification without intent to infringe.

Cataloging-in-Publication Data

Essentials of complementary and alternative medicine / edited by Brendon Gould.
    p. cm.
Includes bibliographical references and index.
ISBN 978-1-68286-480-7
1. Alternative medicine. 2. Medicine, Chinese. 3. Integrative medicine. I. Gould, Brendon.
R733 .E87 2017
615.5--dc23

Printed in the United States of America.

TABLE OF CONTENTS

PREFACE

This book has been an outcome of determined endeavour from a group of educationists in the field. The primary objective was to involve a broad spectrum of professionals from diverse cultural background involved in the field for developing new researches. The book not only targets students but also scholars pursuing higher research for further enhancement of the theoretical and practical applications of the subject.

Alternative medicine or alternative therapies are interventional and pharmaceutical medicine that provide well-being but do not fall under scientific medical procedure. This book on complentary and alternative medicine discusses the innovative concepts of alternative medical practice. Various types of procedures can be classified together as alternative medicine such as traditional Chinese medicine, homeopathy, ayurveda, etc. These medical practices seek to promote a holistic understanding of the human body as well as its overall well-being. The various advancements in alternative medicine are glanced at and their applications as well as ramifications are looked at in detail. This book will serve as a reference to a broad spectrum of readers. It will help the readers in keeping pace with the rapid changes in this field.

It was an honour to edit such a profound book and also a challenging task to compile and examine all the relevant data for accuracy and originality. I wish to acknowledge the efforts of the contributors for submitting such brilliant and diverse chapters in the field and for endlessly working for the completion of the book. Last, but not the least; I thank my family for being a constant source of support in all my research endeavours.

Editor

Steamed and Fermented Ethanolic Extract from *Codonopsis lanceolata* Attenuates Amyloid-β-Induced Memory Impairment in Mice

Jin Bae Weon,[1] Min Rye Eom,[1] Youn Sik Jung,[1] Eun-Hye Hong,[2] Hyun-Jeong Ko,[2] Hyeon Yong Lee,[3] Dong-Sik Park,[4] and Choong Je Ma[1,5]

[1]Department of Medical Biomaterials Engineering, College of Biomedical Science, Kangwon National University, Chuncheon 200-701, Republic of Korea
[2]Laboratory of Microbiology and Immunology, College of Pharmacy, Kangwon National University, Chuncheon 200–701, Republic of Korea
[3]Department of Food Science and Engineering, Seowon University, Cheongju 361-742, Republic of Korea
[4]Functional Food & Nutrition Division, Department of Agro-Food Resources, Suwon 441-853, Republic of Korea
[5]Institute of Bioscience and Biotechnology, Kangwon National University, Chuncheon 200-701, Republic of Korea

Correspondence should be addressed to Choong Je Ma; cjma@kangwon.ac.kr

Academic Editor: Solomon Habtemariam

Codonopsis lanceolata (C. lanceolata) is a traditional medicinal plant used for the treatment of certain inflammatory diseases such as asthma, tonsillitis, and pharyngitis. We evaluated whether steamed and fermented C. lanceolata (SFC) extract improves amyloid-β- (Aβ-) induced learning and memory impairment in mice. The Morris water maze and passive avoidance tests were used to evaluate the effect of SFC extract. Moreover, we investigated acetylcholinesterase (AChE) activity and brain-derived neurotrophic factor (BDNF), cyclic AMP response element-binding protein (CREB), and extracellular signal-regulated kinase (ERK) signaling in the hippocampus of mice to determine a possible mechanism for the cognitive-enhancing effect. Saponin compounds in SFC were identified by Ultra Performance Liquid Chromatography-Quadrupole-Time-of-Flight Mass Spectrometry (UPLC-Q-TOF-MS). SFC extract ameliorated amyloid-β-induced memory impairment in the Morris water maze and passive avoidance tests. SFC extract inhibited AChE activity and also significantly increased the level of CREB phosphorylation, BDNF expression, and ERK activation in hippocampal tissue of amyloid-β-treated mice. Lancemasides A, B, C, D, E, and G and foetidissimoside A compounds present in SFC were determined by UPLC-Q-TOF-MS. These results indicate that SFC extract improves Aβ-induced memory deficits and that AChE inhibition and CREB/BDNF/ERK expression is important for the effect of the SFC extract. In addition, lancemaside A specifically may be responsible for efficacious effect of SFC.

1. Introduction

Alzheimer's disease (AD) is the most common progressive neurodegenerative disorder, causing memory and cognition impairment [1]. There are multiple causes of AD and it is likely that some causes have yet to be discovered. The characteristic pathogenesis of AD is accumulation of amyloid-β- (Aβ-) containing senile plaques and neurofibrillary tangles in the brain that lead to inflammation in surrounding tissue [2]. The presence of neurofibrillary tangles, composed of hyperphosphorylated tau (a microtubule-associated protein), and senile plaques correlate with cellular dysfunction. Aβ plays a significant role in the development of AD [3–5].

Acetylcholine (ACh) is a neurotransmitter involved in memory and learning processing in the cholinergic system. Acetylcholinesterase (AChE) is the enzyme that decreases ACh levels by hydrolysis. High AChE activity is present in the brains of AD patients [6, 7].

cAMP-response element-binding protein (CREB) also plays an essential role in learning and memory formation.

CREB is transcriptionally activated by phosphorylation at Ser-133 [8].

Brain-derived neurotrophic factor (BDNF), a member of the neurotrophin family, has been identified as a target gene of CREB. Downregulation of BDNF expression is associated with memory impairment [9]. CREB and BDNF expressions enhance long-term potentiation in neuronal plasticity [10]. Extracellular signal-regulated kinase (ERK) plays a fundamental role in cell death, cell proliferation, and neuronal plasticity and in activated CREB [11, 12].

Codonopsis lanceolata belongs to the Campanulaceae family and has been used as a traditional herbal medicine for the treatment of hypertension and several inflammatory diseases, such as asthma, tonsillitis, and pharyngitis. *C. lanceolata* contains various compounds such as saponins, alkaloids, tannins, steroids, and polysaccharides [13, 14]. Many previous reports have shown that *C. lanceolata* has antilipogenic, antiobesity, and anti-inflammatory effects, as well as being able to inhibit the production of TNF-α and nitric oxide, the expression of interleukin- (IL-) 3 and IL-6, and LPS-mediated phagocytic uptake in RAW 264.7 cells [15–17].

A cognitive-enhancing effect of steamed and fermented *C. lanceolata* (SFC), against scopolamine-induced memory impairment, has been reported in one of our previous studies [18]. In our present study, we confirm the effect of SFC on Aβ-induced memory deficits in the Morris water maze and passive avoidance tests. Furthermore, the AChE activity and expression of BDNF, CREB, and ERK phosphorylation in the hippocampus of these mice are evaluated.

2. Materials and Methods

2.1. Plant Materials. The roots of *C. lanceolata* were purchased from Hoengseong Deodeok direct outlet (Heongseong, Gangwon-Do of Korea, lines of longitude: 37° and latitude: 127°) and identified by Dr. Young Bae Seo, a professor of the College of Oriental Medicine, Daejeon University, a voucher specimen (LHY-001E). The *C. lanceolata* was dried in the shade at 20–30°C for 2 days and then steamed using a steam device (Dechang Stainless, Seoul, Korea) 5 times, for 8 hours each, at 90°C. The steamed *C. lanceolata* was aseptically inoculated with approximately 10^6 CFU/g of *Bifidobacterium longum* (KACC 20587), *Lactobacillus acidophilus* (KACC 12419), and *Leuconostoc mesenteroides* (KACC 12312) (1 : 1 : 1) in distilled water 8 times and subsequently fermented for 48 hours at 30°C.

600 g fermented *C. lanceolata* was extracted in 60 L with 70% (V/V) ethanol (100 g/10 L) for 24 hours during reflux extraction at 80°C. After evaporation, the fermented *C. lanceolata* (yield: 8.78%) was obtained using spray drying.

2.2. Chemical Material. Carboxymethyl cellulose (CMC), amyloid-β, donepezil, and acetylcholine were supplied by Sigma Aldrich Co. Ltd. (USA).

Primary antibodies (β-actin and BDNF) and secondary antibodies (goat-anti-rabbit IgG HRP and goat-anti-mouse IgG HRP) were purchased from Santa Cruz Biotechnology, Inc. (Dallas, USA).

2.3. Animals. Ten-week-old ICR mice (males weighing 25–30 g; Dae Han Biolink Co., Eumse-ong, Korea) were maintained in a temperature-controlled room (20 ± 3°C) with a 12/12-hour light-dark cycle and allowed access to commercial pellet feed and water *ad libitum*. Mice were housed 7 per cage (high: 13 cm, *W*: 20 cm, *L*: 25 cm) and allowed to adapt for a 1-week period before the *in vivo* test. All animal experiments in this study were approved by Kangwon National University Institutional Animal Care and Use Committee (KIACUC) (IACUC approval number KW-150706-1) and carried out according to the guidelines for laboratory animals.

2.4. Aβ Peptide Injection and Drug Administration. Aβ peptides were dissolved in distilled water and subsequently stored at −20°C. Aβ peptides were incubated at 37°C for 3 days to induce aggregation. Mice were injected in the bregma with a Hamilton microsyringe housing a 26-gauge needle.

SFC (300, 500, and 800 mg/kg) and donepezil (positive control, 1 mg/kg) were dissolved in 0.5% carboxymethylcellulose (CMC) administered orally to mice at a 2 hour before test trial for 4 days with daily for once on the Morris water maze test and the training trial for the passive avoidance test. Sample administration was started 3 days after Aβ peptide injection.

2.5. Morris Water Maze Test. The water maze test was performed as previously described with some modifications [19]. The water maze equipment consisted of a circular pool (90 cm in diameter and 40 cm in height), filled to a depth of 30 cm with water and maintained at a temperature of 20 ± 1°C. Areas of the maze were divided into four equal quadrants, and a white escape platform (10 cm in diameter and 26 cm in height) was submerged 1 cm below the surface of the water in the center of one quadrant. The platform was fixed, and starting points were changed on the outside of the pool each day. Mice were allowed an acquisition session in the absence of the platform for 60 seconds. Mice received a 120-second trial session for 4 consecutive days. The escape latency (seconds), the time to locate the platform, and all swimming behaviors of the mice were recorded and analyzed by the Smart (ver. 2.5.21) video-tracking system. After a 24-hour trial session, the platform was removed for the probe trial, and the time spent in the target quadrant was investigated for 60 seconds to determine the memory of the mice.

2.6. Passive Avoidance Test. The passive avoidance test was carried out as described in our previous study [18]. The passive avoidance apparatus (Gemini, San Francisco, USA) consisted of two equally sized compartments (17 cm × 12 cm × 10 cm), with an electrifiable grid floor, that were divided by a guillotine door. The mice received two trials, a training trial and test trial. On the first day, mice were allowed a training trial and were initially placed in the light compartment. The door between the two compartments was opened 20 seconds later and an electric foot shock (0.1 mA/10 g body weight,

2 sec duration) was delivered through the grid floor when the mice moved to the dark compartment. The latency time, the time that the mice took to move to the dark compartment, was recorded. After 24 hours, the mice were again placed into the light compartment for the test trial and the latency time was measured up to 180 seconds.

2.7. Acetylcholinesterase Activity Determination. Acetylcholinesterase (AChE) activity was measured using the Ellman method with slight modifications [20]. Mice were sacrificed by decapitation. The mouse brain was removed after completion of the behavioral tests, and the hippocampus was dissected from the brain. The hippocampus was rapidly homogenized with sodium phosphate buffer (pH 7.4) and preincubated for 5 minutes at 37°C. The homogenates were stored at −80°C and measured for AChE activity. The reaction mixture contained 33 μL homogenate, 470 μL sodium phosphate buffer, 167 μL DTNB, and 280 μL acetylcholine iodide. Following incubation for 5 minutes, absorbance was measured at 412 nm using a spectrophotometer.

2.8. Tissue Preparation and Western Blot Analysis. Mice were sacrificed by decapitation. Mouse brains were promptly collected and the hippocampus was excised 30 minutes after the behavior tests. Mouse hippocampal tissues were homogenized in ice-cold RIPA buffer containing a protease inhibitor cocktail and centrifuged at 13,000 ×g for 20 minutes to remove particulate matter. The supernatants were stored at −80°C and total protein concentrations were measured using the Bradford assay. The supernatants containing 20–50 μg protein were subjected to 15% SDS-PAGE for 2-3 hours at 100 V and transferred to PVDF membrane at 200 V and 60 mA. After transfer, the membrane was blocked in 5% skimmed milk for 1 hour at room temperature and incubated (overnight at 4°C) with primary antibodies: β-actin (1 : 2000 dilution), BDNF (1 : 1000 dilution), CREB (1 : 1000 dilution), p-CREB (1 : 500 dilution), ERK (1 : 1000 dilution), and p-ERK (1 : 1000 dilution). Following incubation with primary antibody, the membranes were washed with 0.1% PBST and incubated with the corresponding secondary antibody (goat-anti-rabbit IgG HRP 1 : 2000 dilution for BDNF, donkey-anti-goat IgG HRP 1 : 2000 dilution for p-CREB and p-ERK and goat-anti-mouse IgG HRP 1 : 2000 dilution for CREB, ERK and β-actin) for 1 hour at room temperature. Immunoreactive signals were visualized on X-ray with enhanced chemiluminescence (ECL).

2.9. UPLC Analysis of Steamed and Fermented C. lanceolata. Steamed and fermented *C. lanceolata* was analyzed with a Waters ACQUITY UPLC system (Waters, Milford, MA, USA) that was equipped with the Waters Synapt Mass spectrometry system (Waters, Milford, MA, USA) in order to identify saponin compounds. Analysis was performed on an ACQUITY BEH C_{18} (2.1 × 100 mm, 1.7 μm, Waters, Milford, MA, USA) at 35°C. The mobile phase consisted of water with 0.1% formic acid (67%) and acetonitrile (33%) and was applied at a flow rate of 0.2 mL/min during a run time of 15 mins.

The desolvation gas temperature was set at 100 and 400°C with a desolvation gas flow of 30 and 600 L/h. The capillary voltage was set at 2.5 kV and the cone voltage was up to 45 V.

2.10. Statistical Analysis. Statistical analyses were performed using SPSS 1.9. All data from the Morris water maze test, passive avoidance test, and AChE activity values, as well as Western blotting, were performed by one-way ANOVA and Turkey's post hoc test. All experimental data were expressed as the mean ± SEM and $p < 0.05$, $p < 0.01$, and $p < 0.001$ were considered statistically significance.

3. Results

3.1. The Cognitive-Enhancing Effect of SFC Extract on Aβ-Induced Spatial Memory Impairment. The effect of SFC extract on Aβ-induced spatial memory impairment was investigated using the Morris water maze test. The control group showed a decrease in escape latency from day 1 to day 4. The escape latency for the untreated memory impaired group significantly increased after day 1. 500 and 800 mg/kg doses of SFC in the treated group showed significantly reduced escape latency during the 2nd and 4th trial days ($p < 0.005$). The donepezil-treated group, a positive control group, showed a decreased escape latency time during the 4 trial days ($p < 0.005$) (Figure 1). In addition, the SFC-treated group showed a decreased mean swimming distance for 4 days compared with the untreated memory impaired group (Figure 2(a)). However, we confirmed that there was no significant difference with the average swimming speed of mice between the groups during the 4-day test (Figure 2(b)). The results suggest that locomotor activity of the mice did not affect escape latency time. In the probe test, the control group showed a significantly increased swimming time in the target quadrant after the platform was removed. The untreated memory impaired group, however, showed a shorter time spent in the target quadrant than the control group, and the swimming time in the target quadrant by the untreated memory impaired mice was significantly increased when treated with SFC ($p < 0.005$) (Figure 3).

We investigated the effect of SFC extract on Aβ-induced memory deficit in the passive avoidance test to assess long-term memory. The untreated memory impaired group showed an increased latency time compared with the control group. The SFC-treated group (500 and 800 mg/kg doses) significantly ameliorated the shortened latency time of the memory impaired mice in a dose-dependent manner (Figure 4). The donepezil-treated group also showed a significant increase in latency time similar to that with the SFC-treated group.

3.2. Inhibitory Effect of SFC on Acetylcholinesterase Activity. High AChE activity plays an important role in memory impairment. We analyzed the AChE activity in the hippocampus of Aβ-induced memory impaired mice in order to assess the effect of SFC (Table 1). The AChE activity was significantly increased in the hippocampus of these memory impaired mice as compared with the control group. SFC

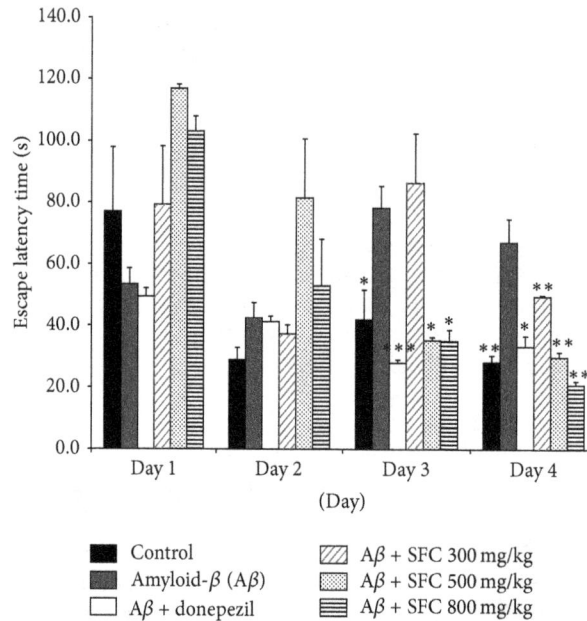

FIGURE 1: The effect of steamed and fermented *C. lanceolata* on escape latency in Aβ-induced memory impaired mice in the Morris water maze test. The donepezil (1 mg/kg body weight, PO) and the steamed and fermented *C. lanceolata* (SFC) groups (300, 500, and 800 mg/kg body weight, PO) are treated for 90 minutes before cognitive impairment by Aβ administration. The escape latency of each groups' training trial session are presented. The values shown are the mean escape latency ± SEM ($n = 7$). (*$p < 0.05$, **$p < 0.01$, and ***$p < 0.001$ versus Aβ-treated mice). SFC: steamed and fermented *C. lanceolata*.

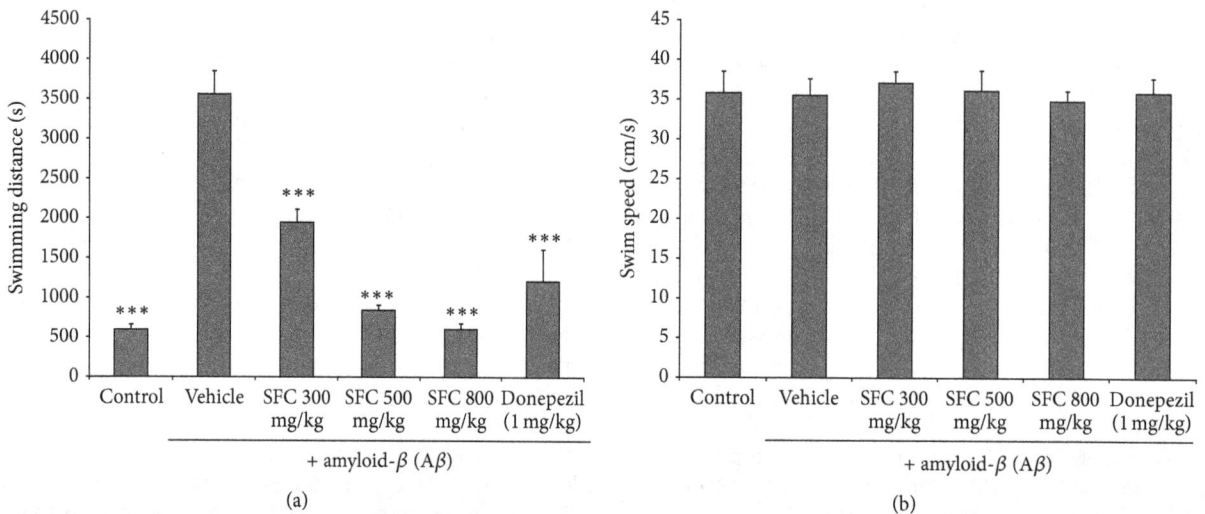

(a)

(b)

FIGURE 2: (a) The mean swimming distance to the platform in the Morris water maze test. (b) The mean swimming speed of each group during the 4 trial days in the Morris water maze test. Results are expressed as the mean ± SEM. ($n = 7$) ***$p < 0.001$ compared with the Aβ-treated group. SFC: steamed and fermented *C. lanceolata*.

treatment significantly inhibited AChE activity at the doses of 500 and 800 mg/kg, when compared with the untreated memory impaired mice. Donepezil, used as positive control, also showed a decrease in the AChE activity of memory impaired mice.

3.3. The Effect of SFC on BDNF Expression, CREB, and ERK Phosphorylation.
The activation of CREB and BDNF improved long-term memory. In addition, the ERK pathway is known to exert memory function. Therefore, in this study we decided to evaluate the effect of SFC on BDNF, p-CREB, and p-ERK expression in the hippocampus using Western blot analysis.

As shown in Figure 5, the hippocampal expression of BDNF, p-CREB, and p-ERK in the untreated memory impaired mice was lower than that of the control group. SFC (300, 500, and 800 mg/kg, PO) treatment significantly increased expression of all three proteins.

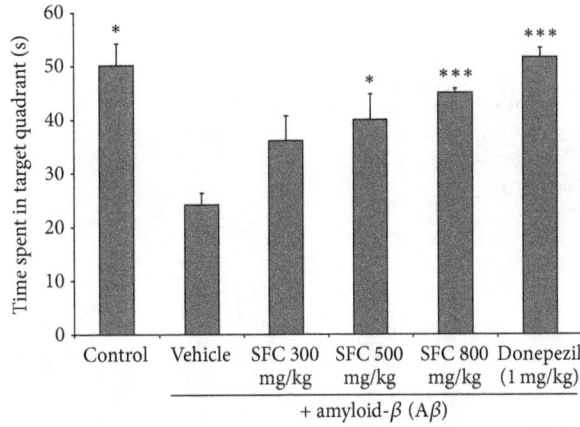

FIGURE 3: The mean escape latency of each group in the probe trial. The time spent in the target quadrant during the probe trial is presented. Data represent the mean ± SEM. $^*p < 0.05$ and $^{***}p < 0.001$ versus the Aβ-treated group. SFC: steamed and fermented C. lanceolata.

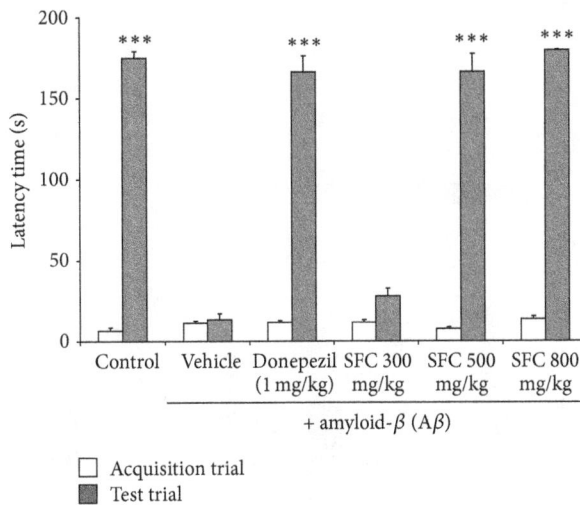

FIGURE 4: The effect of steamed and fermented C. lanceolata on Aβ-induced memory impairment in the passive avoidance test. The latency time to move to the dark compartment was recorded. The mean latency time (s) ± SEM ($n = 7$) $^{***}p < 0.001$ compared with the scopolamine group. SFC: steamed and fermented C. lanceolata.

TABLE 1: The inhibition of steamed and fermented C. lanceolata on acetylcholinesterase (AChE) activity in the hippocampus of mice. Data represent the mean ± SD. $^*p < 0.05$ versus the Aβ-treated group. SFC: steamed and fermented C. lanceolata.

	Groups	U/mg protein
	Control	1.59 ± 0.17*
	Scopolamine	2.54 ± 0.76
	Donepezil	1.85 ± 0.77*
SFC	300 mg/kg	2.29 ± 0.42
	500 mg/kg	1.35 ± 0.25*
	800 mg/kg	1.20 ± 0.37*

p-ERK expression induces CREB phosphorylation with the increase of BDNF activation in the hippocampus. These results indicate that BDNF activation and CREB and ERK phosphorylation can be suppressed by Aβ-treatment of mice and that the SFC-induced increase in BDNF and p-CREB expression may be dependent on p-ERK signaling.

3.4. UPLC-Q-TOF-MS Analysis of Steamed and Fermented C. lanceolata.
Saponin compounds are known to be the main compounds within C. lanceolata. Therefore, SFC extract was analyzed by UPLLC-Q-TOF to identify the specific saponin compounds present. The total ion chromatogram is shown in Figure 6. Compounds were detected within 5 minutes and were identified according to characteristic m/z values of mass spectrometry. Retention time and calculated mass data of the compounds is given in Table 2. The results of the UPLC-Q-TOF-MS analysis indicate that lancemasides A, B, C, D, E, and G and foetidissimoside A are the main compounds contained in SFC. We did not identify the compounds from peaks 5, 7, 8, and 10 and further study by NMR was needed to identify these peaks.

(a)

(b)

(c)

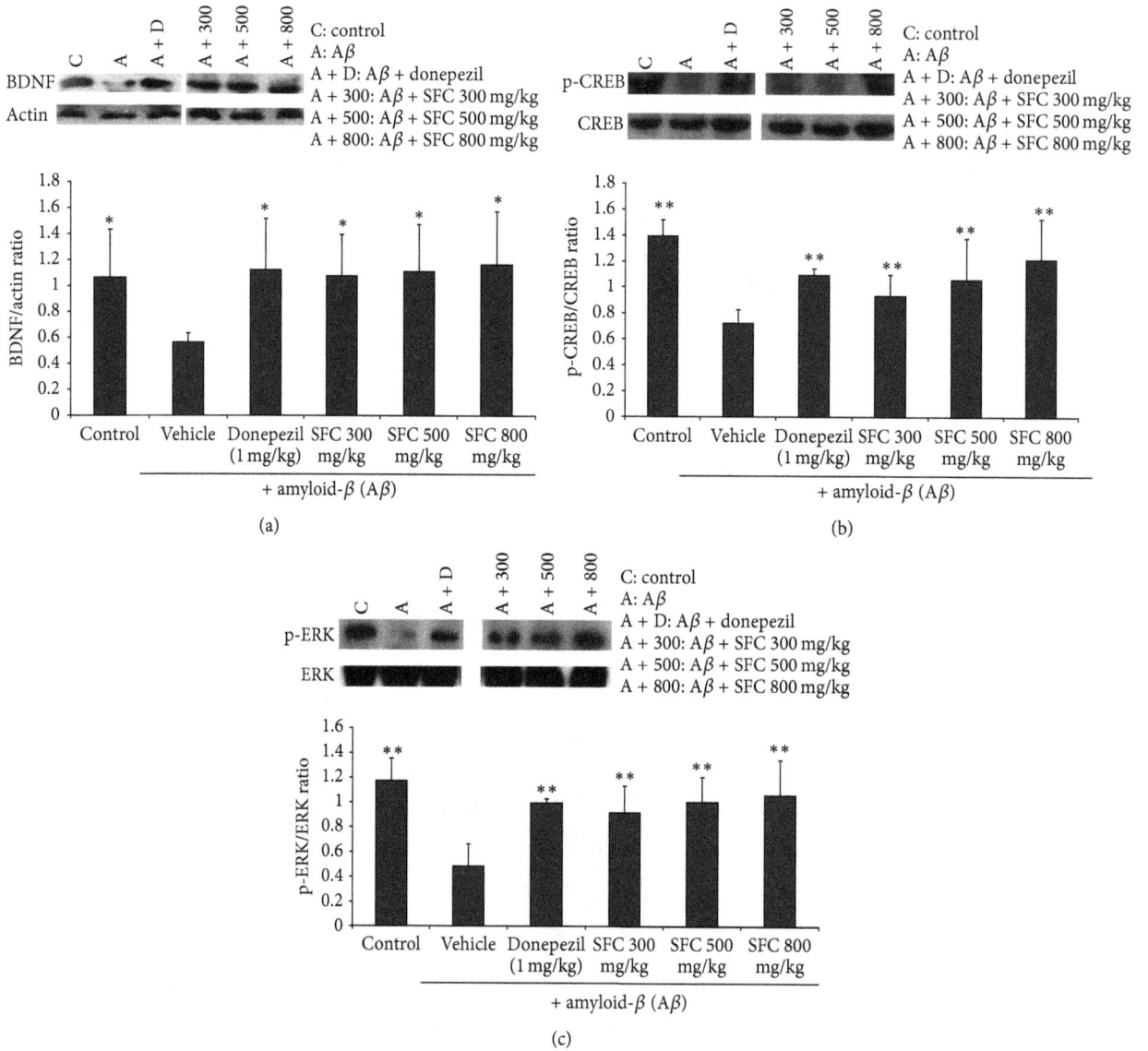

FIGURE 5: The effect of steamed and fermented *C. lanceolata* on BDNF, CREB, and ERK signaling in the hippocampus by Western blot analysis. Data represent the mean ± SD. $^*p < 0.05$ and $^{**}p < 0.01$ versus the Aβ-treated group. SFC: steamed and fermented *C. lanceolata*.

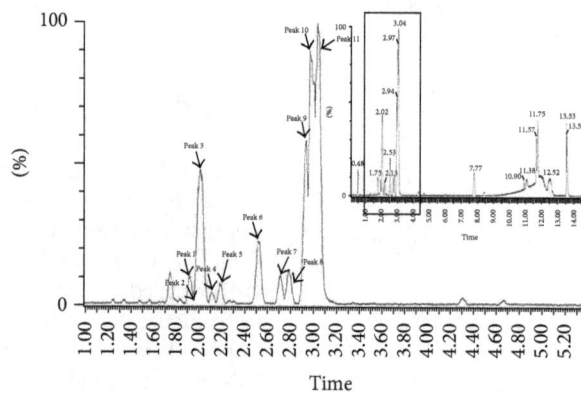

FIGURE 6: Total ion chromatogram of saponin compounds in steamed and fermented *C. lanceolate*: (1) lancemaside C, (2) lancemaside C, (3) lancemaside B, (4) lancemaside D, (5) unknown, (6) lancemaside E, (7) unknown, (8) unknown, (9) foetidissimoside A, (10) unknown, and (11) lancemaside A.

TABLE 2: Characterization of saponin compounds from SFC.

Peak	t_R (min)	m/z ES(−)	Assignment
1	1.93	1219.5748	Lancemaside C
2	1.99	1205.5591	Lancemaside G
3	2.02	1351.617	Lancemaside B
4	2.12	1087.5325	Lancemaside D
5	2.19	1189.5642	Unknown
6	2.53	1351.617	Lancemaside E
7	2.71	1219.5748	Unknown
8	2.78	1189.5642	Unknown
9	2.94	1057.5219	Foetidissimoside A
10	2.98	1189.5642	Unknown
11	3.02	1189.5642	Lancemaside A

4. Discussion

Our previous studies confirmed that SFC attenuates memory impairment induced by scopolamine in mice [18]. Scopolamine inhibits cholinergic activity and produces memory impairment. Pathophysiology of AD includes not only cholinergic blockade but also $A\beta$ deposition in the brain. $A\beta$ is a 40–42 amino acid peptide fragment of amyloid precursor protein (APP). Accumulation of $A\beta$ deposits causes the degeneration of cholinergic neuron function and oxidative stress. In this study, we evaluated the effect of SFC on $A\beta$-induced memory impairment in mice using the Morris water maze and passive avoidance tests. The Morris water maze is the most widely used behavioral test to study hippocampal-dependent spatial learning and memory in mice [19]. The passive avoidance test is also known as a fear-aggravated test to assess long-term memory retention based on the administration of an aversive stimulus such as a foot shock [21].

We confirmed that SFC improves memory and learning in mice with $A\beta$-induced deficits using the Morris water maze and passive avoidance tests. SFC significantly reduced escape latency time from day 2 to day 4, meaning that long-term memory impairment improved in the Morris water maze test. In the passive avoidance test, SFC also increased the latency time shortened by $A\beta$-induced memory impaired mice. These results imply that SFC has a cognitive effect on $A\beta$ treatment-induced memory impairment. Result of mean swimming speed was indirectly suggested that C. lanceolate extract was not affected on health and locomotor of mice. In this study, we did not observe any adverse health effect after administering the drug.

Previous studies have confirmed that $A\beta$ affects AChE activity. Ach was hydrolyzed by AChE at central cholinergic synapses and $A\beta$ increased AChE activity by the reduction of gene expression of muscarinic M1 receptor in hippocampus [22]. The increased neurotoxicity from the $A\beta$-AChE complexes induced an increase in intracellular Ca^{2+} and mitochondrial membrane potential loss in hippocampal neurons [23, 24]. In this study, the hippocampus of memory impaired

mice treated with SFC was observed to have lower AChE activity in a dose-dependent manner. This result suggests that the effect of SFC may be associated with the muscarinic cholinergic receptor and may reverse cognitive impairment by affecting AChE activity in brain.

The high level of $A\beta$ accumulation interfered with neuronal activity by suppressing BDNF expression and phosphorylation of p-CREB [25]. The activation of CREB and BDNF plays an important role in the learning and memory process. Phosphorylation of CREB in order to switch on its transcriptional activity leads to an upregulation of many specific target genes, including BDNF (phosphorylated at Ser-133) [26]. Upregulation of BDNF gene expression enhances LTP and memory formation at hippocampal and cortical synapses [27, 28].

We investigated the effect of SFC on CREB phosphorylation and BDNF expression in $A\beta$-injected mice by Western blot analysis. We confirmed that SFC increases BDNF expression and p-CREB levels in hippocampus of these mice.

Signaling of ERK, a member of the mitogen-activated protein kinase (MAPK) superfamily, also has an important role in learning and memory. ERK1/2 signaling mediates the activation of CREB, which participates in the protein kinase A- (PKA-) dependent LTP. Administration of SFC increased ERK signaling in the hippocampus of $A\beta$-induced memory impaired mice.

In the present study, saponin compounds in SFC were analyzed by UPLC-Q-TOF-MS. Seven compounds present, characterized according to MS data, are lancemasides A, B, C, D, E, and G and foetidissimoside A. Among the seven saponin compounds, lancemaside A is a major saponin that represents the pharmacological activities of Codonopsis lanceolate [29]. Lancemaside A ameliorated scopolamine-induced memory and learning deficits in mice on the passive avoidance, Y-maze, and Morris water maze tasks and lanscemaside A inhibited AChE activity and induced BDNF and p-CREB expression in the brain [30].

The results presented herein suggest that the cognitive-enhancing effect of SFC in behavioral tests correlates with the activation of the p-ERK/p-CREB/BDNF pathway, which plays an important role in learning and memory formation. In addition, the effect of SFC may be associated with the action of the compound lancemaside A contained within.

Steamed and fermented C. lanceolata improved the amyloid-β-induced memory deficit during behavioral tests. In addition, fermented C. lanceolata inhibited AChE activity and increased p-CREB and BDNF expression.

5. Conclusion

In summary, we investigated the cognitive-enhancing effect of steamed and fermented C. lanceolata in the Morris water maze and passive avoidance tests. Steamed and fermented C. lanceolata ameliorated amyloid-β–induced memory impairment and this effect appears to be mediated via the inhibition of AChE activity and the activation of BDNF, p-CREB, and ERK signaling. Further studies will be conducted in order to determine the role of fermented C. lanceolata on the CREB and BDNF expression pathway. Thus, steamed and fermented *C. lanceolata* could be a potential therapeutic agent for the prevention and treatment of neurodegenerative diseases such as AD.

List of Abbreviations

SFC:	Steamed and fermented *C. lanceolata*
AChE:	Acetylcholinesterase
BDNF:	Brain-derived neurotrophic factor
CREB:	Cyclic AMP response element-binding protein
ERK:	Extracellular signal-regulated kinase
UPLC-Q-TOF-MS:	Ultra Performance Liquid Chromatography-Quadrupole-Time-of-Flight Mass Spectrometry.

Competing Interests

The authors have declared that there is no conflict of interests.

Acknowledgments

This work was carried out with the support of "Cooperative Research Program for Agriculture Science & Technology Development (Project no. PJ009001)" Rural Development Administration, Republic of Korea. The authors thank Professor Eun-Joo Shin in Kangwon National University for excellent technical and thoughtful comments.

References

[1] D. R. Crapper and U. DeBoni, "Brain aging and Alzheimer's disease," *Canadian Psychiatric Association Journal*, vol. 23, no. 4, pp. 229–233, 1978.

[2] D. Collerton, "Cholinergic function and intellectual decline in Alzheimer's disease," *Neuroscience*, vol. 19, no. 1, pp. 1–28, 1986.

[3] S. Sadigh-Eteghad, B. Sabermarouf, A. Majdi, M. Talebi, M. Farhoudi, and J. Mahmoudi, "Amyloid-beta: a crucial factor in Alzheimer's disease," *Medical Principles and Practice*, vol. 24, no. 1, pp. 1–10, 2015.

[4] F. S. Esch, P. S. Keim, E. C. Beattie et al., "Cleavage of amyloid β peptide during constitutive processing of its precursor," *Science*, vol. 248, no. 4959, pp. 1122–1124, 1990.

[5] J. J. Palop and L. Mucke, "Amyloid-B-induced neuronal dysfunction in Alzheimer's disease: from synapses toward neural networks," *Nature Neuroscience*, vol. 13, no. 7, pp. 812–818, 2010.

[6] J. T. Coyle, D. L. Price, and M. R. DeLong, "Alzheimer's disease: a disorder of cortical cholinergic innervation," *Science*, vol. 219, no. 4589, pp. 1184–1190, 1983.

[7] C. G. Ballard, "Advances in the treatment of Alzheimer's disease: benefits of dual cholinesterase inhibition," *European Neurology*, vol. 47, no. 1, pp. 64–70, 2002.

[8] C. A. Saura and J. Valero, "The role of CREB signaling in Alzheimer's disease and other cognitive disorders," *Reviews in the Neurosciences*, vol. 22, no. 2, pp. 153–169, 2011.

[9] P. Bekinschtein, M. Cammarota, I. Izquierdo, and J. H. Medina, "Reviews: BDNF and memory formation and storage," *The Neuroscientist*, vol. 14, no. 2, pp. 147–156, 2008.

[10] F. Calabrese, G. Guidotti, G. Racagni, and M. A. Riva, "Reduced neuroplasticity in aged rats: a role for the neurotrophin brain-derived neurotrophic factor," *Neurobiology of Aging*, vol. 34, no. 12, pp. 2768–2776, 2013.

[11] Q.-L. Ma, M. E. Harris-White, O. J. Ubeda et al., "Evidence of Aβ- and transgene-dependent defects in ERK-CREB signaling in Alzheimer's models," *Journal of Neurochemistry*, vol. 103, no. 4, pp. 1594–1607, 2007.

[12] G. Perry, H. Roder, A. Nunomura et al., "Activation of neuronal extracellular receptor kinase (ERK) in Alzheimer disease links oxidative stress to abnormal phosphorylation," *NeuroReport*, vol. 10, no. 11, pp. 2411–2415, 1999.

[13] S. Yongxu and L. Jicheng, "Structural characterization of a water-soluble polysaccharide from the roots of *Codonopsis pilosula* and its immunity activity," *International Journal of Biological Macromolecules*, vol. 43, no. 3, pp. 279–282, 2008.

[14] M. Ushijima, N. Komoto, Y. Sugizono et al., "Triterpene glycosides from the roots of *Codonopsis lanceolata*," *Chemical & Pharmaceutical Bulletin*, vol. 56, no. 3, pp. 308–314, 2008.

[15] S. E. Byeon, W. S. Choi, E. K. Hong et al., "Inhibitory effect of saponin fraction from *Codonopsis lanceolata* on immune cell-mediated inflammatory responses," *Archives of Pharmacal Research*, vol. 32, no. 6, pp. 813–822, 2009.

[16] H. S. Ryu, "Effect of Codonopsis lanceolatae extracts on mouse IL-2, IFN-, IL-10 cytokine production by peritoneal macrophage and the ratio of IFN-, IL-10 cytokine," *The Korean Journal of Food And Nutrition*, vol. 22, no. 1, pp. 69–74, 2009.

[17] J. P. Li, Z. M. Liang, and Z. Yuan, "Triterpenoid saponins and anti-inflammatory activity of *Codonopsis lanceolata*," *Die Pharmazie*, vol. 62, no. 6, pp. 463–466, 2007.

[18] J. B. Weon, B.-R. Yun, J. Lee et al., "Cognitive-enhancing effect of steamed and fermented *Codonopsis lanceolata*: a behavioral and biochemical study," *Evidence-Based Complementary and Alternative Medicine*, vol. 2014, Article ID 319436, 9 pages, 2014.

[19] R. Morris, "Developments of a water-maze procedure for studying spatial learning in the rat," *Journal of Neuroscience Methods*, vol. 11, no. 1, pp. 47–60, 1984.

[20] G. L. Ellman, K. D. Courtney, V. Andres Jr., and R. M. Feather-Stone, "A new and rapid colorimetric determination of acetylcholinesterase activity," *Biochemistry & Pharmacology*, vol. 7, pp. 88–95, 1961.

[21] J. O'Keefe and L. Nadel, *The Hippocampus as a Cognitive Map*, Clarendon Press, Oxford, UK, 1978.

[22] C.-H. Jin, E.-J. Shin, J.-B. Park et al., "Fustin flavonoid attenuates β-amyloid (1–42)-induced learning impairment," *Journal of Neuroscience Research*, vol. 87, no. 16, pp. 3658–3670, 2009.

[23] J. B. Melo, P. Agostinho, and C. R. Oliveira, "Involvement of oxidative stress in the enhancement of acetylcholinesterase activity induced by amyloid beta-peptide," *Neuroscience Research*, vol. 45, no. 1, pp. 117–127, 2003.

[24] A. E. Reyes, M. A. Chacón, M. C. Dinamarca, W. Cerpa, C. Morgan, and N. C. Inestrosa, "Acetylcholinesterase-Aβ complexes are more toxic than Aβ fibrils in rat hippocampus: effect on rat β-amyloid aggregation, laminin expression, reactive astrocytosis, and neuronal cell loss," *American Journal of Pathology*, vol. 164, no. 6, pp. 2163–2174, 2004.

[25] L. Tong, P. L. Thornton, R. Balazs, and C. W. Cotman, "β-amyloid-(1–42) impairs activity-dependent cAMP-response

element-binding protein signaling in neurons at concentrations in which cell survival is not compromised," *The Journal of Biological Chemistry*, vol. 276, no. 20, pp. 17301–17306, 2001.

[26] S. Kida, "A functional role for CREB as a positive regulator of memory formation and LTP," *Experimental Neurobiology*, vol. 21, no. 4, pp. 136–140, 2012.

[27] D. Panja and C. R. Bramham, "BDNF mechanisms in late LTP formation: a synthesis and breakdown," *Neuropharmacology*, vol. 76, pp. 664–676, 2014.

[28] C. R. Bramham and E. Messaoudi, "BDNF function in adult synaptic plasticity: the synaptic consolidation hypothesis," *Progress in Neurobiology*, vol. 76, no. 2, pp. 99–125, 2005.

[29] O. Shirota, K. Nagamatsu, S. Sekita et al., "Preparative separation of the saponin lancemaside A from *Codonopsis lanceolata* by centrifugal partition chromatography," *Phytochemical Analysis*, vol. 19, no. 5, pp. 403–410, 2008.

[30] I.-H. Jung, S.-E. Jang, E.-H. Joh, J. Chung, M. J. Han, and D.-H. Kim, "Lancemaside A isolated from *Codonopsis lanceolata* and its metabolite echinocystic acid ameliorate scopolamine-induced memory and learning deficits in mice," *Phytomedicine*, vol. 20, no. 1, pp. 84–88, 2012.

Evaluating Emotional Well-Being after a Short-Term Traditional Yoga Practice Approach in Yoga Practitioners with an Existing Western-Type Yoga Practice

Maxi Meissner,[1] **Marja H. Cantell,**[2] **Ronald Steiner,**[3] **and Xavier Sanchez**[4]

[1]*Department of Organizational Psychology, Faculty of Behavioural and Social Sciences, University of Groningen, Netherlands*
[2]*Centre for Special Educational Needs and Youth Care, Faculty of Behavioural and Social Sciences,*
 University of Groningen, Netherlands
[3]*Sport- und Rehamedizin Universitätsklinikum Ulm, Germany*
[4]*Department of Medical and Sport Sciences, University of Cumbria, Lancaster, UK*

Correspondence should be addressed to Maxi Meissner; m.meissner@rug.nl

Academic Editor: Lisa A. Conboy

The purpose of the present study was to examine the influence of a traditional yoga practice approach (morning daily practice, TY) compared to that of a Western yoga practice approach (once-twice weekly, evening practice, WY) on determinants of emotional well-being. To that end, in a pre/posttest between-subject design, measures of positive (PA) and negative affect (NA), mindfulness, perceived stress, and arousal states were taken in 24 healthy participants (20 women; mean age: 30.5, SD = 8.1 years) with an already existing WY practice, who either maintained WY or underwent a 2-week, five-times-per-week morning practice (TY). While WY participants maintained baseline values for all measures taken, TY participants showed significant beneficial changes for PA, NA, and mindfulness and a trend for improved ability to cope with stress at the completion of the intervention. Furthermore, TY participants displayed decreased subjective energy and energetic arousal. Altogether, findings indicate that the 2-week TY is beneficial over WY for improving perceived emotional well-being. The present findings (1) undermine and inspire a careful consideration and utilization of yoga practice approach to elicit the best benefits for emotional well-being and (2) support yoga as an evidence-based practice among healthy yoga practitioners.

1. Introduction

Over the twentieth century yoga has become a popular practice in the Western world, with an estimated 30 million people regularly practicing yoga worldwide [1]. The practice of yoga consists of eight limbs (universal moral and ethical principles, individual self-restraint, physical postures, breath control, calming of the senses, concentration, meditation, and pure contemplation) and is thought to facilitate health and well-being [2]. In fact, as substantiated by an ever-growing body of empirical research, yoga is emerging as a complementary practice improving physical, mental, and, especially, emotional health [3].

Parameters associated with emotional health entail affect, mindfulness, perceived stress, and arousal states. Affect is the automatic evaluation of a stimulus as positive (positive affect, PA) or negative (negative affect, NA). While NA is associated with increased subjective stress, aversive mood states, anxiety, depression, low self-esteem, and narrow attention [4, 5], PA is associated with optimism and greater tendencies to cope [6]. Mindfulness has been described as the systematic development of the ability to nonjudgmentally direct attention towards events in the field of consciousness [7]. Perceived stress represents the degree to which one's life is appraised as stressful [8] and furthermore, increased levels of perceived stress are associated with increased emotional distress [9]. Generally speaking, any state of arousal is located on a particular level of two bipolar dimensions, that is, energetic (EA) and tense arousal (TA). EA ranges from tiredness at the low end to energy at the upper end while

TA ranges from calmness at the low end to tension at the upper end [10]. Arousal states have been linked with valence (pleasure versus displeasure); in other words, high energetic arousal (energy) and low tense arousal (calmness) are perceived as pleasant or positive. In contrast, high tense arousal (tension) and low energy (tiredness) are perceived as unpleasant or negative [11].

Altogether, affect, mindfulness, perceived stress, and arousal states have all been demonstrated to change into a beneficial direction when exposing previously yoga-naïve subjects, healthy [12–16] as well as clinical populations [11, 17], to yoga. Notably, most previous research concerning the effect of yoga on parameters of emotional well-being has largely concentrated on previously yoga-naïve participants. The effectiveness of an existing yoga practice on emotional well-being has not yet received much attention.

With regard to yoga practice frequency, previous yoga intervention studies have mostly focused on three different types of yoga practitioners: 1–3-times-weekly practice [18], >3-times-weekly practice [19], or previously yoga-naïve subjects exposed to 1–3-times-weekly yoga practice [11, 13, 14]. These more recreational practice frequencies are in strong disparity to how yoga is traditionally practiced, that is, a daily practice in the morning. This type of frequent practice is advocated to facilitate psychological and physiological health most effectively [20].

Notably, in a cross-sectional study of American Iyengar practitioners average practice frequencies (class attendance combined with home practice) amounted to about 4-5-times-weekly yoga practice [21], paralleling traditional practice frequencies. In this survey, class practice frequency was found an independent predictor of subjective well-being and mindfulness and negatively related to sleep disturbance [21]. Importantly, per day of additional home practice benefits were further increased for subjective well-being and sleep quality. In this cross-sectional survey average practice frequencies (class attendance combined with home practice) amounted to about 4-5-times-weekly yoga practice, altogether providing support for the advocated traditional practice approach. Yet, taking into account the cross-sectional and anonymous survey nature of the previous study, causality cannot be implied. Moreover authors reported a dropout rate of 27% which may have biased the results.

Thus, although cross-sectional data suggests that the traditional way of practicing yoga provides further health outcome benefits compared to the Western practice approach, yoga practice frequency has so far not been directly manipulated in a yoga intervention study. Therefore, the effects of an ongoing and more traditional daily practice have not yet been established.

The aim of the current study was to evaluate the effectiveness of a short-term (two-week) traditional-type yoga practice (five mornings per week, TY) with an ongoing once-to-twice-per-week evening yoga practice (Western yoga approach, WY) on parameters that measure perceived emotional health. More specifically, we compared affect scores using PA and NA (as measured by the Positive Affect and Negative Affect Schedule, PANAS [22]), mindfulness scores

(the Mindful Attention Awareness Scale, MAAS [23]), perceived stress levels (the Perceived Stress Scale, PSS [8]), and arousal states such as energy, tension, tiredness, and calmness (the Activation-Deactivation Adjective Checklist, AD ACL [10]) before and at the end of a 2-week TY intervention. Findings from the current study will in their part help to better understand the psychological health outcomes and effectiveness related to Western and traditional approaches to practicing yoga. Ultimately, results of this study promote specific yoga practice prescriptions to better integrate yoga as an evidence-based alternative and complementary practice for emotional health benefits.

2. Materials and Methods

2.1. Participants. Twenty-four healthy subjects (20 women; mean age: 30.5, SD = 8.1 years) living in the northern part of Netherlands who were already practicing ashtanga yoga once or twice per week for a minimum of at least three months were recruited from a yoga school. Based on personal preference and time availability for the following two weeks, participants chose (convenience sample) to either maintain their regular yoga practice of once or twice per week in the evening time (Western yoga practice approach, WY, $n = 12$) or engage in a yoga practice at a frequency of five times per week between 07:00 h and 08:30 h in the morning (traditional approach to yoga practice, TY, $n = 12$).

2.2. Instruments. The following validated and widely used measures were administered at baseline and at the end of the two-week TY intervention (2-week point): the Positive Affect and Negative Affect Schedule (PANAS) [22], the Mindful Attention Awareness Scale (MAAS [23]), the Perceived Stress Scale (PSS) [8], and the Activation-Deactivation Adjective Checklist (AD ACL) [10].

The PANAS [22] was used to assess participants' mood over the previous week. It comprises 20 items and two subscales of 10 items each: positive affect (PA, score range 1–5; higher values correspond to more positive affect) and negative affect (NA, score range 1–5; higher values correspond to more distress). Cronbach's α was 0.83 and 0.78 for PA, at baseline and the 2-week point, respectively, and 0.88 and 0.88 for NA at baseline and the 2-week point, respectively. The Mindful Attention Awareness Scale (MAAS) [23] assessed participants' core characteristics of dispositional mindfulness over the previous week, specifically, receptive awareness of and attention to what is taking place in the present. It contains 15 items on a scale called mindfulness. Scores range from 1 to 6 and higher scores correspond to more mindfulness. Cronbach's α was 0.85 at baseline and $\alpha = 0.87$ at the 2-week point. Perception of stress was determined by the Perceived Stress Scale [8]. The PSS contains 10 items that assess participants' feelings and thoughts during the previous week and produce one scale: perceived stress. Cronbach's α was 0.87 at baseline and 0.85 at the 2-week point. To evaluate arousal states over the previous week, the 20-item Activation-Deactivation Adjective Checklist (AD ACL) was used [24]. The AD ACL consists of four subscales (5 items each): energy (score range 1–4; higher scores correspond to more energy; Cronbach's α was 0.81 at baseline and 0.86 at the 2-week point), tiredness (score range 1–4; higher scores correspond to more tiredness; Cronbach's α was 0.86 at baseline and 0.88 at the 2-week point), tension (score range 1–4; higher scores correspond to more tension; Cronbach's α was 0.82 at baseline and 0.73 at the 2-week point), and calmness (score range 1–4; higher scores correspond to more calmness; Cronbach's α was 0.70 at baseline and 0.60 at the 2-week point). Combining the subscales energy and tiredness yields energetic arousal (EA) while combining the subscales tension and calmness yields tense arousal (TA).

Moreover, the Measure of Affect Regulation Style (MARS) [25], trait questionnaire, was used to measure participants affect regulation patterns at baseline. The 38 items assess how frequently participants utilize certain affect regulatory strategies. It consists of seven subscales, each scoring from 1 to 7 (higher scores corresponding to increased engagement in each strategy): active distraction (Cronbach's α was 0.73 at baseline), cognitive engagement (Cronbach's α was 0.77), behavioral engagement (Cronbach's α was 0.51), venting and expressing affect (Cronbach's α was 0.74), passive distraction (Cronbach's α was 0.11), rumination and withdrawal (Cronbach's α was 0.43), and waiting and reframing (Cronbach's α was 0.37). It is worth noting that the last three subscales yielded low internal consistency, which appears to be similar to prior work using the MARS [25]. Despite this, all subscales were included for analyses (specially for the passive distraction subscale). A demographic questionnaire was completed by each participant including age, gender, and the number of years/months of yoga practice.

Lastly, a manipulation check was undertaken during the first and the second week of the TY intervention in order to ensure that the perception of the yoga classes and the teacher's performance was similar in both groups. Immediately after each yoga class, participants rated the quality of each yoga class and the performance of the teacher by means of a visual-analogue scale—marking on a 10 cm line where the point at 0 cm corresponded to "very poor" and at 10 cm corresponded to "outstanding."

2.3. *Procedure.* A pre/posttest, between-group study was conducted to test our hypotheses (see Figure 1 for design details). Ethical approval was gained from the Ethics Committee of the Faculty of Behavioural and Social Sciences at the University of Groningen, Netherlands, and participants signed an informed consent form before the study began. After signing the consent form, participants were given unique study identification codes. Identities of the participants were kept confidential. Next, all participants received an e-mail from the researcher with an electronic link to the instructions and questionnaires. The first set of questionnaires served as a baseline measurement and consisted of the demographic questionnaire, the PANAS, MAAS, PSS, AD ACL, and the MARS. Participants were instructed to complete all the questionnaires at the day of their yoga practice, with at least two hours after the yoga

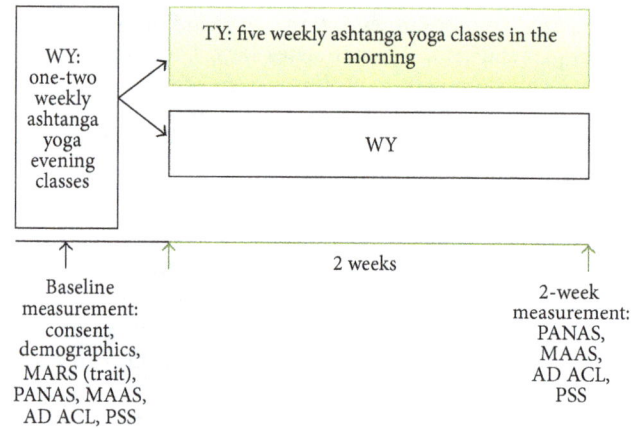

FIGURE 1: Research design. WY = Western yoga practice approach (yoga practice one to two times per week, in the evening), TY = traditional yoga practice approach (yoga practice five times per week in the morning), MARS = Measure of Affect Regulatory Style, PANAS = Positive Affect and Negative Affect Schedule, MAAS = Mindful Attention Awareness Scale, AD ACL = Activation-Deactivation Adjective Checklist, and PSS = Perceived Stress Scale.

practice in order to avoid acute effects of the practice on outcome measures and not more than 6 hours after the yoga practice.

One week after the baseline measurements, participants in the TY group increased their ashtanga yoga practice frequency to five times per week for the following two weeks. All TY participants participated in ten 90-minute long ashtanga yoga morning classes, Monday to Friday (07:00 h–08:30 h) for two weeks; these classes were instructed similarly as the classes they had taken previously in the evening time at their regular yoga school.

TY participants completed the PANAS, MAAS, PSS, and AD ACL at the end of the two weeks of the TY practice (the 2-week point). WY participants completed the same questionnaires during the same week as the TY. All participants completed the 2-week-point questionnaire with at least two hours passing after their yoga practice, but not more than 6 hours. WY participants maintained their evening practice (18:00 h–19:30 h).

We utilized ashtanga-style yoga in this study. Ashtanga yoga is considered a vigorous practice as it is characterized by a combination of physically challenging asanas, practiced as appropriate for each individual practitioner, while attempting to maintain mental focus and awareness to the breath, altogether meant to facilitate a meditative movement practice [26]. In the present study, each 90-minute class followed a similar format: check-in, breath awareness and centering, sun salutations, standing poses, sitting poses, back bends, finishing poses, and relaxation. To accommodate different ranges of physical capabilities, variations to each pose were given and participants were encouraged to consistently monitor sensations in body and mind and practice in a noncompetitive and sensible manner.

TABLE 1: Baseline demographics and affect regulation style.

	WY ($n = 12$)	TY ($n = 12$)	t	p
Demographics				
Age, mean ± SD	30.2 ± 7.9	30.9 ± 8.3	−0.823	0.823
Gender, n (%) female	9 (75.0)	11 (91.7)	−1.076	0.294
Yoga practice experience				
Overall mean ± SD	1.7 ± 1.3	2.00 ± 1.4	−0.616	0.544
n (%)				
2–6 months	2 (16.7)	1 (8.3)		
Up to 1 year	4 (33.3)	4 (33.4)		
Up to 2 years	4 (33.3)	3 (25.0)		
<2 years	2 (16.7)	4 (33.3)		
Affect regulation style,				
mean ± SD				
Active distraction	3.16 ± 0.89	3.04 ± 0.79	−0.339	0.739
Cognitive engagement	3.38 ± 1.42	3.63 ± 0.73	0.540	0.594
Behavioral engagement	3.14 ± 0.98	3.10 ± 0.64	−0.123	0.903
Venting/expressing affect	3.22 ± 1.20	3.43 ± 0.90	0.500	0.622
Passive distraction	1.85 ± 0.25	2.19 ± 0.25	1.080	0.292
Rumination/withdrawal	3.38 ± 0.25	3.04 ± 0.25	0.121	0.383
Waiting/reframing	2.27 ± 0.28	2.77 ± 0.28	0.055	0.957

Baseline demographic characteristics and affect regulation style (Measure of Affect Regulatory Style Score, MARS) in yoga practitioners practicing under a Western approach to practice (WY) and practitioners with an existing WY practice who were about to start the 2-week traditional practice approach (TY). Data are expressed in mean ± SD unless otherwise specified. Independent Student's t-test was performed to compare means between groups. t = t-value, p = p value.

2.4. Data Analysis. For the manipulation check we used an independent samples t-test to check for differences in yoga class perception and teacher rating between WY and TY participants at week 1 and also at week 2 of the TY intervention. An independent t-test was used to examine differences in baseline scores in age, gender, yoga practice experience, PA, NA, MAAS, PSS, AD ACL, and MARS measures between WY and TY participants. We also used independent sample t-tests to examine differences in these variables between WY and TY participants at two weeks. Then, to test the effectiveness of a two-week TY practice in previous WY practitioners, we conducted repeated measures ANOVAs with one related factor on two levels (time: baseline and two-week scores for the dependent variables: PA, NA, MAAS, PSS, and AD ACL scores) and for one unrelated factor (the independent variable: condition, WY and TY). Additionally, we conducted a paired t-test to investigate for differences in PA, NA, MAAS, PSS, and AD ACL measures from baseline to the 2-week point in WY and TY participants.

Furthermore, to investigate the relationships between PA, NA, MAAS, PSS, and AD ACL scores of all participants at the 2-week point, Pearson's coefficient, r, was calculated. Herein, r was considered weak (0.10). All values were expressed as mean (M) ± SD, unless otherwise noted. Alpha was set at 0.05 for all statistical analysis and SPSS 20 software was used for all statistical calculations.

3. Results

There were no differences in age, gender distribution, and duration of yoga practice experience between groups

(Table 1). Furthermore, WY and TY participants utilized similar affect regulatory strategies and no differences in any of the affect regulatory strategies measured were observed (Table 1).

Adherence to the yoga classes in both WY and TY participants was outstanding; all 24 participants completed the study. Only one TY participant missed one class (third day of the TY practice) due to a headache, yet this participant was included in all analyses. The manipulation check revealed that the ashtanga yoga classes and the performance of the teacher were perceived similarly by the TY and WY participants during the 2-week duration of the study (Table 2).

3.1. Positive and Negative Affect. Significant baseline differences were apparent between both groups in PA ($p = 0.007$) and NA ($p = 0.033$) subscales of the PANAS. However, at the 2-week point, no such differences were observed and both groups displayed similar values for PA ($p = 0.663$) and NA ($p = 0.480$). The repeated measures ANOVA for PA showed an effect of time ($F(1, 22) = 26.8$, $p = 0.0001$, Partial Eta Squared = 0.549, and observed power = 0.999) and an interaction of time and condition ($F(1, 22) = 9.3$, $p = 0.006$, Partial Eta Squared = 0.295, and observed power = 0.827, Figure 2(a)). Paired sample t-test revealed that PA scores remained constant in WY participants from baseline to the 2-week point (M = 3.48, SD = 0.48 and M = 3.70, SD = 0.55 at baseline and the 2-week point, resp., $p = 0.160$) while TY practitioners displayed an approximate 27% increase in PA scores from baseline to the 2-week point (M = 2.98, SD = 0.34 and M = 3.78, SD = 0.38 at baseline and the 2-week point, resp., $p = 0.0001$).

(a) Positive affect

(b) Negative affect

(c) Mindfulness

(d) Perceived stress

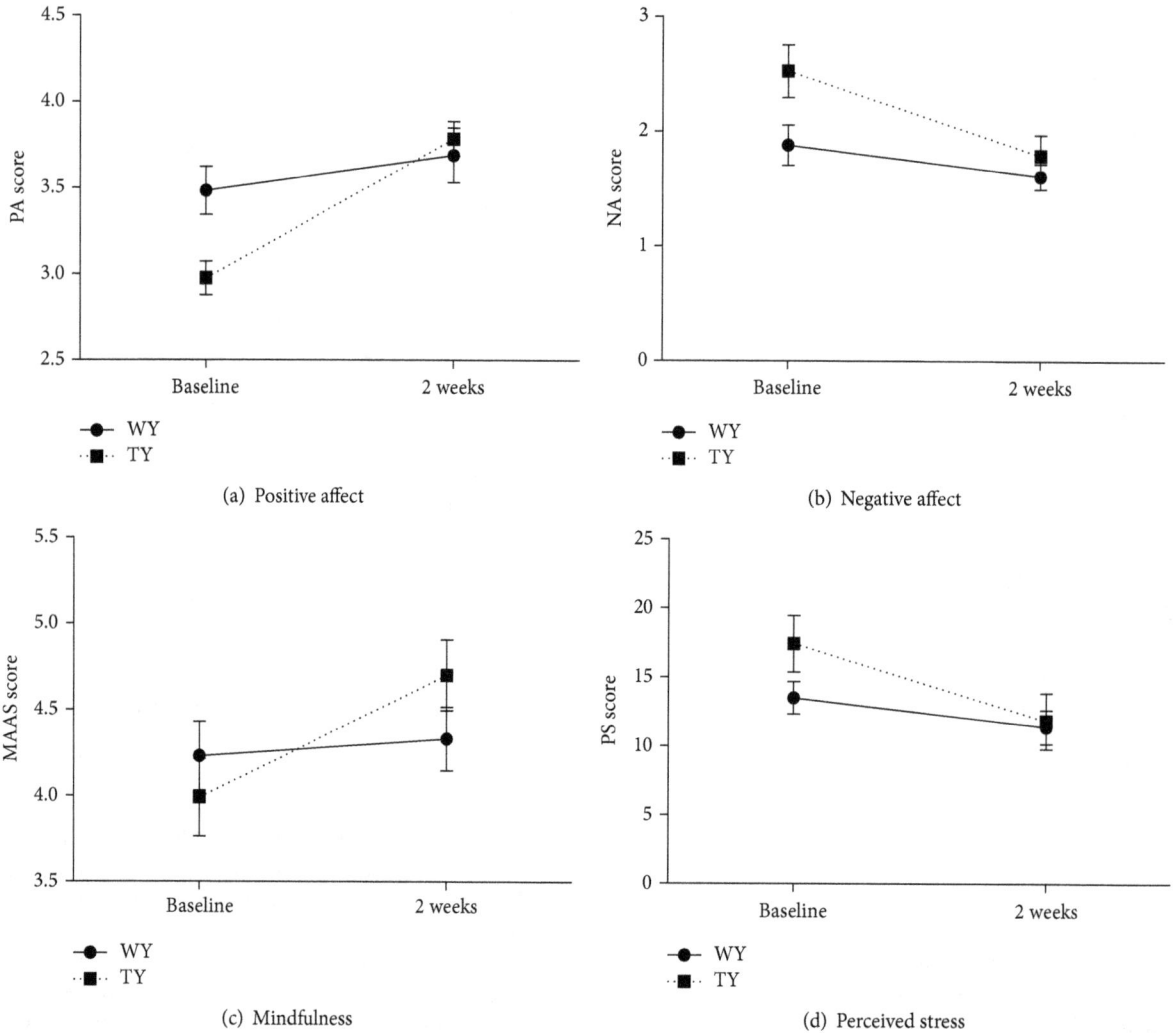

FIGURE 2: Positive affect (a) and negative affect (b) scores as measured by the PANAS, mindfulness scores (measured by MAAS), and perceived stress (measured by PSS) in yoga practitioners practicing under a Western approach to practice (WY) and practitioners with an existing WY practice who underwent the two-week traditional practice approach (TY) at baseline (0 weeks) and at 2-week-point TY practice (2 weeks). Data are represented as mean ± SD.

TABLE 2: Rating of yoga classes and yoga teacher during the intervention.

	WY ($n = 12$)	TY ($n = 12$)	t	p
Rating of yoga class	8.1 ± 1.2	7.9 ± 1.5	−2.943	0.794
Rating of yoga teacher	8.5 ± 1.1	8.9 ± 0.9	0.837	0.234

Overall rating of yoga classes ("How do you feel about class today?") and yoga teacher performance ("How do you rate the performance of the yoga teacher today?") presented in mean ± SD. For yoga practitioners maintaining their Western approach to practice (WY) the average of the two yoga classes that were attended in this two-week period was calculated. For yoga practitioners who underwent the 2-week traditional yoga practice approach (TY), averages of ratings obtained after each of the 10 classes were obtained. Independent Student's t-test was performed to compare means between groups. t = t-value, p = p value.

Moreover, the repeated measures ANOVA for NA revealed an effect of time ($F(1, 22) = 15.0$, $p = 0.001$, Partial Eta Squared = 0.406, and observed power = 9.59)

and a trend for a significant interaction between time and condition ($F(1, 22) = 3.1$, $p = 0.092$, Partial Eta Squared = 0.124, and observed power = 0.392, Figure 2(b)). Notably, the paired sample t-test demonstrated an approximate 29% decrease in NA scores in TY participants from baseline to the 2-week point (M = 2.53, SD = 0.76 and M = 1.80, SD = 0.79 at baseline and the 2-week point, resp., $p = 0.003$). As expected, WY participants maintained the same level of NA from baseline to the 2-week point (M = 1.88, SD = 0.61 and M = 1.61, SD = 0.38 at baseline and the 2-week point, $p = 0.136$).

3.2. Mindfulness. Both groups displayed similar scores for mindfulness at baseline ($p = 0.439$). A time effect ($F(1, 22) = 9.4$, $p = 0.006$, Partial Eta Squared = 0.299, and observed power = 0.83) and interaction between time and condition ($F(1, 22) = 5.3$, $p = 0.031$, Partial Eta Squared = 0.195, and observed power = 0.59) were observed upon repeated measures ANOVA (Figure 2(c)). Although no difference in mindfulness between WY participants was observed at the 2-week point ($p = 0.200$), TY participants displayed a significant increase (by approximately 17.5%) in their mindfulness scores from baseline (M = 4.00, SD = 0.78) to the 2-week point (M = 4.70, SD = 0.64, $p = 0.006$). By contrast, no changes in mindfulness were observed in WY participants from baseline (M = 4.23, SD = 0.54) to the 2-week point (M = 4.33, SD = 0.71, $p = 0.550$). Altogether, these findings indicate that a two-week TY practice is effective in improving one's ability to be present in the moment.

3.3. Perceived Stress. While scores for perceived stress tended to be higher at baseline (by approximately 22%), albeit nonsignificantly ($p = 0.131$) in TY (M = 17.42, SD = 7.08) compared to WY (M = 13.50, SD = 3.69) participants, both groups displayed similar values at the 2-week point (TY: M = 11.83, SD = 7.04; WY: M = 11.40, SD = 3.86, $p = 0.864$). Paired sample t-test analysis demonstrated a trend towards a significant decrease in perceived stress in TY participants from baseline to the 2-week point ($p = 0.063$, Figure 2(d)). This is indicative of a beneficial effect of TY on perceived stress. Repeated measures ANOVA revealed no effect of time (baseline, two-week point) nor an interaction of time and condition.

3.4. Arousal States. Table 3 displays scores for arousal states at baseline and the 2-week point. At baseline TY participants displayed a significantly higher EA value compared to WY participants. This showed as approximately 28% higher energy score in TY compared to WY participants, while tiredness scores were similar between both groups at baseline (Table 3). Repeated measures ANOVA for EA revealed a significant effect of time ($F(1, 22) = 4.18$, $p = 0.048$, Partial Eta Squared = 0.181, and observed power = 0.516) and a significant interaction between time and condition ($F(1, 22) = 7.303$, $p = 0.014$, Partial Eta Squared = 0.267, and observed power = .729). While no differences were observed between both groups at the 2-week point, paired sample t-test showed a ≈15% decrease in EA scores in TY participants from baseline to the 2-week point ($p = 0.004$). This showed as a decrease in energy scores ($p = 0.005$), as scores for tiredness remained unchanged in this period for TY ($p = 0.344$). EA scores for WY participants remained similar from baseline to the 2-week point ($p = 0.702$).

Scores for TA, as well as for its subscales tension and calmness, were all similar for both groups at baseline (Table 3). No effect of time or interaction between condition and time was observed by repeated measures ANOVA for TA or its subcomponents tension and calmness. Also paired t-test did not reveal any change in any of these parameters from baseline to the 2-week point in WY or TY participants.

3.5. Correlations between PA, NA, MAAS, PSS, and AD ACL Scores of All Participants at the 2-Week Point. Several relationships across parameters of emotional well-being were observed at the 2-week point ($n = 24$). A moderate positive relationship was found between PA and mindfulness ($r =$

TABLE 3: Arousal states.

	WY	TY	t	p
Energetic arousal				
Baseline	23.18 ± 5.04	27.33 ± 2.02	2.643	0.015
2-week point	23.18 ± 3.70	23.33 ± 2.87	0.112	0.912
Tense arousal				
Baseline	26.45 ± 2.77	27.08 ± 4.08	0.523	0.673
2-week point	25.82 ± 3.52	26.25 ± 2.34	0.354	0.730
Energy scores				
Baseline	10.27 ± 4.26	14.25 ± 2.52	2.750	0.012
2-week point	11.00 ± 3.52	12.17 ± 3.60	−1.071	0.298
Tiredness scores				
Baseline	12.90 ± 2.34	13.08 ± 1.88	0.189	0.845
2-week point	12.18 ± 2.13	13.92 ± 1.83	2.091	0.298
Tension scores				
Baseline	16.55 ± 2.54	14.92 ± 5.10	−0.963	0.350
2-week point	16.36 ± 3.67	16.00 ± 3.13	−0.262	0.800
Calmness scores				
Baseline	9.91 ± 2.21	12.17 ± 3.61	1.791	0.089
2-week point	9.45 ± 2.01	10.25 ± 2.45	0.843	0.408

Energetic arousal, tense arousal, energy, tiredness, tension, and calmness scores as measured by the AD ACL in yoga practitioners practicing under a Western approach to practice (WY) and practitioners with an existing WY practice who underwent the 2-week traditional practice approach (TY) at baseline (0 weeks) and at the end of the 2-week TY practice (2 weeks). Data are represented as mean ± SD. t = t-value, p = p value.

0.436, $p = 0.017$) indicating that as participants felt more positive, they also experienced more mindfulness. Moreover, strong positive relationships were observed between NA and EA ($r = 0.502$, $p = 0.015$) and NA and perceived stress ($r = 0.633$, $p = 0.000$), as well as a moderate positive relationship between EA and perceived stress ($r = 0.383$, $p = 0.087$). All in all these positive relationships suggest that as participants perceived more stress and energetic arousal, they concurrently felt more negative.

Additionally, a strong negative relationship was observed between PA and perceived stress ($r = −0.503$, $p = 0.017$), illustrating that as participants felt more positive they perceived less stress. Further, strong negative relationships were reported between mindfulness and NA ($r = −0.483$, $p = 0.017$) as well as mindfulness and perceived stress ($r = −0.692$, $p = 0.000$). Moderate negative relationships were found between PA and EA ($r = −0.349$, $p = 0.103$) and NA and TA ($r = −0.362$, $p = 0.089$). In sum, these negative relationships imply that the more mindful the participants were, the less stressed and negative they felt.

4. Discussion

While the benefits of yoga interventions for emotional well-being have been widely explored in previously yoga-naïve participants practicing under a more recreational, Western approach (i.e., 1–3 times weekly [11, 13–15, 17]), the effects of an ongoing and more traditional daily practice approach have so far only been substantiated by cross-sectional survey study with a large dropout rate [21]. We aimed to directly evaluate the effectiveness of a short-term (2-week) traditional yoga practice approach (TY) with an ongoing Western yoga practice approach (WY) on parameters of emotional well-being. Results of the present study demonstrate that several parameters of emotional well-being were improved in TY participants at the completion of the WY intervention suggesting clear benefits of a TY compared to maintaining WY. More precisely, completing a short-term, 2-week, five-times-per-week morning practice in participants who previously practiced yoga in the evenings once or twice a week led to significant improvements in their scores for PA, NA, and mindfulness, alongside a trend for improved levels of perceived stress. Altogether, our results inspire the utilization of a yoga practice approach that is based on careful consideration of the frequency and time of the day to elicit the best benefits for emotional well-being.

In terms of a particular yoga practice approach (frequency and time of practice) and its efficiency in benefiting parameters of emotional well-being, our results are difficult to compare to previous research, as the effects of different yoga practice approaches have not been previously explored directly. Yet, our yoga intervention results undermine Ross et al. [21] findings from their American cross-sectional survey in Iyengar yoga practitioners. The authors of the previous study observed that practice frequency was an independent predictor of subjective well-being and mindfulness, while it was also negatively related to sleep disturbance. Importantly, subjective well-being and sleep quality were further improved by each day of home practice herein.

Moreover, our findings substantiate findings from other exercise studies. In addition, anecdotal observation holds, and well-known yoga teachers recognize, that a committed yoga practice (most days of the week) allows for the positive effects of yoga on parameters of mental and emotional well-being to manifest (Yoga Sutra 1.14 [27]). Furthermore, previous exercise studies highlighted that it is a regular, frequent practice that is associated with mental health benefits, facilitating the prevention of depression and anxiety [28, 29]. For example, Knab et al. found that low reported exercise frequency was significantly associated with several measures of psychopathology (including depression and anxiety) while perceived stress was significantly lowered as reported exercise frequency increased [29]. Altogether, exercise studies underline that a regular and consistent exercise paradigm has significant positive impact on emotional health.

Arguably, it may be that either frequency of practice or switching to a morning practice alone may bring about these favorable changes observed in the present study. From empirical exercise studies, we presuppose that consistency in practice approach, and thereby in frequency and time of practice, is a crucial factor herein. Notably, a recent animal study on scheduled physical activity (in mice) suggests that timing of exercise could help shift physiological rhythms to realign better with external environment [30]. Authors also suggested that regularly scheduled physical activity could potentially delay, or even prevent, development of disease. Herein, a consistent early morning yoga practice may favorably affect physiopsychological parameters, such as

the ones measured in our study and dynamics required to better face the challenges and stressors of daily life.

It is worth noting that we observed baseline differences in PA, NA, and EA between WY and TY participants. Participation in either TY or WY was not randomly assigned; participants were invited to join a group to either maintain their regular WY practice or join the TY for two weeks in order to increase their yoga practice up to 5 times a week. It is possible that TY participants, who as a group initially presented with lower PA and higher NA and EA, were intrinsically more attracted to participate in such a TY intervention. Importantly, such baseline differences appear not to be due to different affect regulatory patterns as both groups reported using similar affect regulatory strategies at baseline. Due to resource limits it was not possible to carry out a randomized controlled study or a crossover design and let WY participants engage in TY. This is a clear limitation for the present study and should be taken into account for the next step.

Nevertheless, our findings are promising as they indicate that healthy individuals presenting with lower PA and higher NA clearly benefit from an even short-term TY intervention. Previous studies already highlighted that introducing middle-aged yoga-naïve participants with symptoms of high distress and anxiety to 1–3-times-per-week yoga led to improved outcomes of emotional well-being including an improvement in affect, mood, perceived stress, anxiety and depression, and mindfulness [13, 14, 17, 31, 32]. In light of our findings, it is intriguing to ponder whether these outcome measures could further improve by increasing the frequency towards daily yoga practice and/or switching to a morning practice. Future research on this area is warranted.

Moreover, TY practitioners initially presented with higher energy scores leading to an increased EA score compared to WY participants at baseline. Unexpectedly, energy scores (as well as EA scores) significantly decreased, reaching similar levels—as displayed by WY participants at 2 weeks. In light of the observed benefits of TY on affect, mindfulness, and perceived stress and the observed strong positive relationship between EA and NA as well as the moderately strong negative relationship between EA and PA (Table 3), this decrease in energy and EA scores appears, at first sight, puzzling. However, taking into account the short-term nature of this intervention (two weeks), it is conceivable that for the TY participants in whom there was the switch from evening to early morning practice and increasing the frequency of the practice, the decreased energy scores undermine an ongoing process of adaptation to new (practice) conditions. It has to be remembered that ashtanga yoga is a physically demanding practice [26]. Although TY participants were encouraged to engage in each practice with awareness to how the body feels and options for adapting the practice were continuously given, increasing the practice frequency from one to five days per week is an exercise increase that requires adaptation. Moreover, participants shifted from an evening to an early morning practice (07:00 h–08:30 h), requiring reorganization of daily schedules. It may well be that more time is required to adapt to such a new routine.

Yoga is a contemplative movement practice, also referred to as mindfulness in motion: it is constituted by inward concentration and awareness of breath and movement while simultaneously monitoring sensations on a physical, mental, and emotional level. Mindfulness is commonly assessed by the MAAS and MAAS scores have established relationships with parameters of emotional well-being [18, 23, 33]. Our data support this as we also observed strong positive relationships between mindfulness scores (obtained by MAAS) and various aspects of well-being, namely, PA, NA, and perceived stress. It would be valuable to follow whether the observed favorable changes in mindfulness, PA, NA, and perceived stress obtained by the 2-week TY intervention would increase by a long-term TY practice and, also, if the changes would be maintained after returning to a WY practice.

5. Conclusion

The present study demonstrates that short-term, 2-week TY compared to ongoing WY led to improved emotional well-being as evidenced by increased PA and mindfulness and decreased NA as well as a trend for decreased perceived stress. Given the increased popularity of yoga in the Western world alongside the already beneficial effects of WY on emotional well-being, our findings lend practical application and promising support to yoga as an evidence-based practice among healthy yoga practitioners.

Competing Interests

The authors declare that they have no competing interests.

References

[1] A. Dangerfield, "Yoga Wars," BBC News Magazine, 2009.

[2] S. Mehta, M. Mehta, and S. Mehta, *Yoga: The Iyengar Way*, A. A. Knopf, New York, NY, USA, 1995.

[3] A. Ross and S. Thomas, "The health benefits of yoga and exercise: a review of comparison studies," *Journal of Alternative & Complementary Medicine*, vol. 16, no. 1, pp. 3–12, 2010.

[4] M. R. Basso, B. K. Schefft, M. Douglas Ris, and W. N. Dember, "Mood and global-local visual processing," *Journal of the International Neuropsychological Society*, vol. 2, no. 3, pp. 249–255, 1996.

[5] D. Watson and J. W. Pennebaker, "Health complaints, stress, and distress: exploring the central role of negative affectivity," *Psychological Review*, vol. 96, no. 2, pp. 234–254, 1989.

[6] K. M. Dillon, B. Minchoff, and K. H. Baker, "Positive emotional states and enhancement of the immune system," *The International Journal of Psychiatry in Medicine*, vol. 15, no. 1, pp. 13–18, 1985.

[7] J. Kabat-Zinn, *Coming to Our Senses: Healing Ourselves and the World through Mindfulness*, Hachette Books, New York, NY, USA, 2005.

[8] S. Cohen, T. Kamarck, and R. Mermelstein, "A global measure of perceived stress," *Journal of Health and Social Behavior*, vol. 24, no. 4, pp. 385–396, 1983.

[9] B. L. Fredrickson, "What good are positive emotions?" *Review of General Psychology*, vol. 2, no. 3, pp. 300–319, 1998.

[10] R. E. Thayer, "Activation-deactivation adjective check list: current overview and structural analysis," *Psychological Reports*, vol. 58, no. 2, pp. 607–614, 1986.

[11] M. J. Mackenzie, L. E. Carlson, P. Ekkekakis, D. M. Paskevich, and S. N. Culos-Reed, "Affect and mindfulness as predictors of change in mood disturbance, stress symptoms, and quality of life in a community-based yoga program for cancer survivors," *Evidence-Based Complementary and Alternative Medicine*, vol. 2013, Article ID 419496, 13 pages, 2013.

[12] N. Hartfiel, J. Havenhand, S. B. Khalsa, G. Clarke, and A. Krayer, "The effectiveness of yoga for the improvement of well-being and resilience to stress in the workplace," *Scandinavian Journal of Work, Environment and Health*, vol. 37, no. 1, pp. 70–76, 2011.

[13] C. C. Streeter, T. H. Whitfield, L. Owen et al., "Effects of yoga versus walking on mood, anxiety, and brain GABA levels: a randomized controlled MRS study," *Journal of Alternative & Complementary Medicine*, vol. 16, no. 11, pp. 1145–1152, 2010.

[14] K. K. F. Rocha, A. M. Ribeiro, K. C. F. Rocha et al., "Improvement in physiological and psychological parameters after 6 months of yoga practice," *Consciousness and Cognition*, vol. 21, no. 2, pp. 843–850, 2012.

[15] S. B. S. Khalsa, S. M. Shorter, S. Cope, G. Wyshak, and E. Sklar, "Yoga ameliorates performance anxiety and mood disturbance in young professional musicians," *Applied Psychophysiology Biofeedback*, vol. 34, no. 4, pp. 279–289, 2009.

[16] J. West, C. Otte, K. Geher, J. Johnson, and D. C. Mohr, "Effects of Hatha yoga and African dance on perceived stress, affect, and salivary cortisol," *Annals of Behavioral Medicine*, vol. 28, no. 2, pp. 114–118, 2004.

[17] A. W. Li and C.-A. W. Goldsmith, "The effects of yoga on anxiety and stress," *Alternative Medicine Review*, vol. 17, no. 1, pp. 21–35, 2012.

[18] N. M. Brisbon and G. A. Lowery, "Mindfulness and levels of stress: a comparison of beginner and advanced hatha yoga practitioners," *Journal of Religion and Health*, vol. 50, no. 4, pp. 931–941, 2011.

[19] L. Gootjes, I. H. A. Franken, and J. W. van Strien, "Cognitive emotion regulation in yogic meditative practitioners: sustained modulation of electrical brain potentials," *Journal of Psychophysiology*, vol. 25, no. 2, pp. 87–94, 2011.

[20] K. B. Smith and C. F. Pukall, "An evidence-based review of yoga as a complementary intervention for patients with cancer," *Psycho-Oncology*, vol. 18, no. 5, pp. 465–475, 2009.

[21] A. Ross, E. Friedmann, M. Bevans, and S. Thomas, "Frequency of yoga practice predicts health: results of a national survey of yoga practitioners," *Evidence-Based Complementary and Alternative Medicine*, vol. 2012, Article ID 983258, 10 pages, 2012.

[22] D. Watson, L. A. Clark, and A. Tellegen, "Development and validation of brief measures of positive and negative affect: the PANAS scales," *Journal of Personality and Social Psychology*, vol. 54, no. 6, pp. 1063–1070, 1988.

[23] K. W. Brown and R. M. Ryan, "The benefits of being present: mindfulness and its role in psychological well-being," *Journal of Personality and Social Psychology*, vol. 84, no. 4, pp. 822–848, 2003.

[24] R. E. Thayer, *The Biopsychology of Mood and Arousal*, Oxford University Press, 1989.

[25] R. J. Larsen and Z. Prizmic, "Affect regulation," in *Handbook of Self-Regulation: Research, Theory, and Applications*, R. Baumeister and K. Vohs, Eds., pp. 40–61, Guilford Press, New York, NY, USA, 2004.

[26] B. R. Smith, "Body, mind and spirit? Towards an analysis of the practice of yoga," *Body and Society*, vol. 13, no. 2, pp. 25–46, 2007.

[27] B. K. S. Iyengar, "Samadhi Pada," in *Light on the Yoga Sutras of Patanjali*, pp. 43–97, 2010.

[28] D. Garcia, T. Archer, S. Moradi, and A. Andersson-Arntén, "Exercise frequency, high activation positive affect, and psychological well-being: beyond age, gender, and occupation," *Psychology*, vol. 3, no. 4, pp. 328–336, 2012.

[29] A. M. Knab, D. C. Nieman, W. Sha, J. J. Broman-Fulks, and W. H. Canu, "Exercise frequency is related to psychopathology but not neurocognitive function," *Medicine and Science in Sports & Exercise*, vol. 44, no. 7, pp. 1395–1400, 2012.

[30] A. M. Schroeder, D. Truong, D. H. Loh, M. C. Jordan, K. P. Roos, and C. S. Colwell, "Voluntary scheduled exercise alters diurnal rhythms of behaviour, physiology and gene expression in wild-type and vasoactive intestinal peptide-deficient mice," *The Journal of Physiology*, vol. 590, no. 23, pp. 6213–6226, 2012.

[31] R. M. Raghavendra, H. S. Vadiraja, R. Nagarathna et al., "Effects of a yoga program on cortisol rhythm and mood states in early breast cancer patients undergoing adjuvant radiotherapy: a randomized controlled trial," *Integrative Cancer Therapies*, vol. 8, no. 1, pp. 37–46, 2009.

[32] A. Michalsen, M. Jeitler, S. Brunnhuber et al., "Iyengar yoga for distressed women: a 3-armed randomized controlled trial," *Evidence-based Complementary and Alternative Medicine*, vol. 2012, Article ID 408727, 9 pages, 2012.

[33] S. Jain, S. L. Shapiro, S. Swanick et al., "A randomized controlled trial of mindfulness meditation versus relaxation training: effects on distress, positive states of mind, rumination, and distraction," *Annals of Behavioral Medicine*, vol. 33, no. 1, pp. 11–21, 2007.

3

Effect of Catnip Charcoal on the *In Vivo* Pharmacokinetics of the Main Alkaloids of Rhizoma Coptidis

Yanfei He, Siyu Chen, Hai Yu, Long Zhu, Yayun Liu, Chunyang Han, and Cuiyan Liu

College of Animal Science and Technology, Anhui Agricultural University, 130 Changjiang West Road, Hefei, Anhui 230036, China

Correspondence should be addressed to Cuiyan Liu; cyliu@ahau.edu.cn

Academic Editor: Kamal D. Moudgil

This study aims to explore the effect of catnip *Nepeta cataria* (CNC) charcoal on the pharmacokinetics of the main alkaloids of Rhizoma Coptidis *in vivo*. Twenty-four rabbits were randomly divided into four groups and given oral administration of an aqueous extract of Rhizoma Coptidis (RCAE), RCAE plus CNC, RCAE plus activated carbon (AC), or distilled water, respectively. Plasma samples were collected after administration. The concentrations of berberine, coptisine, palmatine, and epiberberine in plasma were measured by high-performance liquid chromatography (HPLC). The pharmacokinetics data were calculated using pharmacokinetic DAS 2.0 software. The results showed that the area under the concentration-time curve (AUC) of berberine increased, while the AUC of coptisine, palmatine, and epiberberine decreased in the rabbits that received RCAE plus CNC. Meanwhile, the AUC of berberine, coptisine, palmatine, and epiberberine decreased in the group given RCAE plus AC. The difference of main pharmacokinetics parameters among the four groups was significant ($P < 0.05$). This study showed that CNC improved the bioavailability of berberine in comparison to AC and prolonged its release in comparison to RCAE alone. However, it decreased the bioavailability of coptisine, palmatine, and epiberberine. In comparison, AC uniformly declined the bioavailability of berberine, coptisine, palmatine, and epiberberine.

1. Introduction

Herbal charcoals have been used traditionally in Chinese medicine for many years, being one of the most characteristic processing methods of Chinese herbal medicines with the purpose of changing the herbal nature, enhancing the astringency, hemostasis, and antidiarrheal activities, and also reducing toxicity of some herbals [1, 2]. The catnip *Nepeta cataria* (CNC) charcoal is typically made from cut pieces of CNC, which are carbonized until coke-black on a strong fire. Catnip *Nepeta cataria* (CNC) charcoal has been shown to exhibit better effects than the noncharcoal form in the treatment of hematochezia, metrorrhagia, and postpartum anemic fainting [3]. Notably, although in charcoal form, various charcoals of Chinese herbs partially retain the inherent nature of the raw herbal [4].

Pharmacological research has indicated that the charcoal form of Chinese herbal medicines could enhance the astringency, hemostasis, and antidiarrheal activity of herbs due to the absorption and astringency of activated carbon (AC),

which is generated during the processing of charcoals [5, 6]. It was unclear, however, whether the carbonized herbs subsequently absorbed the active components of other herbals when used in combination, thus decreasing their therapeutic effects due to nonselective absorption of AC. In addition, Mullins et al. found that AC could accelerate the excretion of other drugs from the body and decrease the bioavailability of some drugs due to the interruption of drug recirculation following reabsorption from the gastrointestinal tract or the promotion of vasoconstriction of the capillaries in the intestinal wall [7]. In summary, no common consensus has been reached with regard to the mechanisms of carbonized Chinese herbal medicines and their effects on other drugs taken concomitantly.

Nepeta cataria has an acrid and bitter taste. From a traditional Chinese medicinal perspective, it is slightly warm in nature and often used to expel pathogenic wind from the body surface. Clinically, it may be used to treat exanthema and as a hemostatic. On the other hand, Rhizoma Coptidis (RC) has been used in traditional Chinese medicine to clear

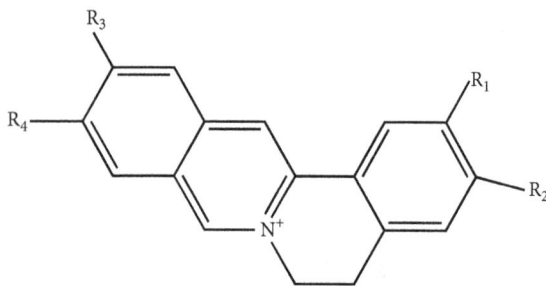

FIGURE 1: The molecular structure of berberine, epiberberine, coptisine, and palmatine. Note: berberine (R_1-R_2 = –O–CH_3–O–; R_3 = –OCH_3; R_4 = –OCH_3); epiberberine (R_1 = –OCH_3; R_2 = –OCH_3; R_3-R_4 = –O–CH_3–O–); coptisine (R_1-R_2 = –O–CH_3–O–; R_3-R_4 = –O–CH_3–O–); palmatine (R_1 = –OCH_3; R_2 = –OCH_3; R_3 = –OCH_3; R_4 = –OCH_3).

heat, purge intense heat, and dry dampness and it may also be used in detoxification. *Nepeta cataria* and RC have been used together to clear "heat evil," eliminate wind, and relieve liver conditions, as a part of the Jingjielianqiao decoction [8]. The purpose of this study was to clarify the effect of carbonized Chinese herbal medicines on the absorption of other drugs taken concomitantly. As such, to provide a basis for the clinical application of carbonized Chinese herbal medicines, the effect of CNC on the pharmacokinetics of berberine, coptisine, palmatine, and epiberberine, which are the main alkaloids in RC (showed in Figure 1), was investigated.

2. Materials and Methods

2.1. Agilent 1100 Series HPLC System. The Agilent 1100 Series LC consists of Agilent 1100 Series Quaternary Pump (G1311A), Agilent 1100 Series Autosampler (G1313A), Agilent 1100 Series Thermostatted Column Compartment (G1316A), Agilent 1100 Series Vacuum Degasser (G1379A), and Agilent 1100 Series variable wavelength UV detector (G1314A).

2.2. Herbal Medicines and Reagents. RC and CNC were purchased from Hefei Lejia Herbal Pieces Co. Ltd. (Anhui, China) and authenticated by Professor Shunxin Guo (Chinese Academy of Medical Science, Peking Union Medical College Institution of Medicinal Plant Development) in accordance with the *Chinese Pharmacopoeia*, 2010 edition. Medicinal AC was purchased from Sinopharm Chemical Reagent Co. Ltd. (China). Berberine, coptisine, palmatine, and epiberberine were purchased from the National Institutes for Food and Drug Control (China). High-performance liquid chromatography (HPLC) grade methanol and acetonitrile were provided by J. T. Baker Co. Ltd. (USA). Potassium dihydrogen phosphate and sodium lauryl sulfate were obtained from Anaqua Chemicals Supply (USA).

2.3. Animals. Twenty-four clean-grade adult male New Zealand rabbits (scxk (Shandong) 2014-0006) weighing 3.1 ± 0.6 kg were purchased from Jinan Jinfeng Experimental Animal Co. Ltd. Animals were treated humanely according to the National Research Council's guidelines.

2.4. Preparation of Stock Solutions and Herbal Medicines

2.4.1. Preparation of Standardized Solution. Stock solutions were prepared by dissolving the accurately weighed four standard reference compounds in methanol (28 μg/mL for coptisine, 20 μg/mL for epiberberine, 11 μg/mL for palmatine, and 28 μg/mL for berberine).

2.4.2. Preparation of Aqueous Extract of RC (RCAE). Fifty g RC was soaked in 600 mL water for 30 min and then boiled over a strong flame prior to simmering for 30 min and the decoction liquid was collected. The remaining herbal residue was mixed with 300 mL water and boiled for a second time. After filtration, the two filtrates were mixed and concentrated to 500 mL to attain a final concentration of 0.1 gram of raw herb in 1 mL (0.1 g/mL) using a rotary evaporator at 45°C. Then they were divided into three equal parts (a, b, and c): part b was mixed with CNC at the ratio of 0.5 percent, and part c was mixed with AC at the ratio of 0.5 percent.

2.4.3. Preparation of Powdered CNC and AC. CNC and AC were pulverized and sieved using 80-mesh and 120-mesh strainers, respectively. The resulting fine powders were kept for use in this study.

2.5. HPLC Analysis for Charred Nepeta cataria and Nepeta cataria. According to the stipulation of Chinese Pharmacopoeia (2015), the condition of HPLC was set and detecting solution was prepared. A ZOBAX C18 chromatography column (250 mm × 4.6 mm, 5 μm) was used in this study. The mobile phase was a mixture of water (A) and methol (B). The elution of p-menthone was performed using an isocratic method of 80% A. The flow rate was set at 0.8 mL/min. The injection volume was 10 μL, temperature of the column oven was set at T = 25°C during all experiment, and the wavelength for detection was 252 nm. The reference solution of p-menthone was prepared by dissolving the accurately weighed p-menthone in methanol.

2.6. Establishment of HPLC Method for Detecting Four Alkaloids in Rhizoma Coptidis. A ZOBAX C18 (250 mm × 4.6 mm, 5 μm) chromatography column was used in this study. The mobile phase consisted of water containing 0.05 mol/L potassium dihydrogen phosphate (A) and acetonitrile (B) at a ratio of 50 : 50 (v/v). The injection volume was 10 μL, the flow rate was 0.8 mL/min, the column temperature was 25°C, and the wavelength for detection was 345 nm.

2.7. HPLC Method Validation. The specificity was tested by comparison of the plasma sample to blank rabbit plasma and blank plasma spiked with the four analytes using established HPLC methods to observe the interference from endogenous substances contained in the analyte. Six samples were tested for specificity.

Calibration curves were prepared using standard plasma samples with different concentrations of the four analytes, the standard concentrations of berberine were 7.0, 17.5, 35, 70, 100, and 140 ng/mL, the standard concentrations of coptisine were 1.4, 8.75, 17.5, 35, 70, and 140 ng/mL, the standard concentrations of palmatine were 13.5, 27, 56.25,

112.5, 225, and 550 ng/mL, and the standard concentrations of epiberberine were 5, 12.5, 25, 50, 80, and 100 ng/mL. The peak area of the analyte was set as the vertical coordinate and the concentration of the analyte was set along the x-axis.

The precision and accuracy were evaluated by assaying six sample replicates with low, medium, and high concentrations during a single day and measuring six sample replicates with low, medium, and high concentrations once a day for five days. The precision was measured by the relative standard deviation (RSD) and the accuracy was described by the relative error (RE).

The extraction recovery and matrix effects of the four analytes were determined at three levels with six replicates. The extraction recoveries were evaluated by comparing the peak area obtained from the plasma sample spiked before extraction with the plasma sample spiked after extraction. The matrix effect was investigated by comparing the peak area of the analyte added to the preextracted plasma from untreated rats with that of the analyte dissolved in matrix component-free reconstitution solvent.

2.8. Pharmacokinetics Experiments. Twenty-four New Zealand rabbits were randomly divided into four groups, labeled Group A, Group B, Group C, and Group D. Group A received RCAE orally, Group B received RCAE and CNC orally, Group C received RCAE and AC orally, and Group D was administrated distilled water orally. The dosage of Groups A, B, and C was 15 mL/kg. All rabbits were fasted 24 h before administration and had free access to water. Before and immediately after oral treatment, rabbit blood samples (2.0 mL) were obtained from the auricular vein and samples were subsequently taken 0.25, 0.5, 0.75, 1, 1.5, 2, 2.5, 3, 4, 6, 8, 10, 12, 14, 18, 24, 36, and 72 h after administration. The blood samples were immediately heparinized and centrifuged at 4000 rpm for 10 min at 4°C. Prepared plasma samples were stored at −20°C until analysis. All of the pharmacokinetic parameters were processed by noncompartmental analysis using DAS 2.0 software (Mathematical Pharmacology Professional Committee of China, Shanghai, China) and all animal studies were performed according to the *Guide for the Care and Use of Laboratory Animals*.

2.9. Plasma Sample Preparation. Plasma samples (200 μL) were placed in Eppendorf tubes and extracted with 0.8 mL acetonitrile by vortex mixing for 3 min and ultrasonic extraction for 30 min. After centrifugation at 12000 rpm for 10 min, the supernatant (0.8 mL) was pipette-transferred to another Eppendorf tube. Then, the residue was extracted via the same procedure for a second time. The supernatant was combined for each sample and evaporated to dryness under nitrogen at 45°C. The residue was redissolved in 80 μL of the HPLC mobile phase and the solution was filtrated through a microporous filter membrane (0.22 μm) prior to analysis. All samples were measured within a week. Interday precision and accuracy of the assay reached the standard of quantitative analysis, and the standard samples in low, medium, and high concentration of four analyses were measured to assure the accuracy every day.

TABLE 1: Calibration curves, correlation coefficients (r), and linear ranges of the four analytes in RCAE.

Compound	Calibration curve	r value	Linear range (ng/mL^{-1})
Epiberberine	$y = 178.99x + 2.6353$	0.9992	5.0–100
Coptisine	$y = 508.97x + 3.9844$	0.9990	1.4–140
Palmatine	$y = 368.91x - 5.9279$	0.9950	13.5–550
Berberine	$y = 332.46x - 0.2947$	0.9997	7.0–140

2.10. Statistical Analysis. Data were represented in the mean ± standard deviation of the mean. Comparisons between different groups were carried out by Turkey's test. The level of significance was set at $P < 0.05$. SPSS software (version 19.0, IBM, Inc., USA) was used in statistical analysis.

3. Results

3.1. HPLC Analysis for Charred Nepeta cataria and Nepeta cataria. The retention time of p-menthone was 5.037 min under the stipulated HPLC condition, and the calibration curve was $y = 12135x + 641.5$ ($r = 0.9999$), as shown in Figure 2; (a) showed the HPLC image of p-menthone, (b) showed the HPLC image of charred *Nepeta cataria*, and (c) showed the HPLC image of *Nepeta cataria*. The results of the accuracy, precision, and extraction recovery showed that the extraction recovery was more than 90%, and both the RSD and reproducibility met the measure requirements. The results showed that the content of p-menthone of *Nepeta cataria* was 0.96 mg/g which was higher than 0.08% stipulated in *Chinese Pharmacopoeia* (2015) and the content of p-menthone of charred *Nepeta cataria* was 0.43 mg/g.

3.2. Specificity of the HPLC Method. The retention times of berberine, coptisine, palmatine, and epiberberine were 9.94, 11.10, 13.501, and 14.99 min, respectively. As shown in Figure 3, (a) showed the HPLC trace for the plasma sample after administration of RC, (b) showed the blank plasma spiked with the four analytes, and (c) showed the trace for blank plasma. There was no obvious interference from endogenous substances contained in the analytes according to the HPLC trace of blank rabbit plasma, blank plasma spiked with the four analytes, and the plasma sample after administration.

3.3. Calibration Curves. The standard curves of the four analytes all exhibited good linearity and good coefficients of correlation ($r > 0.993$). The limit of quantitation was appropriate for the quantitative detection of the four analytes in the plasma samples. The linear ranges, regression equations, and correlation coefficients were shown in Table 1.

3.4. Accuracy, Precision, and Extraction Replicates. The results of the specificity of the HPLC method showed that the matrix effect of the plasma taken from rabbits in the control group would not disturb measurement of the four alkaloids. The results of the accuracy, precision, and extraction recovery showed that the extraction recovery was more than 90%, and both the RSD and reproducibility met the measure

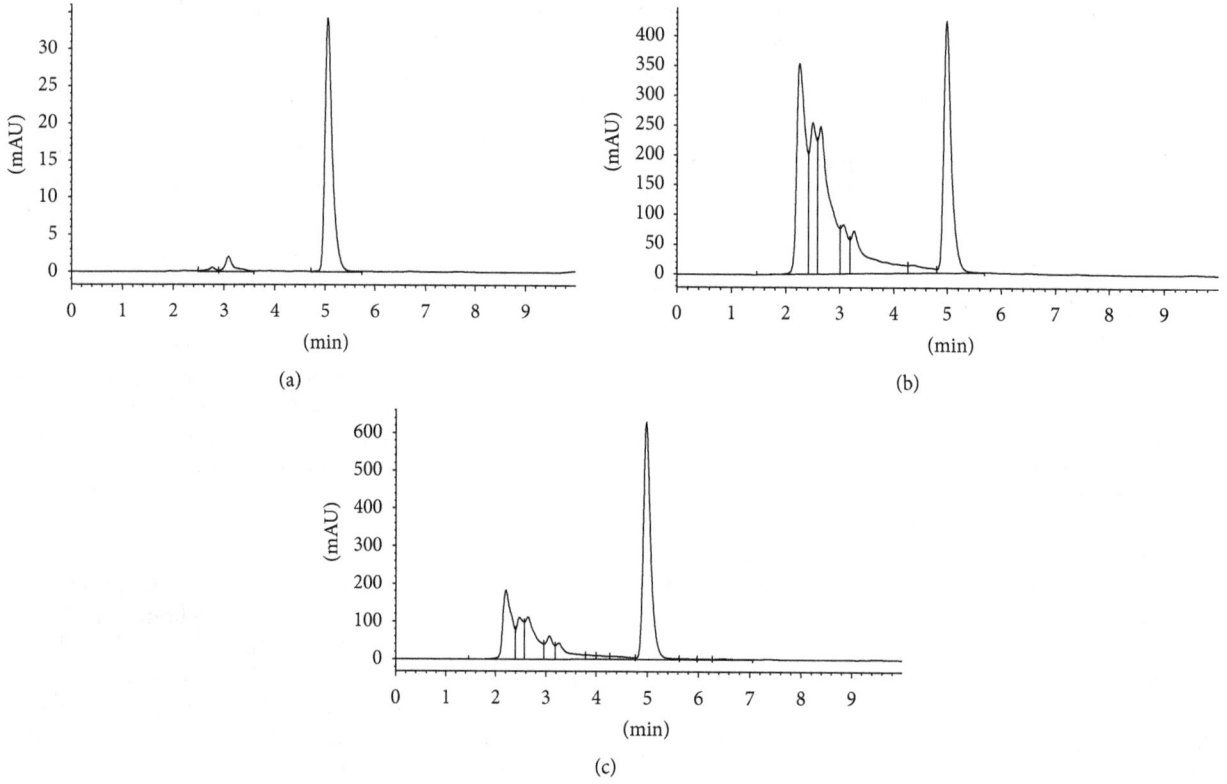

FIGURE 2: (a) shows the HPLC image of menthone, (b) shows the HPLC image of charred *Nepeta cataria*, and (c) shows the HPLC image of *Nepeta cataria*.

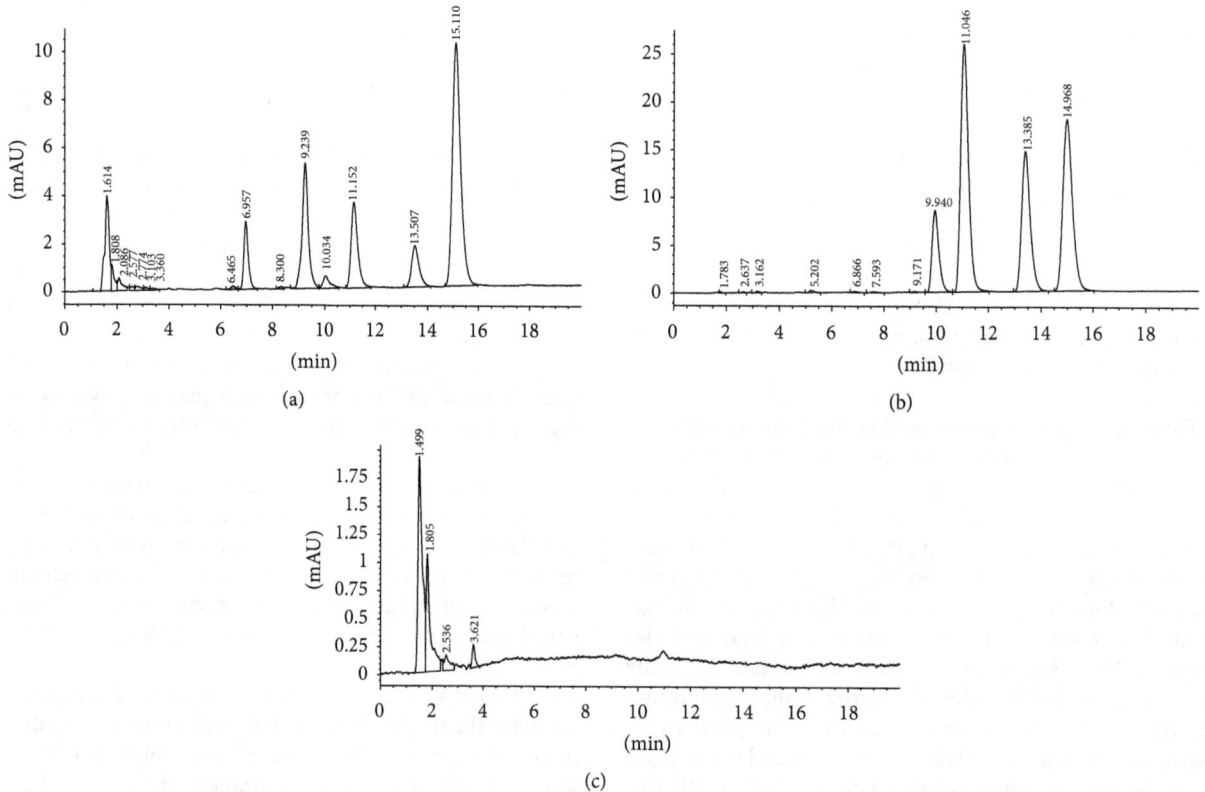

FIGURE 3: HPLC chromatogram of a plasma sample after administration (a), blank plasma spiked with the four analytes (b), and blank rabbit plasma (c).

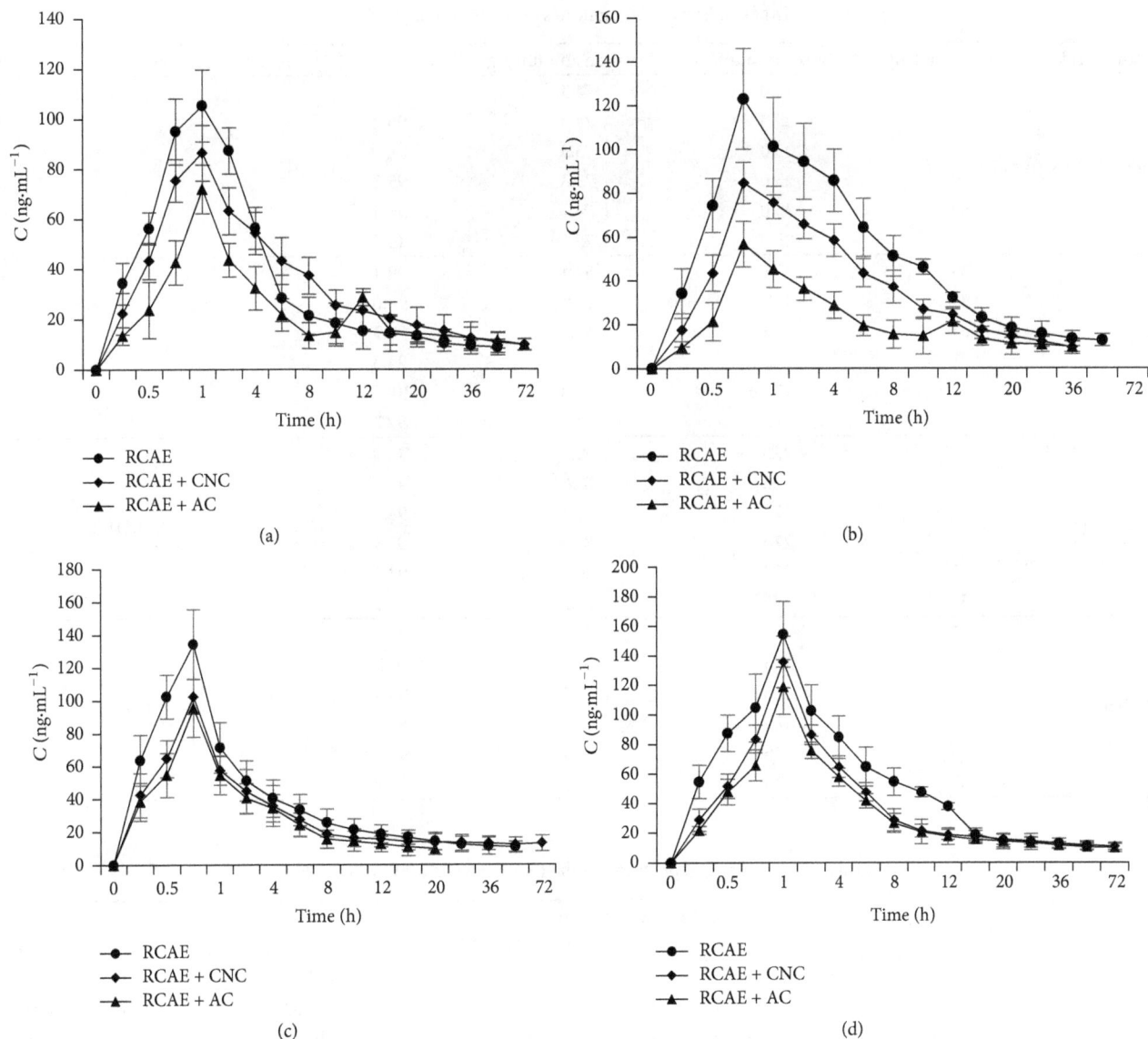

FIGURE 4: Concentration-time profile in plasma for berberine (a), coptisine (b), palmatine (c), and epiberberine (d).

requirements. All results showed that the HPLC method was reliable (Tables 2 and 3).

3.5. Concentration-Time Profile

3.5.1. Concentration-Time Profile of Berberine in Plasma. Figure 4(a) showed the concentration changes of berberine in plasma extracted from rabbits in Groups A–C. The concentration of plasma berberine in Group A was higher than in Group B from the point of administration to 2 h after administration. However, at 4 h after administration, the concentration in Group B exceeded that of Group A and this trend continued up until 72 h after administration. Meanwhile, the concentration of plasma berberine in Group C was lower than in Groups A and B, although the berberine concentration of Group C did increase again at 10 h after

administration, showing a second peak in the concentration profile at 12 h after administration.

3.5.2. Concentration-Time Profile of Coptisine in Plasma. Figure 4(b) showed the concentration changes for coptisine in plasma for Groups A–C, indicating that the concentration in Group B was lower than in Group A during the study, while the concentration in Group C was lower than in Groups A and B. Again, the profile for Group C showed a second peak at 12 h after administration.

3.5.3. Concentration-Time Profile of Palmatine in Plasma. Figure 4(c) showed the concentration changes of plasma palmatine in Groups A–C. As can be seen from the figure, the concentration of plasma palmatine in Group B was lower than in Group A during the study, but the concentration of plasma

TABLE 2: Extraction replicates of the four analytes.

Compound	Origin amount/ng	Addition amount/ng	Measured amount/ng	Recovery rate (%)	Average recovery rate (%) (RSD%)
Epiberberine	50	25.0	74.3	97.2	98.5 (2.3)
	50	25.0	74.8	99.2	
	50	25.0	75.3	101.2	
	50	25.0	73.8	95.2	
	50	25.0	74.1	96.4	
	50	25.0	75.5	102.0	
Coptisine	35	17.5	52.4	99.4	98.0 (2.04)
	35	17.5	51.8	96.0	
	35	17.5	52.3	98.9	
	35	17.5	51.5	94.3	
	35	17.5	52.8	101.7	
	35	17.5	52.1	97.7	
Palmatine	55	27.5	81.1	94.9	96.2 (1.51)
	55	27.5	81.6	96.7	
	55	27.5	82.1	98.5	
	55	27.5	81.9	97.8	
	55	27.5	80.8	93.8	
	55	27.5	81.3	96.7	
Berberine	35	17.5	51.9	96.5	97.1 (0.98)
	35	17.5	52.1	97.7	
	35	17.5	51.7	95.4	
	35	17.5	52.1	97.7	
	35	17.5	51.9	96.6	
	35	17.5	52.3	98.8	

TABLE 3: Accuracy and precision of the four analytes in RCAE ($n = 6$).

Compound	Concentration (ng/mL)	Intraday precision Measured amount ($\overline{x} \pm s$)	RSD (%)	RE (%)	Interday precision Measured amount ($\overline{x} \pm s$)	RSD (%)	RE (%)
Coptisine	2.0	1.98 ± 0.033	0.41	1.0	1.97 ± 0.33	1.61	1.5
	35	34.950 ± 0.122	0.35	0.14	35.017 ± 0.213	0.61	0.048
	110	109.667 ± 0.314	0.28	0.30	109.967 ± 0.829	0.75	0.03
Berberine	10.0	9.932 ± 0.073	0.74	0.68	9.968 ± 0.117	1.17	0.032
	50.0	49.968 ± 0.084	0.17	0.11	50.050 ± 0.139	0.28	0.10
	110.0	109.93 ± 0.125	0.11	0.064	110.110 ± 0.827	0.75	0.12
Palmatine	16	15.888 ± 0.085	0.53	0.70	15.922 ± 0.164	1.03	0.49
	200	199.682 ± 0.226	0.11	0.17	200.328 ± 0.839	0.42	0.164
	400	397.182 ± 1.594	0.40	0.71	399.945 ± 2.468	0.62	0.013
Epiberberine	6.0	5.96 ± 0.025	0.42	0.68	6.02 ± 0.052	0.87	0.33
	50.0	49.785 ± 0.093	0.19	0.43	50.047 ± 0.592	1.18	0.094
	80.0	79.713 ± 0.294	0.37	0.36	79.823 ± 0.356	0.45	0.22

palmatine in Group C was lower than in Group B. However, the difference between Groups B and C was not significant.

3.5.4. *Concentration-Time Profile of Epiberberine in Plasma.* Figure 4(d) showed the concentration changes of epiberberine in plasma for Groups A–C. Akin to the results for palmatine, the concentration of plasma epiberberine in Group B was lower than in Group A during the study, while

the concentration of plasma epiberberine in Group C was lower than in Group B. Again, the difference between Groups B and C was not significant.

3.6. *Maximum Plasma Concentration, Time to Reach the Maximum Concentration, Area under Curve, and Drug Half-Life.* Table 4 and Figures 5 and 6 showed the maximum plasma concentration ($C_{\max}$), the time required to reach

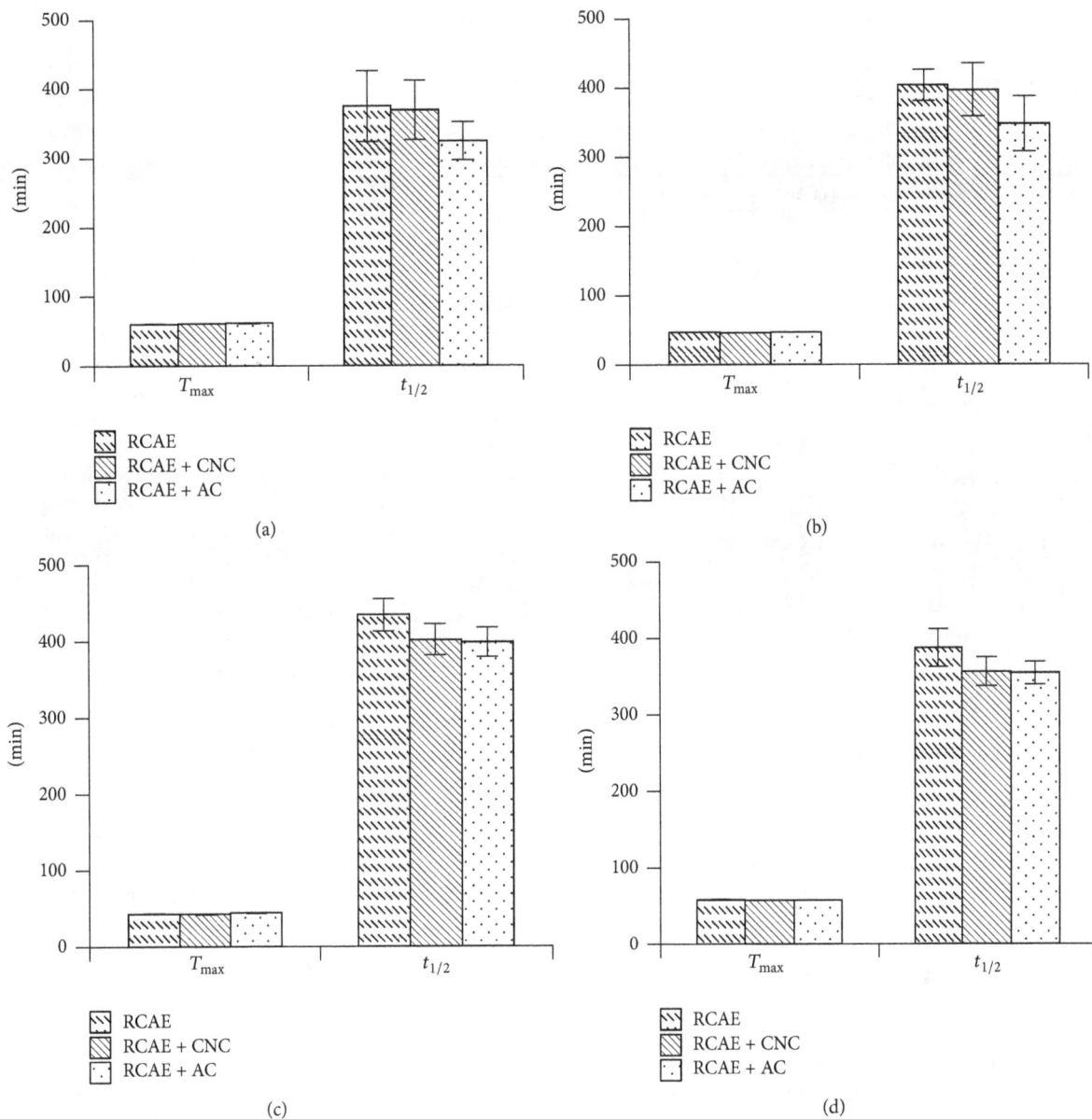

FIGURE 5: The time required to reach the maximum concentration (T_{max}) and the half-life ($t_{1/2}$) for berberine (a), coptisine (b), palmatine (c), and epiberberine (d).

the maximum concentration (T_{max}), the area under the concentration-time curve (AUC_{0-t}), and the half-life ($t_{1/2}$) for berberine (Figure 5(a)), coptisine (Figure 5(b)), palmatine (Figure 5(c)), and epiberberine (Figure 5(d)).

There was a significant difference with regard to C_{max} of berberine between the groups, whereby Group A > Group B > Group C. However, there was no significant difference with regard to T_{max} among the three groups ($P > 0.05$). $t_{1/2}$ of berberine in Group C was significantly lower than those of Groups A and B. The differences with regard to the AUC_{0-t} among the three groups were significant ($P < 0.05$), whereby Group B > Group A > Group C (Table 4). All of the above results (Figure 3(a)) indicated that CNC enhanced

the bioavailability of berberine in comparison to AC, which decreased the bioavailability. The results also suggested that CNC may prolong the release of berberine in comparison to RCAE alone.

There was a significant difference with regard to C_{max} of coptisine among the groups, whereby Group A > Group B > Group C. However, there was no significant difference with regard to T_{max} among the three groups ($P > 0.05$). Meanwhile, $t_{1/2}$ of coptisine for Group C was significantly lower than those of Groups A and B ($P < 0.05$). The difference with regard to the AUC_{0-t} among the three groups was significant ($P < 0.05$), with Group A > Group B > Group C (Table 4). All of the above results (Figure 3(b)) indicated that

TABLE 4: Area under concentration-time curve (AUC_{0-t}) for the four analytes in Groups A–C.

Group	Berberine	Coptisine	Palmatine	Epiberberine
Group A	8123.2 ± 1734.1^b	8092.3 ± 1423.7^a	8674.3 ± 1534.7^a	8415.1 ± 1434.2^a
Group B	8432.21 ± 1831.3^a	7532.4 ± 1231.4^b	8347.2 ± 1617.4^b	8117.4 ± 1534.3^b
Group C	5472.41 ± 1041.7^c	5317.3 ± 1047.4^c	8274.7 ± 1537.8^b	8074.2 ± 1374.5^b

Note: "a, b, and c" indicated the difference of AUC_{0-t} among three groups.

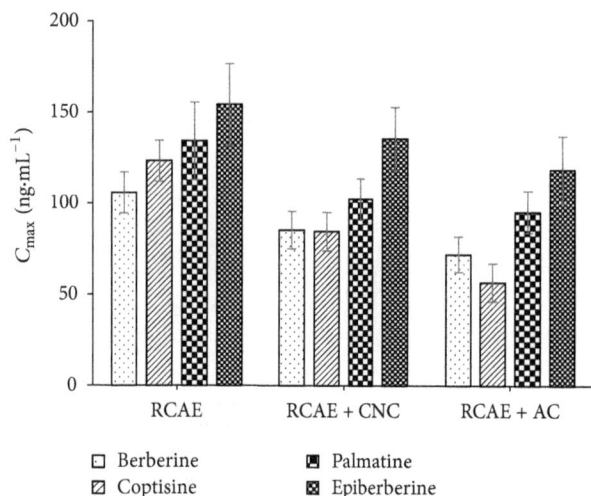

FIGURE 6: Maximum plasma concentration (C_{max}) for berberine, coptisine, palmatine, and epiberberine.

both CNC and AC decreased the bioavailability of coptisine in comparison to RCAE alone; however, CNC had a less significant effect compared to AC.

The C_{max} of palmatine in Group A was significantly higher than those of Groups B and C ($P < 0.05$), but the difference in C_{max} values between Groups B and C was not significant ($P > 0.05$). The differences with regard to T_{max} and $t_{1/2}$ of palmatine among the three groups were not significant. Meanwhile, the AUC_{0-t} of Group A was higher than Groups B and C, whereby Group A > Group B > Group C (Table 4); however, the differences were not significant. These results (Figure 3(c)) indicated that both CNC and AC may decrease the bioavailability of palmatine in comparison to RCAE alone.

With regard to C_{max} of epiberberine, Group A showed a significantly higher concentration than Groups B and C ($P < 0.05$), but the difference between Groups B and C was not significant ($P > 0.05$). With regard to T_{max} and $t_{1/2}$ of epiberberine, differences between the three groups were not significant. Furthermore, differences in the AUC_{0-t} between the groups were not significant (Table 3). These results indicated that CNC and AC may decrease the concentration of epiberberine in plasma in comparison to RCAE alone, although other parameters appear to be less affected.

4. Discussion

Carbonized herbal medicines have traditionally been used in Chinese medicine, with their use being first recorded 2000 years ago in *Prescriptions for Fifty-Two Diseases*. Recent researches have suggested that carbonized drugs may indeed have clinically relevant, curative effects [9–11]. However, investigation of the mechanism of action for carbonized Chinese herbal medicines has largely fallen behind their clinical applications and has mainly focused on the various chemical components and trace elements contained therein [12–15]. To address this shortfall, in this study the mechanism of carbonized herbal medicines was investigated via the effects of CNC on the pharmacokinetics of berberine, coptisine, palmatine, and epiberberine *in vivo*, which are the main alkaloids contained in RC. The results indicated that orally administered CNC in combination with RCAE enhanced the bioavailability of the alkaloids in comparison to RCAE and AC, and CNC prolonged the release of berberine in comparison to RCAE alone. However, CNC with RCAE resulted in decreased bioavailability of coptisine, palmatine, and epiberberine. The reason why CNC enhanced the bioavailability of some compounds over AC and prolonged the release of berberine may be due to the presence of CNC micropowder, which may adsorb alkaloids, thus prolonging their retention in the small intestine, from where they can be reabsorbed. However, this adsorption capacity may be strong, resulting in the decreased release of some alkaloids from CNC prior to excretion. This mechanism would account for the differences found here between the alkaloids as some may adhere more strongly to the micropowdered CS, hindering their release in the small intestine.

The bioavailability of berberine, coptisine, palmatine, and epiberberine decreased when RCAE was orally administered with AC. This result is in accordance with the accelerated clearance of drugs as a result of AC, with a concomitant decline of bioavailability [16, 17]. This is one of the reasons why AC has been used for the treatment of intoxication as a result of some drugs [7, 18]. However, the reason for the second peak in the concentration-time profiles of berberine and coptisine for Group C (Figure 2) is not well understood. However, similar secondary peaks have been observed in the concentration-time profiles of aconitine, hypaconitine, and mesaconine following administration of prepared Radix Glycyrrhizae and prepared *Aconitum carmichaelii* Debx. [19]. Typically, there are five reasons for a double peak concentration-time profile in pharmacology. Firstly, the drug may arrive at the small intestine in two (or more) batches due to nonuniform gastric emptying. The second reason may be that two different parts of the gastrointestinal tract are involved in drug absorption with different rates. The third possible explanation is due to the enterohepatic cycle. The fourth reason relates to pharmaceutics containing ingredients that delay release or promote fast release, and the fifth and final reason is due to the liposolubility of the drug distributed throughout the tissue, which may allow release of the drug into the blood again when the component in blood has declined to a certain extent. In this study the double peak concentration-time profile for some alkaloids in Group C may arise mainly as a result of pharmaceutic agents, with the aqueous extract providing fast release while the addition of AC resulted in delayed release.

5. Conclusions

The results of this research have shown that there was a significant difference between the effect of AC and CNC on the transportation of RC alkaloids *in vivo*, whereby AC results in a double peak concentration-time profile for some alkaloids. It was noteworthy that while CNC decreased the bioavailability of RC alkaloids in comparison to RCAE administered alone, it increased their bioavailability in comparison to AC and it prolonged the release of berberine.

Further investigations will be required to elucidate the precise mechanism of action of carbonized Chinese herbal medicines *in vivo*.

Competing Interests

The authors declare that there are no competing interests regarding the publication of this paper.

Authors' Contributions

Yanfei He and Siyu Chen made equal contribution.

Acknowledgments

This work was supported by the National Natural Science Foundation of China (Grant no. 31172358) and the Open Fund of State Key Laboratory of Tea Plant Biology and Utilization (Grant no. SKLTOF20150203). The authors thank Jingang Gu, associate research fellow, for his kind help, and they also thank the Key Laboratory of Microbial Resource Collection and Preservation for providing the conditions for the investigation.

References

[1] Y. Chen, "Primary analysis of six carbon soupapplied by famous specialist of traditional Chinese medicine," *Guangming Journal of Chinese Medicine*, vol. 29, no. 1, pp. 151–153, 2014.

[2] T. Zhang, X. M. Dang, and W. Z. Huang, "Application of carbon in the treatment of idiopathic thrombocytopenic purpura," *Sichuan Journal of Traditional Chinese Medicine*, vol. 20, no. 11, pp. 16–17, 2002.

[3] M.-Q. Shan, L. Zhang, and A.-W. Ding, "Advances in studies on carbonic herbs," *Chinese Traditional and Herbal Drugs*, vol. 39, no. 4, pp. 631–634, 2008.

[4] J. Meng, S. Y. Xu, L. Chen et al., "Study on quality standard of dried ginger for 'carbonizing drug characteristic'," *China Journal Chinese Materia Medica*, vol. 37, no. 4, pp. 453–456, 2012.

[5] D. Wang, "Discussion on the factor of the effect on the hemostasis of the Chinese medicinal herbs after the charcoal," *Hubei Journal of Traditional Chinese Medicine*, vol. 36, no. 1, pp. 70–71, 2014.

[6] Y. Wu, Q. Liu, Y. Wang, G. L. Chen, and X. Y. Liang, "Adsorption performances of active carbon spheres of small pore diameters," *Chinese Journal of Pharmaceuticals*, vol. 39, no. 4, pp. 288–293, 2008.

[7] M. Mullins, B. R. Froelke, and M. R.-P. Rivera, "Effect of delayed activated charcoal on acetaminophen concentration after simulated overdose of oxycodone and acetaminophen," *Clinical Toxicology*, vol. 47, no. 2, pp. 112–115, 2009.

[8] M. S. Lai, S. B. Chong, and H. M. Lan, "Preventive effect of oral JJLQT on rat acute radioactive dermatitis," *China Journal of Dermato Venereologica*, vol. 28, no. 8, pp. 843–845, 854, 2014.

[9] G. H. Ma, "Modern cognition of the theory of Chinese traditional medicine for the hemostasis of carbonizing," *Traditional Chinese Medicine Research*, vol. 17, no. 5, pp. 15–18, 2004.

[10] Z. Liu and H. G. Yu, "Elaboration on the functions of carbonized herbs," *Shanghai Journal of Traditional Chinese Medicine*, vol. 38, no. 10, pp. 54–55, 2004.

[11] Y. Zhou and Z. L. Zhang, "Discussion on the theory of 'fried carbon and hemostasis' in Chinese Medicine," *Heilongjiang Science and Technology Information*, vol. 22, p. 253, 2007.

[12] Q. Huang, J. Meng, D. L. Wu et al., "Content of the tannin and the absorption capacity of carbon between scutellaria radix and charred scutellaria radix," *Chinese Journal of Experiment Traditional Medicine Formula*, vol. 19, no. 22, pp. 82–85, 2013.

[13] D. Y. Guo, Y. Q. Shi, and X. Wang, "Determination of tannin content in different processed rhubarb," *Modern Traditional Chinese Medicine*, vol. 32, no. 4, pp. 76–79, 2012.

[14] L.-X. Li, B. Qiao, Y.-B. Li et al., "Changes of chemical constituents in Phellodendri Chinensis Cortex before and after charing based on RPLC/Q-TOF-MS technology," *Chinese Traditional and Herbal Drugs*, vol. 43, no. 7, pp. 1314–1319, 2012.

[15] B.-H. Bao, L. Zhang, W.-F. Yao, and Q. Zhu, "Changes of 2-furoic acid in *Celosia cristata* after carbon-fried processing," *Chinese Traditional and Herbal Drugs*, vol. 42, no. 12, pp. 2462–2464, 2011.

[16] X. Wang, S. Mondal, J. Wang et al., "Effect of activated charcoal on apixaban pharmacokinetics in healthy subjects," *American Journal of Cardiovascular Drugs*, vol. 14, no. 2, pp. 147–154, 2014.

[17] F. van Gorp, S. Duffull, L. P. Hackett, and G. K. Isbister, "Population pharmacokinetics and pharmacodynamics of escitalopram in overdose and the effect of activated charcoal," *British Journal of Clinical Pharmacology*, vol. 73, no. 3, pp. 402–410, 2012.

[18] R. Neijzen, P. V. Ardenne, M. Sikma, A. Egas, T. Ververs, and E. V. Maarseveen, "Activated charcoal for GHB intoxication: an in vitro study," *European Journal of Pharmaceutical Sciences*, vol. 47, no. 5, pp. 801–803, 2012.

[19] L.-P. He, B. Di, Y.-X. Du, F. Yan, and H.-Q. Liu, "Comparative pharmacokinetics of aconitine, mesaconitine and hypaconitine in rats after oral administration of four decoctions composed with Radix Aconiti Lateralis," *Journal of China Pharmaceutical University*, vol. 41, no. 1, pp. 55–59, 2010.

Ultrastructural Changes and Death of *Leishmania infantum* Promastigotes Induced by *Morinda citrifolia* Linn. Fruit (Noni) Juice Treatment

Fernando Almeida-Souza,[1,2] Noemi Nosomi Taniwaki,[3] Ana Cláudia Fernandes Amaral,[4] Celeste da Silva Freitas de Souza,[1] Kátia da Silva Calabrese,[1] and Ana Lúcia Abreu-Silva[2]

[1]*Laboratório de Imunomodulação e Protozoologia, Instituto Oswaldo Cruz, Fiocruz, 21040-900 Rio de Janeiro, RJ, Brazil*
[2]*Departamento de Patologia, Universidade Estadual do Maranhão, 65055-310 São Luís, MA, Brazil*
[3]*Unidade de Microscopia Eletrônica, Instituto Adolf Lutz, 01246-000 São Paulo, SP, Brazil*
[4]*Laboratório de Plantas Medicinais e Derivados, Farmanguinhos, Fiocruz, 21041-250 Rio de Janeiro, RJ, Brazil*

Correspondence should be addressed to Kátia da Silva Calabrese; calabrese@ioc.fiocruz.br

Academic Editor: Kang-Ju Kim

The search for new treatments against leishmaniasis has increased due to high frequency of drug resistance registered in endemics areas, side effects, and complications caused by coinfection with HIV. *Morinda citrifolia* Linn., commonly known as Noni, has a rich chemical composition and various therapeutic effects have been described in the literature. Studies have shown the leishmanicidal activity of *M. citrifolia*; however, its action on the parasite has not yet been elucidated. In this work, we analyzed leishmanicidal activity and ultrastructural changes in *Leishmania infantum* promastigotes caused by *M. citrifolia* fruit juice treatment. *M. citrifolia* fruit extract showed a yield of 6.31% and high performance liquid chromatography identified phenolic and aromatic compounds as the major constituents. IC_{50} values were 260.5 μg/mL for promastigotes and 201.3 μg/mL for intracellular amastigotes of *L. infantum* treated with *M. citrifolia*. Cytotoxicity assay with J774.G8 macrophages showed that *M. citrifolia* fruit juice was not toxic up to 2 mg/mL. Transmission electron microscopy showed cytoplasmic vacuolization, lipid inclusion, increased exocytosis activity, and autophagosome-like vesicles in *L. infantum* promastigotes treated with *M. citrifolia* fruit juice. *M. citrifolia* fruit juice was active against *L. infantum* in the *in vitro* model used here causing ultrastructural changes and has a future potential for treatment against leishmaniasis.

1. Introduction

Due to the continental dimensions of Brazil there are various parts of its territory with difficult access. Consequently, there is a limit to public health resources and a tendency for the inhabitants of these remote regions not to get the necessary government health benefits. This geographical isolation contributes to strengthening the local traditional medical practices and other natural resources to treat diseases, including parasitic diseases such as leishmaniasis [1].

Leishmaniasis is caused by protozoan parasites transmitted through the bites of infected female sandflies (usually *Phlebotomus* or *Lutzomyia*). The disease appears in three clinical forms: the visceral form, also known as kala-azar, is usually fatal within 2 years if left untreated; the cutaneous form, causing skin ulcers; and the mucocutaneous form, which invades the mucous membranes of the upper respiratory tract, causing gross mutilation by destroying soft tissues in the nose, mouth, and throat [2]. The disease, which is prevalent in 98 countries and 3 territories on 5 continents, has approximately 1.3 million new cases annually, of which 300,000 are visceral and 1 million are cutaneous or mucocutaneous. These numbers show the importance of this disease in public health, including Brazil [3].

Treatment for leishmaniasis was first introduced by Vianna in 1912. Organic compounds of antimony are the drugs of choice in treating this disease, and amphotericin B was introduced recently. Both treatments present several side effects, are highly toxicity, and have an elevated cost which has led to the search for new alternatives. The search for a leishmanicidal agent of low toxicity and high efficiency is a challenge and has involved several research groups around the world [4]. Herbal remedies have gained a lot of attention in this area as a potential source to obtain new compounds with therapeutic activities.

Morinda citrifolia Linn. is a small plant native to Southeast Asia, commonly known as Noni, and one of the most significant sources of traditional medicine in those countries. Due to the various ethnopharmacological activities associated with this plant, it is now cultivated all over the world, including Brazil. Studies have shown the efficacy of Noni in the treatment of pain and inflammatory reactions [5] and antitumoral activity [6]. Activity against bacteria [7] and fungi [8] has also been observed. Recently, the *in vitro* activity of morindicone and morinthone isolated from the stem of *M. citrifolia* was described against *L. major*. Moreover, a clinical study was carried out to determine the efficiency of a topical ointment with *M. citrifolia* stem extract against cutaneous leishmaniasis, and there was an excellent response in 50% and a good improvement in 30% of the 40 patients evaluated [9]. Therefore, to demonstrate the action of *M. citrifolia* against promastigotes of *Leishmania* and evaluate the ultrastructural changes caused by such treatment, this study evaluated promastigotes forms of *Leishmania infantum* treated with *M. citrifolia* fruit juice by electron microscopy.

2. Materials and Methods

2.1. Plant Material. M. *citrifolia* fruits were collected in November 2011 from São Luís (S2°31 W44°16), Maranhão, in the Brazilian Legal Amazon at 24 m above sea level. Fruits were collected when the exocarp was translucent. The plant material was identified by Ana Maria Maciel Leite, and the voucher specimen number 2000346 was deposited at the Herbário Professora Rosa Mochel, Universidade Estadual do Maranhão. In the laboratory, the fruits were washed with distilled and sterilized water, dried at 25°C, and placed in sterile glass bottles for 3 days to drain off the extract released. This liquid was centrifuged twice at 4000 rpm for 15 minutes; the supernatant was lyophilized and stored at −20°C [8]. The lyophilized *M. citrifolia* fruit juice was dissolved in DMSO and dilutions with different concentrations in culture medium were made immediately before use. The concentration of DMSO in medium did not exceed 1%.

2.2. High Performance Liquid Chromatography Coupled with Diode Array and Evaporative Light Scattering Detectors (HPLC-DAD-ELSD). The HPLC chromatographic profile of the *M. citrifolia* fruit juice was performed on a Shimadzu LC-10Avp equipped with two LC-8Avp pumps, controlled by a CBM-10A interface module, an automatic injector with two detectors, a diode array detector SPD-M10A (DAD), and an evaporative light scattering detector (ELSD) with a drift tube temperature setting of 40°C, using nitrogen as the nebulizer gas and gain at 4.0. HPLC grade solvents and Milli-Q water were used and the analysis was performed on a reversed phase LiChrospher C18 column (4.6 mm × 250 mm; 5 μm, Waters).

The mobile phase was water (A) and methanol (B), with the following gradient composition: (0–20 min) 5–20% (B), (20–30 min) 20%–35% (B), and (30–35 min) 35% (B). The UV chromatogram was obtained at 365 nm. The sample injection volume was 10 μL. A constant flow of 1 mL/min was used during the analysis. Before analysis 5.0 mg of the extract was dissolved in 1.0 mL of Milli-Q water and the mixture was centrifuged.

2.3. Parasites. Promastigote forms of *L. infantum* (MCAN/BR/2008/1112) were cultured at 26°C in Schneider's Insect medium (Sigma-USA) supplemented with 10% fetal bovine sera (Gibco-USA), 100 U/mL of penicillin (Gibco-USA), and 100 μg/mL of streptomycin. The cultures used had a maximum of ten *in vitro* passages.

2.4. Animals. Female BALB/c mice of 4–6 years old were purchased from Centro de Criação de Animais de Laboratório do Instituto Oswaldo Cruz, Rio de Janeiro, and maintained under pathogen-free conditions. The animals were handled in accordance with Guidelines for Animal Experimentation of the Colégio Brasileiro de Experimentação Animal. The local Ethics Committee on Animal Care and Utilization approved all procedures involving the animals (CEUA FIOCRUZ-LW72/12).

2.5. Cells Culture. The macrophage J774.G8 line was cultured in RPMI 1640 medium (Sigma, USA) supplemented with 10% fetal bovine sera, penicillin (100 U/mL), and (100 μg/mL) streptomycin, at 37°C and 5% CO_2. Female BALB/c mice were inoculated with 3 mL of sodium thioglycolate 3% and after 72 hours peritoneal macrophages were harvested with PBS solution. The harvest was centrifuged at 4000 rpm and the cells suspended in RPMI medium supplemented as described before and cultured at 37°C and 5% CO_2.

2.6. Activity against Promastigote Forms. Promastigote forms of *L. infantum* (10^6 parasites/mL) from a 2–4-day-old culture were placed in 96-well plates in the presence of different concentrations of *M. citrifolia* fruit juice (960–30 μg/mL), in a final volume of 200 μL per well, for 72 hours. Wells without parasites were used as blank and wells with only parasites were used as control. After the treatment, the viability of parasites was evaluated by the tetrazolium-dye (MTT) colorimetric modified method [10]. MTT (5 mg/mL), a volume equal to 10% of the total, was added to each well. After 2 hours, the plate was centrifuged at 4000 rpm; then the supernatant was removed from each well and 100 μL of DMSO was added to dissolve the formazan. The absorbance was analyzed on a spectrophotometer at a wavelength of 540 nm. The data was normalized according to the formula

$$\% \text{ survival} = \text{DO sample} - \frac{\text{DO blank}}{\text{DO control}} - \text{DO blank} \times 100. \tag{1}$$

The results were used to calculate IC_{50} (50% inhibition of parasite growth). Amphotericin B was used as the reference drug.

TABLE 1: Activity against promastigotes and intracellular amastigotes of *Leishmania infantum*, cytotoxicity in peritoneal macrophages from BALB/c and selectivity index of *Morinda citrifolia* fruit extract treatment and amphotericin B.

Compounds	IC$_{50}$ (μg/mL)		CC$_{50}$	SI
	Promastigote	Intracellular amastigote	J774.G8	
Morinda citrifolia fruit juice	260.5 ± 0.044	201.3 ± 0.175	>2000	>9.9
Amphotericin B	3.1 ± 0.230	0.9 ± 0.121	2.7 ± 0.156	3.0

IC$_{50}$: inhibitory concentration of 50% parasites. CC$_{50}$: cytotoxicity concentration of 50% cells. SI: selectivity index. Data are presented as the mean $\pm$ SD of three independent experiments realized at least in triplicate.

2.7. Activity against Intracellular Amastigotes.

Peritoneal macrophages were cultured in 24-well plates (10^5 cells/well), with coverslips, at 37°C and 5% CO_2. The cells were infected with promastigote forms of *L. infantum* using a ratio of 10 : 1 parasite/cell, and after 2 hours the cells were washed three times with PBS to remove free parasites. The infected cells were treated with different concentrations of *M. citrifolia* fruit juice (480–30 μg/mL) in triplicate for 24 hours. The coverslips with the infected and treated cells were fixed with Bouin, stained with Giemsa, and examined by light microscopy. The inhibition percentage was calculated and IC$_{50}$ was calculated with the GraphPad Prism software. Amphotericin was used as the reference drug.

2.8. Cytotoxicity Assay.

J774.G8 macrophages were cultured in 96-well plates (5×10^5 cells/mL) with different concentrations of *M. citrifolia* fruit juice (2000–1.8 μg/mL) to a final volume of 200 μL per well, at 37°C and 5% CO_2. Wells without cells were used as blank and wells with only cells were used as control. After 24 hours, the cells were fixed with 10% trichloroacetic acid for 1 hour at 4°C, stained with Sulforhodamine B (Sigma, USA) solution 0.4% in 1% acetic acid for 30 minutes, and washed with 1% acetic acid solution. Sulforhodamine B was solubilized in 200 μL of 10 mM tris-base solution and the plate was read in a spectrophotometer at 540 nm wavelength [11]. The data was normalized following the formula described earlier. The results were used to calculate the cell cytotoxicity by 50% (CC$_{50}$) with the GraphPad Prism 5.

2.9. Transmission Electron Microscopy.

Promastigote forms of *L. infantum* were treated with *M. citrifolia* fruit juice at concentrations of 480, 240, 120, 60, and 30 μg/mL for 24 hours. The parasites were fixed with 2.5% glutaraldehyde (Sigma, USA) in 0.1 M sodium-cacodylate buffer, pH 7.2 overnight. Parasites were washed three times with 0.1 M sodium-cacodylate buffer and postfixed in a solution containing 1% osmium tetroxide, 0.8% ferrocyanide, and 5 mM calcium chloride, washed in 0.1 M sodium-cacodylate buffer, dehydrated in graded acetone, and embedded in epoxy resin. Ultrathin sections were stained with uranyl acetate and lead citrate and examined in a transmission electron microscope JEM-1011 (JEOL, Japan).

2.10. Statistical Analysis.

The values were expressed as mean $\pm$ SD. The results were analyzed statistically by Analysis of Variance (ANOVA) followed by the Tukey test. The analyses were performed with the software GraphPad Prism 5.0.4. Differences were considered significant when $p < 0.05$.

3. Results and Discussion

The *M. citrifolia* fruit juice was brown, translucent, and of medium viscosity, with its characteristic odor and pH 3.94. After lyophilization, the juice yielded 6.31% of a highly hygroscopic powder. The constituents of *M. citrifolia* fruit juice were analyzed by HPLC-DAD-ELSD and the analysis of the chromatograms obtained from both detectors showed peaks related to compounds with sensitivity in the UV region. The LC-DAD and LC-ELSD chromatograms are presented in Figure 1. The major peaks of the UV-365 nm chromatogram were associated with the characteristic UV spectra of flavonoid (peak 8) and anthraquinones (peak 11). The ELSD fingerprint showed an intense peak at 3.2 min which was not observed in the DAD chromatogram. This signal could be related to the polysaccharides previously reported in *M. citrifolia* that have significant antitumoral activity [12]. Polysaccharides from *Echinacea purpurea* showed activity against *Leishmania enriettii* [13] and the presence of these substances in the phytochemical fingerprint showed the probable chemical potential of the fruit extract against protozoa such as the *Leishmania* genus. This potential was demonstrated through in vitro leishmanicidal activity of the *M. citrifolia* fruit juice against *L. infantum*.

The effect of *M. citrifolia* fruit juice on the promastigote forms of *L. infantum* was monitored for 72 hours. *M. citrifolia* fruit juice produced a dose-dependent reduction in the proliferation of the parasite (Figure 2(a)), with growth inhibition of 50% of the promastigotes at a concentration of 260.5 μg/mL (Table 1). The values are considered promising when compared with other fruit extracts. The crude extract from the fruit *Momordica charantia* showed an IC$_{50}$ under 600 μg/mL for *L. donovani* promastigotes [14].

There are few data about in vitro leishmanicidal activity of *M. citrifolia* constituents in the literature. A clinical trial on the antileishmanial activity of *M. citrifolia* showed good activity for two anthraquinones isolated from stem extract, morindicone and morinthone [9]. Anthraquinones also have been isolated from *M. lucida*, a plant of same gender of *M. citrifolia*, and presented activity against the growth of *Plasmodium falciparum* and promastigotes of *L. major in vitro* [15].

Trying to find compounds responsible for in vitro leishmanicidal activity, the *M. citrifolia* fruit juice was submitted to a column partition and, interestingly, the partitions showed IC$_{50}$ values above the value obtained for the full juice (data not shown). This result indicates that various substances present in the *M. citrifolia* fruit juice contribute to the leishmanicidal activity, probably, synergistically, corroborating

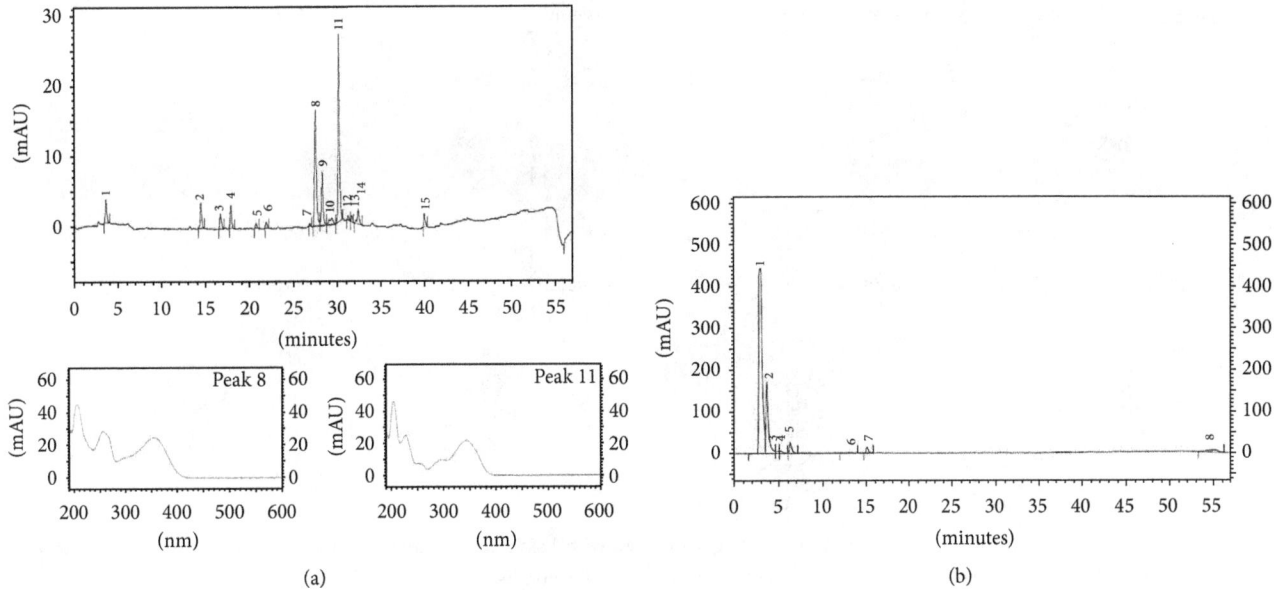

FIGURE 1: High Performance Liquid Chromatography coupled with diode array detector (a) and evaporative light scattering detector (b) of *Morinda citrifolia* fruit juice at 365 nm. (a) Peaks 8 and 11: highlight of the UV spectra.

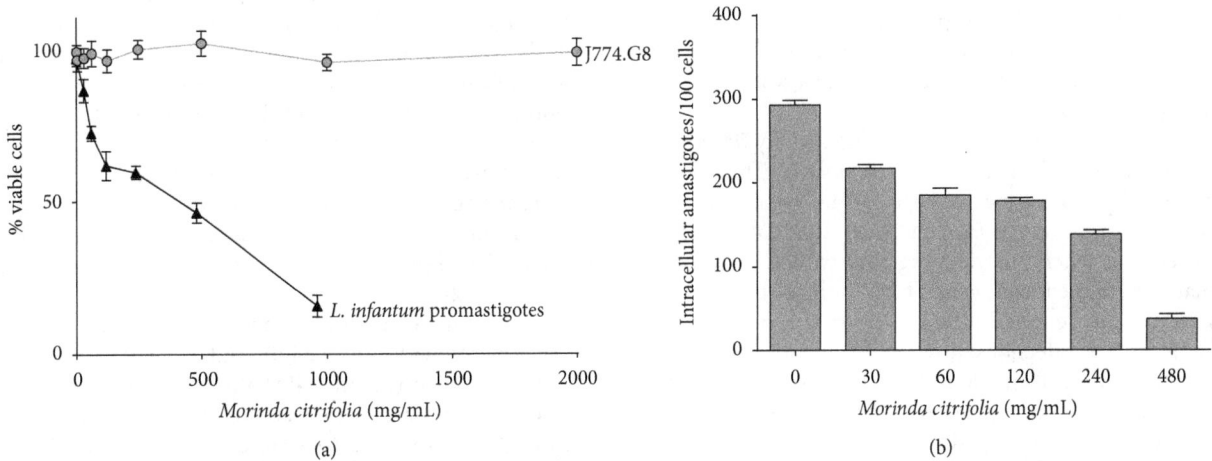

FIGURE 2: Leishmanicidal activity and *in vitro* cytotoxicity of *Morinda citrifolia* fruit juice. (a) Viability of *Leishmania infantum* promastigotes and J774.G8 macrophages treated with *M. citrifolia* for 72 and 24 hours, respectively. (b) Intracellular amastigotes in BALB/c peritoneal macrophages treated for 24 hours. Data represent mean ± SD of at least three independent experiments realized in quintuplicate.

previous studies where more than one molecule presented biological activity [16, 17].

Although the leishmanicidal activity *in vitro* against promastigotes is used by many researchers as a screening test to search for new drugs for the treatment of leishmaniasis, the positive result of this test alone cannot be considered as an indicator of potential drug action. Activity against intracellular amastigotes is necessary and is perhaps the most effective way to relate the *in vitro* activity of a substance with its possible effectiveness *in vivo*. Thus we also evaluated *M. citrifolia* activity against intracellular amastigotes (Figure 2(b)).

As shown in Table 1, there is an increase in activity of the *M. citrifolia* fruit juice against intracellular amastigotes

compared with the activity against promastigotes. The IC_{50} value decreased for intracellular amastigotes with a value of 201.3 μg/mL. When observed by light microscopy, macrophages showed vacuoles with probable remains of intracellular amastigotes (Figure 3). This result indicates the possible action of the *M. citrifolia* fruit juice on macrophage activation and modulation, as already shown in previous works, such as the decreased production of IL-4 and increased production of TNF-α, IL-1β [12], INF-γ, and NO [18].

To ensure that *M. citrifolia* fruit juice was only acting on intracellular amastigotes, without causing damage to the host cell, the cytotoxicity in J774.G8 lineage macrophages was investigated by the Sulforhodamine B method (Figure 2(a)).

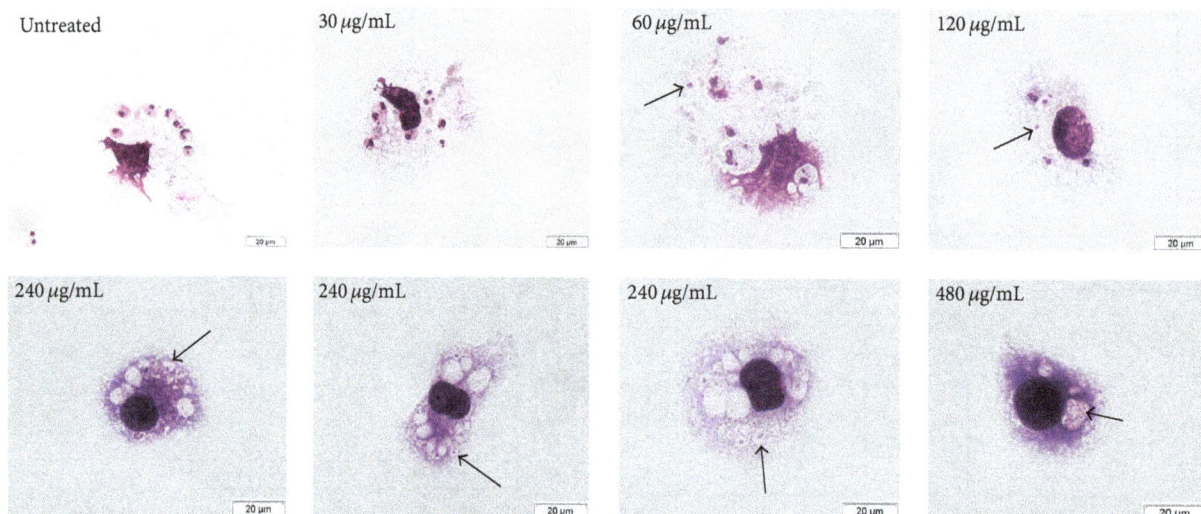

FIGURE 3: Light microscopy of BALB/c peritoneal macrophages infected with *Leishmania amazonensis* and treated with *Morinda citrifolia* fruit juice. Arrows indicate vacuoles with probable remains of intracellular amastigotes.

This colorimetric method is based on the quantification of total protein by binding anionic Sulforhodamine B electrostatic crystals with cellular proteins. No cytotoxicity was observed at the concentrations analyzed and the selectivity index for *M. citrifolia* fruit juice was at least 3.3-fold higher than amphotericin B (Table 1).

Macrophages were used to assess the toxicity *in vitro* for being target cells of infection by *Leishmania*. The analysis of cytotoxicity against macrophages J774.G8 shows the low cytotoxicity of *M. citrifolia* fruit juice. This data becomes more relevant when analyzed together with IC_{50} to intracellular amastigote forms, generating SI higher than 9.9 that falls within the generic hit selection criteria of SI to new compounds for infectious diseases from Japanese Global Health Innovative Technology [19]. Indeed, as the generic hit criteria must be applied to phytotherapy with some reservations, the selective index is the most reliable criterion to assess the safety of extracts, essential oils, or others natural products. Besides, the leishmanicidal activity of *M. citrifolia* must be analyzed in addition to immunomodulatory effects and toxicity in posterior studies.

The transmission electron microscopy analysis of *L. infantum* promastigotes treated with the *M. citrifolia* fruit juice was performed to determine the ultrastructural changes. Photomicrographs of promastigotes (Figures 4, 5, 6, and 7) showed the degree of damage after 24 hours of treatment. The parasites without treatment showed normal morphology (Figure 4(a)).

The observation of *L. infantum* promastigotes treated with 30 μg/mL of juice showed vacuolization of the cytoplasm, some with electron-dense regions inside, and this became more evident at higher concentrations (Figures 4(b) and 4(c)). Similar structural changes have also been described in *L. amazonensis* treated with essential oils [20]. In these, the vacuoles are associated with entry of substances by simple diffusion, caused by increased permeability of the membrane due to the compounds in the essential oils.

Vesicles in the flagellar pocket were observed in promastigotes treated with 30 and 60 μg/mL of *M. citrifolia* fruit juice (Figures 4(d), 5(b), and 5(c)). The presence of vesicles in flagellar pockets indicates an intense exocytic activity in the region of the flagellar pocket. These changes have also been reported in promastigotes of *L. amazonensis* treated with inhibitors of ergosterol synthesis, such as 22,26-azasterol [21]. The increased activity in the region of the exocytic flagellar pocket may be the result of an abnormal secretion of lipids, which accumulate as a consequence of drug action or indicate an exacerbated production of proteins by cells in an attempt to survive [22].

Membrane structures in the cytoplasm were observed in treatments with 30, 60, 120, and 240 μg/mL of *M. citrifolia* fruit juice (Figures 4(b)–4(d), 5(a), 6(a) and 6(b)). These structures are membranes of the endoplasmic reticulum dispersed in the cytoplasm and are probably involved in the recycling of abnormal organelles. The presence of autophagosome-like vesicle material in promastigotes treated with 240 μg/mL of *M. citrifolia* fruit juice shows an autophagic process (Figures 6(c) and 6(d)), suggesting a remodeling of organelles irreversibly damaged by the treatment. Autophagy can serve as a protective mechanism by recycling macromolecules and removing damaged organelles, but excessive autophagy can result in cell death [23]. To try to survive the effects caused by *M. citrifolia* fruit juice treatment, parasites may react triggering autophagic events, and this exacerbated autophagic response could lead to death, as observed in parasites treated with the 480 μg/mL of juice.

The treatment with 480 μg/mL of *M. citrifolia* fruit juice for 24 hours induced severe cellular damage (Figures 7(a) and 7(b)), with the extravasation of cytoplasmic contents and loss of cellular integrity. The progression of ultrastructural changes is related to increasing drug concentrations, reaching its apex with parasite destruction at higher drug concentrations, and showing the direct action of *M. citrifolia*

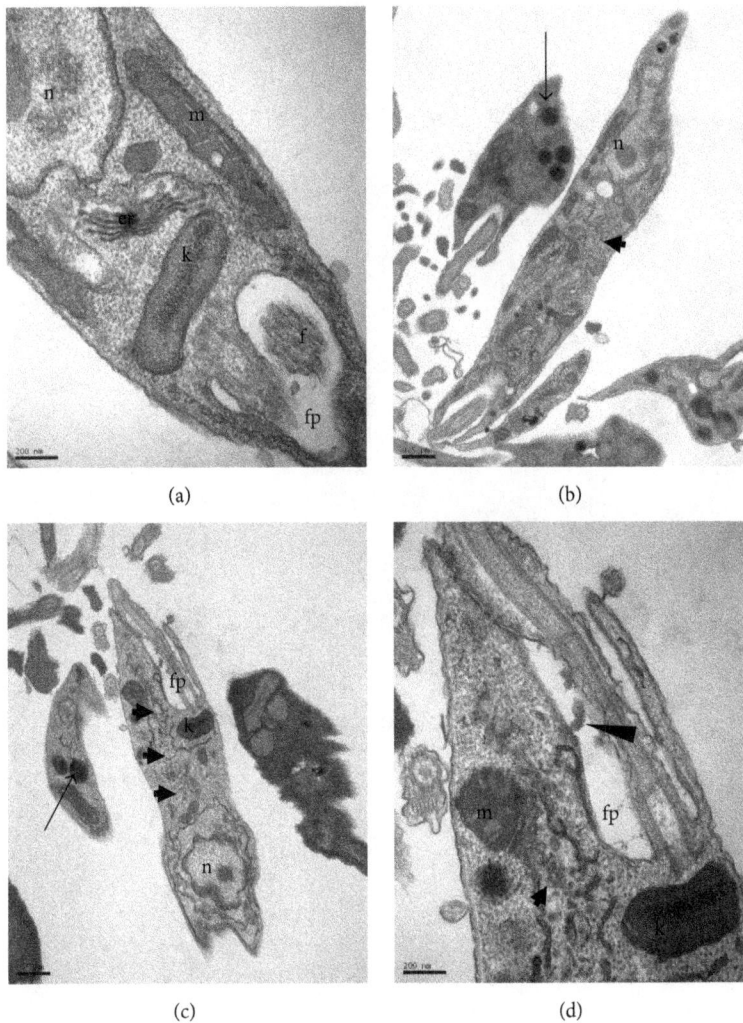

(a)   (b)

(c)   (d)

FIGURE 4: Ultrastructure of *Leishmania infantum* promastigotes incubated for 24 hours, at 26°C, with *Morinda citrifolia* fruit juice. (a) Control. (b–d) Promastigote treated with 30 μg/mL. (b-c) Electron-dense vesicles (arrows) and granular material throughout the cytoplasm (block arrows). (d) Membranes in flagellar pocket (arrowhead). k: kinetoplast, m: mitochondria, n: nucleus, pf: flagellar pocket, f: flagellum, and er: endoplasmic reticulum.

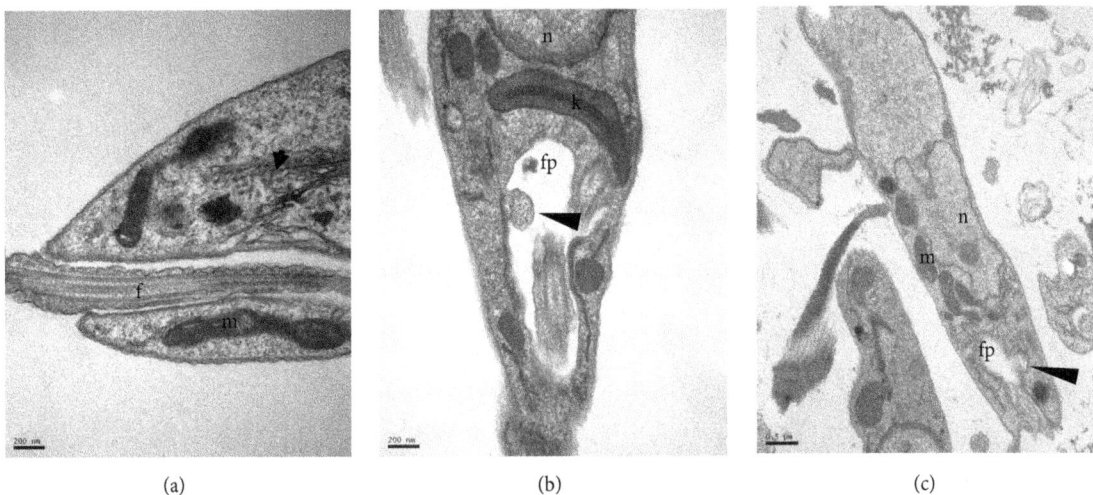

(a)   (b)   (c)

FIGURE 5: Ultrastructure of *Leishmania infantum* promastigotes incubated for 24 hours, at 26°C, with *Morinda citrifolia* fruit juice. (a–c) Promastigote treated with 60 μg/mL. Electron-dense vesicles (arrows) and granular material throughout the cytoplasm (block arrows). Vesicles breaking up in flagellar pocket (arrowhead). k: kinetoplast, m: mitochondria, n: nucleus, pf: flagellar pocket, and f: flagellum.

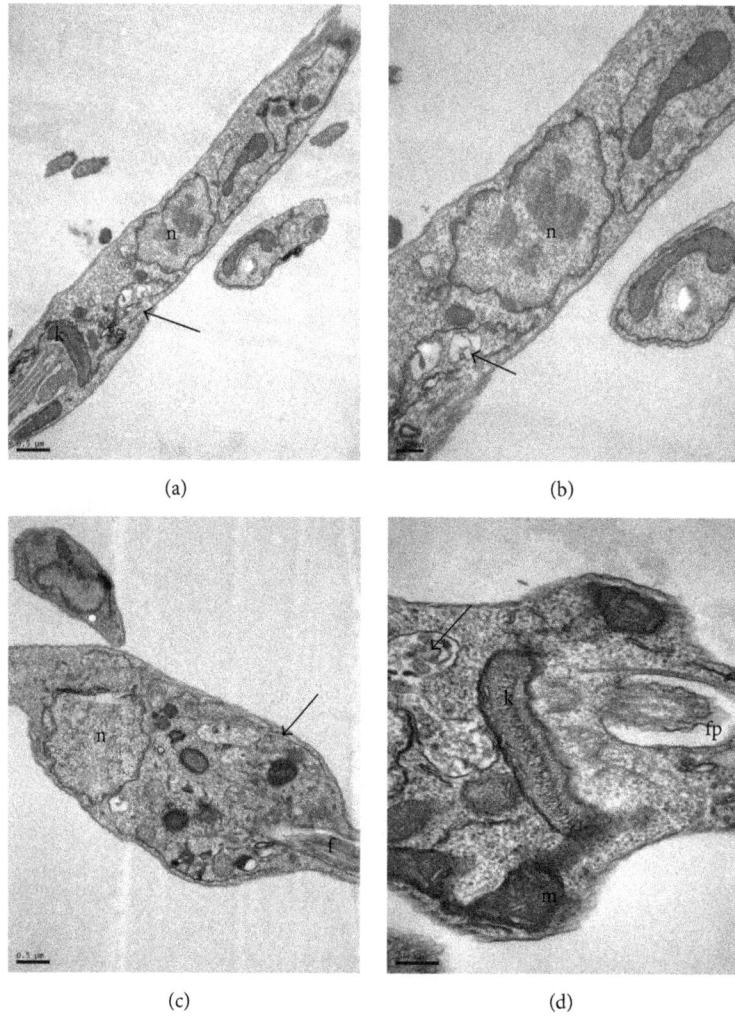

FIGURE 6: Ultrastructure of *Leishmania infantum* promastigotes incubated for 24 hours, at 26°C, with *Morinda citrifolia* fruit juice. (a-b) Promastigotes treated with 120 μg/mL. (c-d) Promastigotes treated with 240 μg/mL. Vesicles with granular material throughout the cytoplasm (arrows). Vesicles with autophagosome-like material (asterisks). k: kinetoplast, m: mitochondria, n: nucleus, pf: flagellar pocket, and f: flagellum.

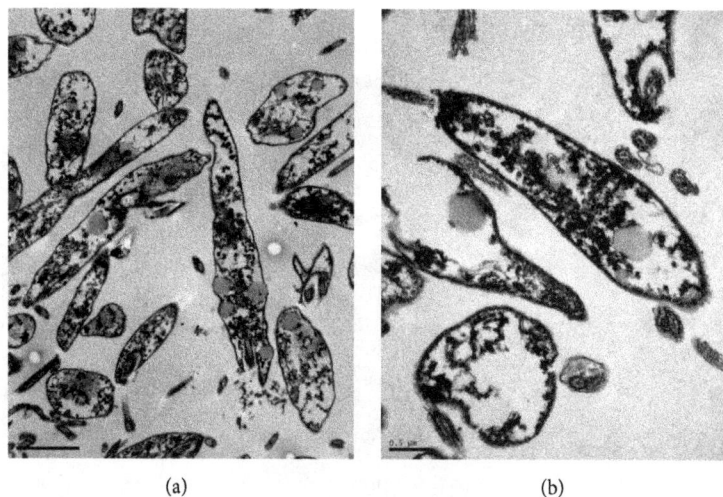

FIGURE 7: Ultrastructure of *Leishmania infantum* promastigotes incubated for 24 hours, at 26°C, with 480 μg/mL of *Morinda citrifolia* fruit juice. (a-b) Promastigotes with loss of membrane integrity.

fruit juice on the parasite and its dose-dependent action. No changes were observed in the nucleus, the mitochondria, the flagellum, the kinetoplast, or the subpellicular microtubules.

4. Conclusion

M. citrifolia fruit juice showed leishmanicidal activity against *L. infantum* promastigote, causing ultrastructural changes such as cytoplasmic vacuolization, lipid inclusion, increased exocytosis activity, autophagosome-like vesicles, loss of cellular integrity, and death of the parasite. Considering the activity and the alterations observed against promastigote forms of *L. infantum*, further studies must be conducted to evaluate the potential of *M. citrifolia* fruit juice in leishmaniasis treatment.

Disclosure

Ana Lúcia Abreu-Silva (CNPq no. 306218/2010-0) is senior researcher.

Competing Interests

The authors report no conflict of interests.

Authors' Contributions

Kátia da Silva Calabrese and Ana Lúcia Abreu-Silva contributed equally to this work.

Acknowledgments

This work was supported by FAPEMA (APP-00844/09), CNPq (407831/2012.6), and IOC.

References

[1] E. Rodrigues, "Plants and animals utilized as medicines in the Jaú National Park (JNP), Brazilian Amazon," *Phytotherapy Research*, vol. 20, no. 5, pp. 378–391, 2006.

[2] WHO, *Sustaining the Drive to Overcome the Global Impact of Neglected Tropical Diseases: Second Who Report on Neglected Diseases*, World Health Organization, Lyon, France, 2013.

[3] J. Alvar, I. D. Vélez, C. Bern et al., "Leishmaniasis worldwide and global estimates of its incidence," *PLoS ONE*, vol. 7, no. 5, Article ID e35671, 2012.

[4] H. A. Miot, L. D. Miot, A. L. Costa, C. Y. Matsuo, and L. H. O'Dwyer, "Avaliação do efeito antiparasitário do omeprazol na prevenção do desenvolvimento de lesões cutâneas em hamsters infectados por *Leishmania brasiliensis*," *Anais Brasileiros de Dermatologia*, vol. 80, supplement 3, article 4, pp. S329–S332, 2005.

[5] S. Basar, K. Uhlenhut, P. Högger, F. Schöne, and J. Westendorf, "Analgesic and antiinflammatory activity of Morinda citrifolia L. (Noni) fruit," *Phytotherapy Research*, vol. 24, no. 1, pp. 38–42, 2010.

[6] T. Hiramatsu, M. Imoto, T. Koyano, and K. Umezawa, "Induction of normal phenotypes in ras-transformed cells by damnacanthal from *Morinda citrifolia*," *Cancer Letters*, vol. 73, no. 2-3, pp. 161–166, 1993.

[7] D. Kandaswamy, N. Venkateshbabu, D. Gogulnath, and A. J. Kindo, "Dentinal tubule disinfection with 2% chlorhexidine gel, propolis, morinda citrifolia juice, 2% povidone iodine, and calcium hydroxide," *International Endodontic Journal*, vol. 43, no. 5, pp. 419–423, 2010.

[8] A. Jainkittivong, T. Butsarakamruha, and R. P. Langlais, "Antifungal activity of Morinda citrifolia fruit extract against Candida albicans," *Oral Surgery, Oral Medicine, Oral Pathology, Oral Radiology and Endodontology*, vol. 108, no. 3, pp. 394–398, 2009.

[9] F. A. Sattar, F. Ahmed, N. Ahmed, S. A. Sattar, M. A. K. Malghani, and M. I. Choudhary, "A double-blind, randomized, clinical trial on the antileishmanial activity of a *Morinda citrifolia* (Noni) stem extract and its major constituents," *Natural Product Communications*, vol. 7, no. 2, pp. 195–196, 2012.

[10] T. Mosmann, "Rapid colorimetric assay for cellular growth and survival: application to proliferation and cytotoxicity assays," *Journal of Immunological Methods*, vol. 65, no. 1-2, pp. 55–63, 1983.

[11] P. Skehan, R. Storeng, D. Scudiero et al., "New colorimetric cytotoxicity assay for anticancer-drug screening," *Journal of the National Cancer Institute*, vol. 82, no. 13, pp. 1107–1112, 1990.

[12] A. Hirazumi and E. Furusawa, "An immunomodulatory polysaccharide-rich substance from the fruit juice of Morinda citrifolia (noni) with antitumour activity," *Phytotherapy Research*, vol. 13, no. 5, pp. 380–387, 1999.

[13] C. Steinmüller, J. Roesler, E. Gröttrup, G. Franke, H. Wagner, and M.-L. Lohmann-Matthes, "Polysaccharides isolated from plant cell cultures of *Echinacea purpurea* enhance the resistance of immunosuppressed mice against systemic infections with *Candida albicans* and *Listeria monocytogenes*," *International Journal of Immunopharmacology*, vol. 15, no. 5, pp. 605–614, 1993.

[14] S. Gupta, B. Raychaudhuri, S. Banerjee, B. Das, S. Mukhopadhaya, and S. C. Datta, "Momordicatin purified from fruits of *Momordica charantia* is effective to act as a potent antileishmania agent," *Parasitology International*, vol. 59, no. 2, pp. 192–197, 2010.

[15] A. A. Sittie, E. Lemmich, C. E. Olsen et al., "Structure-activity studies: *in vitro* antileishmanial and antimalarial activities of anthraquinones from *Morinda lucida*," *Planta Medica*, vol. 65, no. 3, pp. 259–261, 1999.

[16] C.-H. Liu, Y.-R. Xue, Y.-H. Ye, F.-F. Yuan, J.-Y. Liu, and J.-L. Shuang, "Extraction and characterization of antioxidant compositions from fermented fruit juice of Morinda citrifolia (Noni)," *Agricultural Sciences in China*, vol. 6, no. 12, pp. 1494–1501, 2007.

[17] E. Furusawa, A. Hirazumi, S. Story, and J. Jensen, "Antitumour potential of a polysaccharide-rich substance from the fruit juice of *Morinda citrifolia* (Noni) on sarcoma 180 ascites tumour in mice," *Phytotherapy Research*, vol. 17, no. 10, pp. 1158–1164, 2003.

[18] A. K. Palu, A. H. Kim, B. J. West, S. Deng, J. Jensen, and L. White, "The effects of *Morinda citrifolia* L. (noni) on the immune system: its molecular mechanisms of action," *Journal of Ethnopharmacology*, vol. 115, no. 3, pp. 502–506, 2007.

[19] K. Katsuno, J. N. Burrows, K. Duncan et al., "Hit and lead criteria in drug discovery for infectious diseases of the developing world," *Nature Reviews Drug Discovery*, vol. 14, no. 11, pp. 751–758, 2015.

[20] V. C. S. Oliveira, D. M. S. Moura, J. A. D. Lopes, P. P. de Andrade, N. H. da Silva, and R. C. B. Q. Figueiredo, "Effects of essential oils from *Cymbopogon citratus* (DC) Stapf., *Lippia sidoides* Cham., and *Ocimum gratissimum* L. on growth and

ultrastructure of *Leishmania chagasi* promastigotes," *Parasitology Research*, vol. 104, no. 5, pp. 1053–1059, 2009.

[21] J. C. F. Rodrigues, M. Attias, C. Rodriguez, J. A. Urbina, and W. De Souza, "Ultrastructural and biochemical alterations induced by 22,26-azasterol, a Δ24(25)-sterol methyltransferase inhibitor, on promastigote and amastigote forms of Leishmania amazonensis," *Antimicrobial Agents and Chemotherapy*, vol. 46, no. 2, pp. 487–499, 2002.

[22] T. S. Tiuman, T. Ueda-Nakamura, D. A. Garcia Cortez et al., "Antileishmanial activity of parthenolide, a sesquiterpene lactone isolated from *Tanacetum parthenium*," *Antimicrobial Agents and Chemotherapy*, vol. 49, no. 1, pp. 176–182, 2005.

[23] T. Nishikawa, N. H. Tsuno, Y. Okaji et al., "Inhibition of autophagy potentiates sulforaphane-induced apoptosis in human colon cancer cells," *Annals of Surgical Oncology*, vol. 17, no. 2, pp. 592–602, 2010.

5

Preliminary Screening of Antioxidant and Antibacterial Activities and Establishment of an Efficient Callus Induction in *Curculigo latifolia* Dryand (Lemba)

Reza Farzinebrahimi,[1] **Rosna Mat Taha,**[1] **Kamaludin A. Rashid,**[2] **Bakrudeen Ali Ahmed,**[1] **Mahmoud Danaee,**[3] **and Shahril Efzueni Rozali**[2]

[1]*Institute of Biological Sciences (IBS), Faculty of Science, University of Malaya, 50603 Kuala Lumpur, Malaysia*
[2]*Biology Division, Center for Foundation Studies in Science, University of Malaya, 50603 Kuala Lumpur, Malaysia*
[3]*Academic Development Centre (AdeC), Wisma R&D, University of Malaya, 59990 Kuala Lumpur, Malaysia*

Correspondence should be addressed to Reza Farzinebrahimi; rfebrahimi@siswa.um.edu.my

Academic Editor: Nunziatina De Tommasi

Leaf, seed, and tuber explants of *C. latifolia* were inoculated on MS medium supplemented with various concentrations of BAP and IBA, alone or in combinations, to achieve *in vitro* plant regeneration. Subsequently, antioxidant and antibacterial activities were determined from *in vitro* and *in vivo* plant developed. No response was observed from seed culture on MS media with various concentrations of PGRs. The highest percentage of callus was observed on tuber explants (94%) and leaf explants (89%) when cultured on MS media supplemented with IBA in combination with BAP. A maximum of 88% shoots per tuber explant, with a mean number of shoots (8.8 ± 1.0), were obtained on MS medium supplemented with combinations of BAP and IBA ($2.5 \, \mathrm{mg \, L^{-1}}$). The best root induction (92%) and mean number (7.6 ± 0.5) from tuber explants were recorded on $2.5 \, \mathrm{mg \, L^{-1}}$ IBA alone supplemented to MS medium. The higher antioxidant content (80%) was observed from *in vivo* tuber. However, tuber part from the intact plant showed higher inhibition zone in antibacterial activity compared to other *in vitro* and *in vivo* tested parts.

1. Introduction

There are more than 20 species in the family Hypoxidaceae where *Curculigo* and *Hypoxis* are the two main genera of this family. The genus *Curculigo* is distributed in the tropical region of Africa and Asia rainforest's, particularly Malaysia and Singapore [1]. The four main species of this genus include *C. latifolia*, *C. capitulations*, *C. racemes*, and *C. orchioides* [2].

 Curculigo latifolia Dryand, Lemba in Malaysia, is one of the important traditional Chinese medicinal plants. These species are propagated by rhizomes [3] and may be found abundantly in highland areas (with 1500–2000-meter altitude) and normally on slopes and forests. The leaf fibres can be used for making the fishing net, rope, and twines in Borneo and Malaysia. The leaves and flowers can treat a high fever. Flower and root concoctions are used to ease stomach-ache and frequent urination [4]. However, the rhizome dressing is applied externally to cure the cut and wounds [5]. In addition, it is reported to have an inhibitory effect on hepatitis B virus by rhizome extract [6]. Yamashita et al. [7] revealed two unique sweet proteins in the fruit such as Curculin and Neoculin that exhibit both sweet-tasting and taste-modifying characteristics at the same time. These proteins have been proven 500 times sweeter than sucrose by weight [8, 9] which could be employed as a low-calorie sweetener for diabetes or obesity [2]. To date, more than hundred compounds of secondary metabolites (such as phenols and phenolic glycosides), two polysaccharides (COPb-1 and COPf-1), and three proteins (Curculin, Neoculin, and β-amylase) have been known and extracted from this species. However, the phenols and phenolic glycosides from this plant are categorised as benzyl benzoate glycosides, followed by phenol glycosides and simple phenol. The 20 unique saponins are cycloartane triterpenoids and could be found in this species [10].

Grzegorczyk et al. [11] reported the *in vitro* acetone extract of *Salvia officinalis* exhibited antioxidant properties. However, many authors stated that *in vitro* and *in vivo* plant extracts showed antioxidant activities [12–15].

The increase in demands of this plant for commercial use requires an alternative rate of proliferation. During these years, *in vitro* technique is being widely applied to produce identical quality and disease-free plants [16]. There is no evidence on propagation of *C. latifolia* from seeds, but we reported that it is being propagated through rhizome [3]. However, due to high medicinal, industrial, and unique value of its compounds and low productivity and failed attempts for plantation of this species by conventional methods in nurseries, propagation of this plant by *in vitro* or tissue culture technique is mandatory.

An *in vitro* method for propagation of the species *C. orchioides* was established as a rare and endangered species in India [17–20]. However, some success of *in vitro* culture of this species has been reported [21].

The present study is advancement over the earlier protocol, because it describes the PGRs regulation, *in vitro* plant regeneration, and the role of regeneration plantlets in antioxidant and antibacterial effects to compare with *in vivo* *C. latifolia* and the subsequent transplantation of the plantlets to natural environmental conditions.

2. Plant Materials and Sterilization

The fresh mature fruits of *C. latifolia*, grown at Genting Highlands, Malaysia, were collected in the middle of September 2014. The tiny black seeds were obtained from dry fruits. Some botanists identified the plant materials and some pots were deposited at The University of Malaya (Green House, Institute Biological Sciences). The seed explants of *C. latifolia* were surface sterilized according to Taha [22] with some modifications.

The seeds were treated with 70%, 50%, 20%, and 10% (v/v) commercial bleach (Clorox) for 1 min at each concentration. The treated seeds were submerged in 70% (v/v) ethanol and finally by 3 times rinsing with sterile distilled water. Two drops of Tween-20 were also added during the treatment with 100% (v/v) Clorox to facilitate the sterilization process and reduce surface tensions.

Leaves and tubers were collected from (5-6 months old) seedlings, which were grown in Genting Highlands, Malaysia. Both types of explants were washed thoroughly under running tap water for 20 min. The leaves were soaked with commercial bleach or Clorox (70%) for 3 min under laminar flow and were rinsed 2 times with sterile distilled water. Treated leaves were submerged in 70% (v/v) ethanol and finally were rinsed 5 times with sterile distilled water.

The tubers were dipped in 30% citric acid to remove phenolic content and were immersed in 75% Clorox for 10 min. The tubers were sterilized by ethanol 100% (v/v) containing 0.1% (V/V) Tween 20 for 5 min and finally were rinsed five times with sterile distilled water.

3. Medium, Plant Growth Regulators (PGRs), and Callus Induction

For all treatments, MS basal medium [23] containing 3% sucrose was solidified with 2.5 g L^{-1} Gelrite (Duchefa brand, Netherland) and supplemented with various concentrations of IBA either alone or in combination with BAP $(0.5–4 \text{ mg L}^{-1})$.

All the media were adjusted to pH of 5.7 ± 0.1 with 0.1 N KOH prior to autoclaving at $121°C$ for 20 min. The media were dispensed into 60 mL specimen presterilized containers under laminar flow in aseptic condition.

The leaves were further cut into approximately 0.5 cm^2 pieces, removing leaf ribs, and any other major leaf veins before being placed on the culture medium. The explants (3 per plate) were arranged horizontally and were pressed lightly into the surface of the culture medium.

Tubers (3 per plate) were cut into 2 cm^2 and placed on the surface of the culture medium. In order to avoid the death of explants due to phenolic exudation, the tuber explants were subcultured three times every 3 days to the same media and PGRs.

The leaves and tuber explants were inoculated on MS basal media and supplemented either alone or in combination with IBA and BAP. The cultures were maintained at $25°C$ under a 16–8-hour photoperiod at a photon flux rate of $60 \mu\text{mol m}^{-2} \text{ s}^{-1}$ provided by cool daylight fluorescent lamps.

3.1. In Vitro Callus Growth. Callus cultures were optimized and measured for its biomass and secondary metabolic content. By applying various concentrations of PGRs, fresh and dry weights of the callus were determined at 8 weeks. At the end of the period, for all the treatments, each callus was harvested by careful separation from media using metal spatulas, and fresh and dry weight were promptly recorded.

3.2. Acclimatization. The regenerated plantlets were transplanted to 6 cm plastic pots filled with perlite and pit (3 : 1) and were kept in a controlled condition chamber with 80–90% relative humidity under a 16/8 h (light/dark) of photoperiod at a photon flux rate of $60 \mu\text{mol m}^{-2} \text{ s}^{-1}$ provided by cool daylight fluorescent for 8 weeks. The plantlets were transferred to greenhouse conditions after 8 weeks.

3.3. Plant Extraction. *In vivo* samples from young and healthy leaves and tuber (5-6 months old) were collected. The *in vitro* developed friable callus (without roots and shoots) from leaf and tuber explants was collected and both *in vivo* and *in vitro* samples were dried separately at room temperature for 4 days. To produce a fine homogenous powder, the samples were ground by electric blender. The 5 g of dried *in vivo* sample and *in vitro* regenerated callus of *C. latifolia* was extracted five times with ethanol [24]. The ethanol extract was centrifuged for 5 min at 5000 rpm. The supernatant was carefully pipetted into Eppendorf tubes. The plant extract (10 g L^{-1}) was dissolved in phosphate buffered saline (PBS) and was kept at $4°C$.

4. Antioxidant Activity

In order to study antioxidant properties, radical scavenging and superoxide dismutase assay were applied and the obtained results were compared.

4.1. Radical Scavenging Capacity Assay. DPPH* (2, 2-diphenyl-1-picrylhydrazyl) free radical scavenging capacity assay was achieved using the protocol described by Rafat et al. [15]. DPPH (950 μL) at a concentration of 90 μM was mixed with 50 μL plant extract (10 g L^{-1}), and the volume was adjusted to 4 mL using ethanol (95%). The solution was incubated for 120 min at room temperature in the dark condition. Scavenging of DPPH reduced the color of the solution and was measured using a spectrophotometer at 515 nm.

Comparison of the reduction of color in the examined samples with the blank (solution without plant extract) was used to measure the potential of scavenging capacity of the plant extracts using the following formula [15]:

$$\text{Radical scavenging capacity (\%)} = \left[\frac{\text{blank} - \text{sample}_A}{\text{blank}}\right] \times 100. \quad (1)$$

4.2. Superoxide Dismutase Assay. Superoxide dismutase (SOD) determination kit (19160), ascorbic acid (A4544) from Sigma-Aldrich (St. Louis, Mo), and Tert-butylated hydroxytoluene (34750) from Fluka (Spain), were used for this part of the study. Plant extracts with a concentration of 10 g L^{-1} were added to 200 μL of the kit working solution. The mixture, after gentle shaking, was incubated at 37°C for 20 min after adding 20 μL of the kit enzyme working solution. The absorbance of the mixtures was measured at 450 nm using a microplate reader (BIO-RAD Model 550, USA) and the SOD activity was calculated based on the following equation [11]. Ascorbic acid (1 g L^{-1}) and BHT or tert-butylated hydroxytoluene (1 g L^{-1}) were employed as the positive controls in this study:

$$\text{Inhibition\% (SOD activity)}$$
$$= \frac{(\text{blank}_1 - \text{blank}_2) - (\text{sample}_A - \text{blank}_{\text{sample}_A})}{(\text{blank}_1 - \text{blank}_2)} \quad (2)$$
$$\times 100,$$

where blank$_1$ = blank of mixture working solution + enzyme working solution + double distilled water, blank$_2$ = blank of mixture plant extract + working solution + dilution buffer + double distilled water, blank$_{\text{sample}_A}$ = blank of mixture plant extract + working solution + dilution buffer.

5. Antibacterial Activity Assay (Disk Diffusion Method)

The antibacterial potential of *C. latifolia* was investigated based on the paper disc diffusion method adopted from

Farzinebrahimi et al. [12] with minor modification. Two gram-positive bacteria (*Staphylococcus aureus* and *Bacillus cereus*) and two gram-negative pathogenic bacteria (*Pseudomonas aeruginosa* and *Klebsiella* sp.) were obtained from Microbiology Division of Institute of Biological Sciences, University of Malaya, and maintained in a nutrient broth medium to produce a final concentration of 107 colony forming units (CFU) per mL. The test bacteria (0.1 mL) were streaked by sterile cotton swab on Mueller Hinton medium (MH) plates. Sterilized filter paper discs were soaked in extracts (10 g L^{-1}) and then placed at the centre of test bacteria plates. The diameters of the inhibition zones were recorded after 24 hours of incubation at a temperature of 37°C overnight. Ampicillin (30 μg) was applied as positive and negative controls, respectively. Sterile paper disks were put in samples; sterile distilled water and kanamycin antibiotic were as control for two hours.

6. Statistical Analysis

The experiments were conducted in a factorial based on randomized completely design with 4 blocks and 16 treatments. For all treatments, the mean and standard error were calculated. The data were analyzed by ANOVA followed by mean comparison using Duncan multiple range test (DMRT) [25]. Data were subjected to normality test using one sample Kolmogorov-Smirnov. All data analysis was done using SPSS ver. 21.

7. Results

7.1. Callus Induction. The seeds did not respond to MS media and different PGRs either alone or in combination after eight weeks of seed inoculation. It may be due to the hard seed coat, immature embryo, rudimentary embryo, and inhibitor substances. However, the callus initiation did not form without PGRs (plant growth regulators, control) in tuber and leaf explants.

The best callus induction from tuber explants was recorded in MS media with combinations of IBA and BAP (94%), whereas the same media supplemented with IBA and BAP alone produced 71% and 79% callus, respectively. This pattern was observed in callus formation from leaf explants, when combination of IBA and BAP produced higher percentage of callus (89%) as compared with IBA (82%) and BAP (83%).

Among the various concentrations of applied PGRs in callus induction from tuber explants, IBA (3.5 and 4 mg L^{-1}) and BAP (4.0 mg L^{-1}) induced nature callus with a maximum of fresh and dry weight. However, the highest callus was formed in leaf explants when IBA and BAP (4.0 mg L^{-1}) were applied alone or in combination (Figures 1 and 2).

7.2. Regeneration. The root and shoot formation were observed after 21 and 28 days of tuber inoculation and 16 and 21 days after leaf culture, respectively. The shoot and root formation were found in both tuber and leaf explants. However, the shoots formed in all concentrations of BAP alone or in combination with different concentrations of

TABLE 1: Mean number of shoots and roots' formation from tuber explants of *C. latifolia* Dryand cultured on MS media supplemented with BAP alone or in combination with IBA (IBA+BAP) at various concentrations after 8 weeks of culture ($\rho < 0.05$, $n = 4$). Different letters in the same column represent a significant difference at the 5% level in Duncan's multiple range tests.

PGRs	Mean number of shoots per leaf explant $\pm$ SE	Mean number of roots per leaf explant $\pm$ SE
Control	0^f	0^g
0.5 IBA	0^f	2.3 ± 0.6^{ef}
0.5 BAP	1 ± 0.2^e	0^g
0.5 (BAP+IBA)	1.3 ± 0.4^e	4.3 ± 0.2^{de}
1 IBA	0^f	4.4 ± 0.4^{de}
1 BAP	2.4 ± 0.8^d	0.9 ± 0.2^f
1 (BAP+IBA)	3.6 ± 0.6^d	4.6 ± 0.9^{de}
1.5 IBA	0^f	5.5 ± 0.3^d
1.5 BAP	4.4 ± 0.6^c	0.9 ± 0.2^f
1.5 (BAP+IBA)	4.5 ± 0.9^c	5.9 ± 0.7^{bc}
2 IBA	0	6.7 ± 0.1^{ab}
2 BAP	5.4 ± 0.1^b	0.9 ± 0.5^f
2 (BAP+IBA)	6.8 ± 0.5^a	6.9 ± 0.3^a
2.5 IBA	0^f	7.6 ± 0.5^a
2.5 BAP	6.9 ± 0.3^a	4.2 ± 0.8^{de}
2.5 (BAP+IBA)	8.8 ± 1.0^a	7.4 ± 1.0^a
3 IBA	0^f	5.4 ± 0.5^d
3 BAP	6.8 ± 0.5^a	3.2 ± 0.4^{ef}
3 (BAP+IBA)	6.3 ± 0.1^{ab}	5.5 ± 0.1^d
3.5 IBA	0^f	5.6 ± 0.8^d
3.5 BAP	4.3 ± 0.4^c	5.8 ± 0.6^{cd}
3.5 (BAP+IBA)	3.5 ± 0.3^d	5.1 ± 0.2^d
4 IBA	0^f	4.6 ± 0.4^{de}
4 BAP	4.6 ± 0.3^c	2.4 ± 0.2^{ef}
4 (BAP+IBA)	3.4 ± 0.9^d	1.3 ± 0.4^f

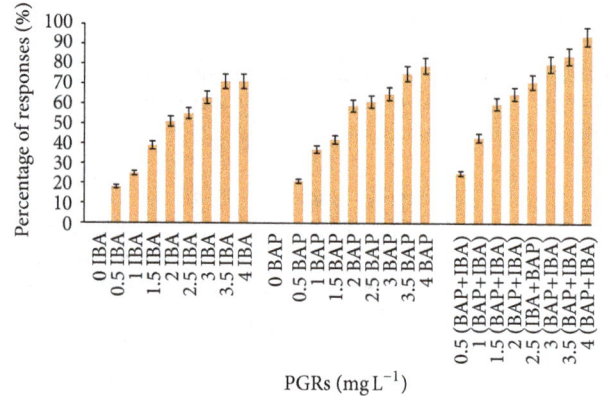

FIGURE 1: Callus formation from tuber explants of *C. latifolia* Dryand cultured on MS media supplemented with BAP alone or in combination with IBA (IBA+BAP) at various concentrations after 8 weeks of culture. No response was observed in IBA or BAP alone.

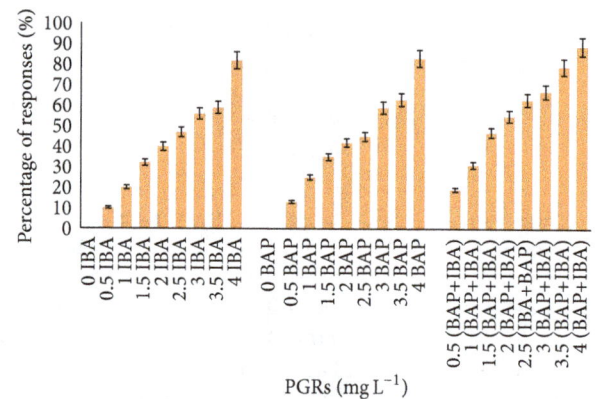

FIGURE 2: Callus formation from leaf explants of *C. latifolia* Dryand cultured on MS media supplemented with BAP alone or in combination with IBA (IBA+BAP) at various concentrations after 8 weeks of culture. No response was observed in IBA or BAP alone.

IBA with regard to the mean number of shoots and roots' elongation per explants. Control treatments involving no plant growth regulators, as well as those treatments that did not use IBA alone, produced no shoots at all in either the tuber or the leaf explants.

7.3. Root and Shoot Formation

7.3.1. Tuber Explants. As illustrated in Table 1, the tuber explants inoculated in MS media supplemented with combinations of IBA and BAP ($2.5 \, \text{mg L}^{-1}$) showed the highest number of shoots (8.8 ± 1.0). However, the best root numbers (7.6 ± 0.5) were formed in the same media added with IBA ($2.5 \, \text{mg L}^{-1}$) alone after eight weeks of culture.

7.3.2. Leaf Explants. The highest number of roots/explants was obtained from leaves (7.3 ± 0.1), when leaf explants were cultured on MS media supplemented with $2 \, \text{mg L}^{-1}$ IBA

alone. However, combinations of BAP and IBA ($2 \, \text{mg L}^{-1}$) produced 5.7 ± 0.8 shoots/explants (Table 2).

7.4. Root and Shoot Elongation

7.4.1. Leaf Explants. The leaf explants cultured in MS media supplemented with combination of IBA and BAP ($2 \, \text{mg L}^{-1}$) showed the optimum result of root and shoot length ($6.61 \pm 0.68 \, \text{cm}$ and $5.35 \pm 1.31 \, \text{cm}$), respectively (Figure 3). The lengths of roots and shoots from tuber explants were increased ($8.2 \pm 1.12 \, \text{cm}$ and $7.7 \pm 0.28 \, \text{cm}$) when the explants were cultured on the same media with a combination of $2.5 \, \text{mg L}^{-1}$ IBA and BAP (Figure 4).

Based on the obtained results shown in Figure 5, tuber explants inoculated on MS media supplemented with combinations of $4 \, \text{mg L}^{-1}$ IBA and BAP showed the higher weight based on fresh ($45.589 \pm 1.45 \, \text{g}$) and dry weight ($12.805 \pm 0.57 \, \text{g}$). The leaf explants inoculated on the same media and PGRs showed higher fresh and dry weight ($53.82 \pm 1.45 \, \text{g}$, $16.818 \pm 0.87 \, \text{g}$), respectively (Figure 6).

TABLE 2: Mean number of shoots and roots' formation from leaf explants of *C. latifolia* Dryand cultured on MS media supplemented with BAP alone or in combination with IBA (IBA+BAP) at various concentrations after 8 weeks of culture ($\rho < 0.05$, $n = 4$). Different letters in the same column represent a significant difference at the 5% level in Duncan's multiple range tests.

PGRs	Mean number of shoots per leaf explant ± SE	Mean number of roots per leaf explant ± SE
Control	0[f]	0[e]
0.5 IBA	0[f]	3.3 ± 0.9[d]
0.5 BAP	1.4 ± 0.1[e]	0.9 ± 0.4[e]
0.5 (BAP+IBA)	1.0 ± 0.2[ef]	3.5 ± 0.5[d]
1 IBA	0[f]	4.9 ± 1.0[c]
1 BAP	1.8 ± 0.1[de]	1.0 ± 0.1[e]
1 (BAP+IBA)	2.4 ± 0.4[d]	5.8 ± 0.5[b]
1.5 IBA	0[f]	6.1 ± 0.4[b]
1.5 BAP	3.09 ± 0.3[bc]	1.4 ± 0.4[de]
1.5 (BAP+IBA)	4.4 ± 0.2[b]	6.7 ± 0.8[a]
2 IBA	0[f]	7.3 ± 0.1[a]
2 BAP	5.5 ± 0.4[a]	2.1 ± 0.1[d]
2 (BAP+IBA)	5.7 ± 0.8[a]	7.1 ± 0.5[a]
2.5 IBA	0[f]	6.6 ± 0.4[ab]
2.5 BAP	4.3 ± 0.6[b]	2.1 ± 0.8[d]
2.5 (BAP+IBA)	4.8 ± 0.5[ba]	6.8 ± 0.2[ab]
3 IBA	0[f]	6.1 ± 0.5[b]
3 BAP	3.9 ± 0.4[bc]	1.1 ± 0.4[e]
3 (BAP+IBA)	4.8 ± 0.7[ba]	5.8 ± 0.6[b]
3.5 IBA	0[f]	4.3 ± 0.8[bc]
3.5 BAP	3.7 ± 0.3[cb]	1.0 ± 0.7[e]
3.5 (BAP+IBA)	3.2 ± 0.2[c]	5.6 ± 1.0[b]
4 IBA	0[f]	5.1 ± 0.2[c]
4 BAP	2.4 ± 0.3[cd]	0.8 ± 0.5[e]
4 (BAP+IBA)	1.3 ± 0.1[de]	1.8 ± 0.3[d]

7.5. Acclimatization. The regenerated plants were kept for six weeks in the rooting medium and transferred to MS medium free of PGRs for two weeks. The plantlets were maintained under normal room temperature for 7-8 days before transplantation under semicontrolled temperature ($30 \pm 2°C$) in a chamber with 80% humidity. The plants were transferred to the open place and gradually were acclimated to outdoor condition. The survival rate was measured as 89%.

7.6. Antioxidant Properties. The antioxidant activity of plant extracts (callus from leaf and tuber, resp.) of *C. latifolia* was compared with leaves from *in vivo* plants, butylated hydroxyl toluene (BHT) and ascorbic acid or vitamin C (1 mg L^{-1}) as a positive control.

Based on the results in Figure 7, the free radical scavenging potential of callus from tuber extracts (70%) was higher than callus from leaf extracts (65%). In addition, *in vivo* tuber and leaf extract showed 80% and 60%, respectively. The

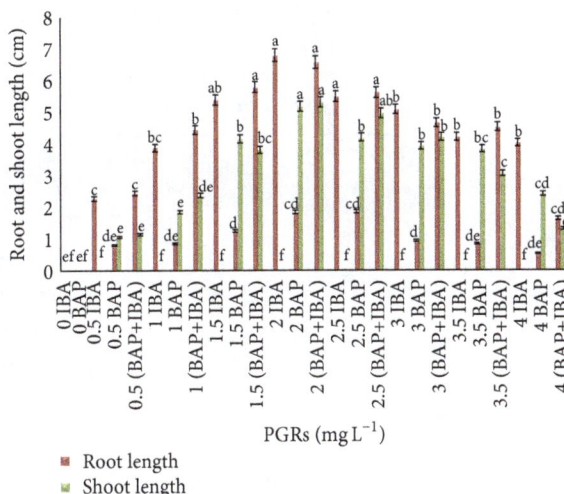

FIGURE 3: Root and shoot length from leaf explants of *C. latifolia* Dryand cultured on MS media supplemented with BAP and IBA alone or in combination (IBA+BAP) at various concentrations after 8 weeks of culture ($\rho < 0.05$, $n = 4$). The columns and bars represent mean + SE. The different letters at the top of columns in the same color indicate significant differences based on Duncan's multiple range tests.

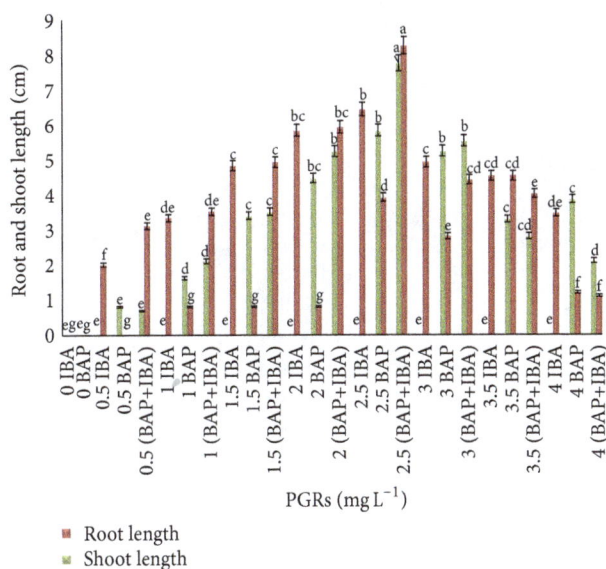

FIGURE 4: Root and shoot length from tuber explants of *C. latifolia* Dryand cultured on MS media supplemented with BAP and IBA alone or in combination (IBA+BAP) at various concentrations after 8 weeks of culture ($\rho < 0.05$, $n = 4$). The columns and bars represent mean + SE. The different letters at the top of columns in the same color indicate significant differences based on Duncan's multiple range tests.

same pattern was observed when SOD activity was applied (Figure 8).

7.7. Antibacterial Activities. The value of various *C. latifolia* extracts was investigated, quantitatively, by measuring the diameter of the inhibition zones around the discs.

TABLE 3: Inhibition effect of 10 g L^{-1} of *C.latifolia* ethanoic extracts (leaf and tuber *in vitro* and *in vivo* generated) against the growth of four pathogenic bacteria.

	Tested microorganisms	Types of plants	Inhibitory zone (mm) ± standard deviation	Ampicillin (30 μg) ± standard deviation
Gram-positive bacteria	S. aureus	Leaf extracts *in vitro*	7.1 ± 1.54[d]	18 ± 2.84[a]
		Tuber extract *in vitro*	12.1 ± 1.14[b]	18 ± 2.57[a]
		Tuber extract *in vivo*	13.8 ± 1.24[b]	18.2 ± 1.14[a]
		Leaf extracts *in vivo*	7.8 ± 1.47[c]	18.7 ± 2.64[a]
	Bacillus cereus	Leaf extracts *in vitro*	7.0 ± 1.30[e]	25 ± 3.60[a]
		Tuber extract *in vitro*	12.5 ± 1.10[c]	25 ± 3.10[a]
		Tuber extract *in vivo*	17.3 ± 1.24[b]	25 ± 3.10[a]
		Leaf extracts *in vivo*	7.2 ± 1.10[d]	25 ± 1.60[a]
Gram-negative bacteria	Klebsiella sp.	Leaf extracts *in vitro*	7.1 ± 1.30[d]	24 ± 3.20[a]
		Tuber extract *in vitro*	17.4 ± 1.10[b]	24 ± 4.30[a]
		Tuber extract *in vivo*	22.3 ± 1.24[ab]	24 ± 3.20[a]
		Leaf extracts *in vivo*	7.4 ± 1.10[c]	24 ± 3.20[a]
	P. aeruginosa	Leaf extracts *in vitro*	10.2 ± 1.50[c]	31 ± 2.10[a]
		Tuber extract *in vitro*	18.8 ± 1.7[b]	30.1 ± 1.80[a]
		Tuber extract *in vivo*	25.4 ± 1.01[ab]	30.1 ± 1.80[a]
		Leaf extracts *in vivo*	10.7 ± 1.10[bc]	30.2 ± 1.10[a]

Inhibition zone in mm (5 mm diameter of disk) as the means of triplicate of experiments. The data were analysed by one-way ANOVA and the inhibition means of samples were compared using Duncan's multiple comparison test (DMCT). Different letters in the same column represent a significant difference at the 5% level in Duncan's multiple range tests.

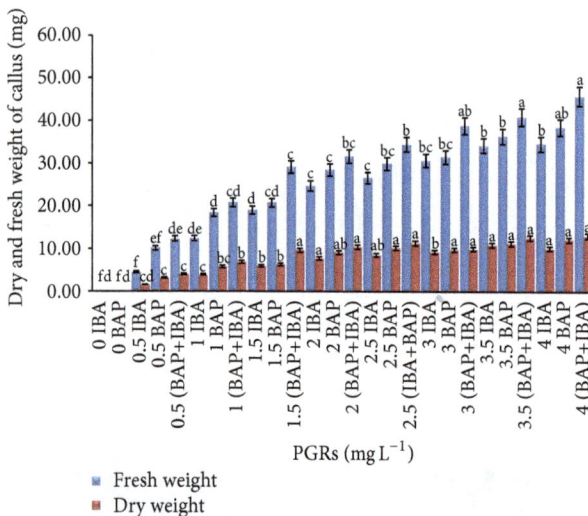

FIGURE 5: Fresh and dry matter yield from tuber explants of *C. latifolia* Dryand on MS media supplemented with BAP and IBA alone or in combination (IBA+BAP) at various concentrations after 8 weeks of culture. The columns and bars represent mean + SE. The different letters at the top of columns in the same color indicate significant differences based on Duncan's multiple range tests.

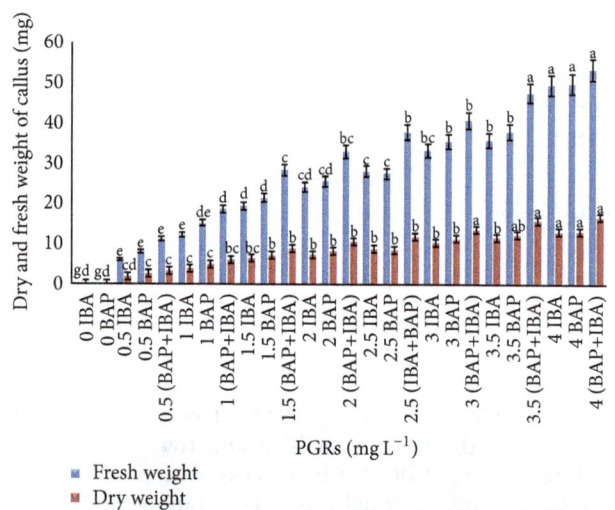

FIGURE 6: Fresh and dry matter yield from leaf explants of *C. latifolia* Dryand on MS media supplemented with BAP and IBA alone or in combination (IBA+BAP) at various concentrations after 8 weeks of culture. The columns and bars represent mean + SE. The different letters at the top of columns in the same color indicate significant differences based on Duncan's multiple range tests.

The various extract of *C. latifolia* exhibited considerable antibacterial activity against both gram-negative and gram-positive bacteria at a concentration of 10 g L^{-1} (Table 3). However, tuber and leaf extracts from the intact plant (*in vivo*) and callus (*in vitro*) showed higher inhibition zone compared to other extracts on gram-negative bacteria, especially against *Klebsiella* spp. and *P. aeruginosa*.

8. Discussion

It is well known that *in vitro* establishment and regeneration of plants are influenced by various factors, such as explants

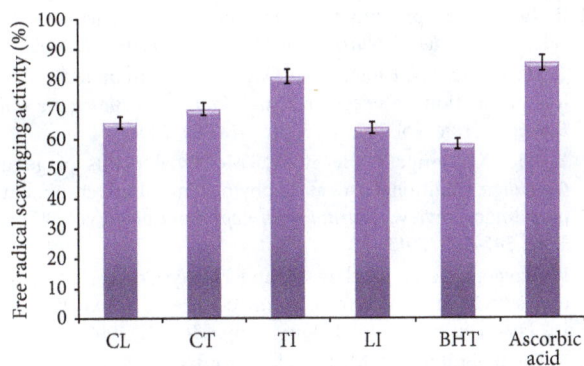

FIGURE 7: CL: callus from leaf, CT: callus from tuber, TI: tuber from intact plant (*in vivo*), and LI: leaf from intact plant (*in vivo*). Antioxidant activity of examining plant extracts (leaves from *in vivo* plants compared to callus from leaf and tuber, resp.) of *C. latifolia* Dryand ($10\,g\,L^{-1}$) measured using a DPPH* scavenging activity assay presented as a percentage value. Ascorbic acid and BHT (butylated hydroxyl toluene $1\,mg\,L^{-1}$) were applied as the positive controls. All the values are average of triplicates. The data were analyzed by one-way ANOVA and the DPPH* scavenging activity percentage means of samples were compared using Duncan's Multiple comparison test $p < 0.05$ (DMCT).

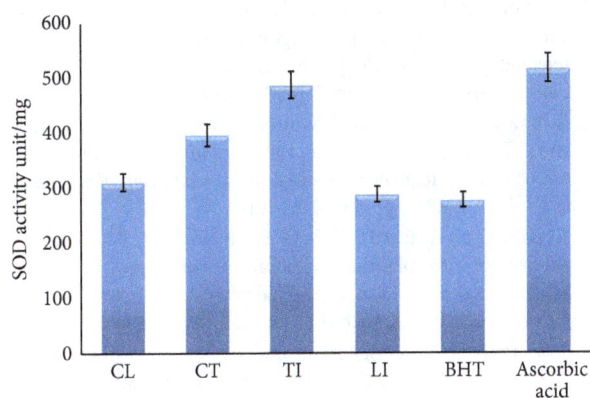

FIGURE 8: CL: callus from leaf, CT: callus from tuber, TI: tuber from intact plant (*in vivo*), and LI: leaf from intact plant (*in vivo*). Superoxide dismutase (SOD) was applied according to the kit protocol to examine SOD activities in plant extracts (leaves from *in vivo* plants compared to callus from leaf and tuber, resp.) of *C. latifolia* Dryand ($10\,g\,L^{-1}$). Ascorbic acid and BHT (butylated hydroxyl toluene $1\,mg\,L^{-1}$) were applied as the positive controls. All the values are average of triplicates. The data were analyzed by one-way ANOVA and the results of samples were compared using Duncan's Multiple comparison test $p < 0.05$ (DMCT).

type, the physiological status of *in vivo* plants, genotype, species, and media composition, type and combination of plant growth regulators, and culturing conditions.

In this study, among the different types of explants such as leaf, tuber, and seed, *in vitro* regeneration was only obtained from leaf and tuber explants. The explants cultured in MS medium in the absence of PGRs have showed no response to shoot and root induction. The response of tuber explants

to *in vitro* regeneration in Hypoxidaceae species varied considerably.

Vinesi et al. [26] reported successful rhizome culture of *H. obtusa* (Hypoxidaceae) on MS medium supplemented with ($1\,mg\,L^{-1}$) BAP. Based on Page and Van Staden [27], more than 70% of shoot and root from corn explants of *H. rooperi* (Hypoxidaceae) were formed on MS media added with ($1\,mg\,L^{-1}$) BAP between six and ten weeks, respectively.

However, the best in multiplication response of *H. colchicifolia* reported on MS medium containing $2\,mg\,L^{-1}$ BAP compared to other PGRs [28].

Appleton and van Staden [29] and Nsibande [30] reported regeneration in Hypoxidaceae family is varied with respect to the growth regulators requirement, shoot multiplication, and callus production. The leaf explants inoculated on MS media supplemented with various concentrations of BAP showed only a small amount of shoot formation in the absence of IBA. However, the shoot and root were induced when explants inoculated on MS medium with a combination of IBA and BAP. Nsibande [30] reported similar results on this family.

Based on our research, the antioxidant activities of this plant from leaves and tubers have not been reported. Even then, slight differences in the antioxidant activities do occur that solely depend on varieties, location, and growth conditions. Overall, in the estimation of the antioxidant capacities and the free radical scavenging assays showed positive results. The percent of inhibition in the DPPH assay and SOD activity were found more from tuber and leaf extraction (*in vivo*). According to Farzinebrahimi et al. [12], Farzinebrahimi et al. [13], and Khorasani et al. [14] different parts of the plants produced different antioxidant compounds or different amount of compounds possibly due to their degree of differences in gene expression. The ethanolic extracts of *H. hemerocallidea* from this family showed antioxidant properties via hydroxyl scavenging ability [10]. *In vitro* studies indicated good ability to scavenge free radicals (hydroxyl ions) [31]. The antibacterial activity of the tuber may be due to presence of phenolic active compounds in [32] *C. latifolia*. Antibacterial effect against gram-negative and gram-positive bacteria could be as natural source for producing pharmacological products. The results of the current study supported the traditional treatment by medicinal plants and proposed antibacterial agents from plant extracts with antibacterial properties.

The maximum activity was observed against gram-negative and gram-positive bacteria for *C. latifolia* tuber extracts *in vivo* and *in vitro* as compared with leaf extract, respectively.

Antimicrobial properties of medicinal plants are being increasingly stated from various parts of the world. Based on The World Health Organization report, the plant active constituents are used as folk medicine in traditional therapies of 80% of the world's population. In this study, the tuber extracts obtained from *C. latifolia* (*in vivo* and *in vitro*) showed strong activity against most of the tested bacterial strains. The results were compared with standard antibiotic drug.

The effect of antibacterial in medicinal plants varies intensely depending on the phytochemical features of plant families and subfamilies and even the grown area [33, 34]. Our results revealed that the tuber of *Curculigo latifolia* Dryand has the most effective antibiotics against all the studied bacteria compared with other explants.

9. Conclusion

Combinations of BAP and IBA in MS media exhibited the highest average numbers of root and shoot formation from leaf and tuber explants. Our data revealed that frequent subculture was effective in reducing phenolic exudation; also, pretreatment of tubers with citric acid could eliminate browning during culture period. This study also showed that tuber extracts from *in vivo* gave higher results for antioxidant activity and inhibition zone against gram-negative bacteria compared to the same concentration of callus extract from tuber and leaf.

Further and more specific studies, *in vivo* or *in vitro*, are recommended to determine the characteristics of this species.

Competing Interests

The authors declare that there are no competing interests regarding the publication of this paper.

Acknowledgments

The authors would like to thank The University of Malaya for the facilities and financial assistance provided (IPPP Grant no. PG091-2013A) and bright spark unit to carry out the research.

References

[1] A. Kocyan, "The discovery of polyandry in Curculigo (Hypoxidaceae): implications for androecium evolution of asparagoid monocotyledons," *Annals of Botany*, vol. 100, no. 2, pp. 241–248, 2007.

[2] M. F. Ismail, N. Psyquay Abdulla, G. B. Saleh, and M. Ismail, "Anthesis and flower visitors in Curculigo latifolia dryand," *Journal of Biology and Life Science*, vol. 1, pp. 13–15, 2010.

[3] R. Farzinebrahimi, R. M. Taha, and K. A. Rashid, "Effect of light intensity and soil media on establishment and growth of Curculigo latifolia Dryand," *Journal of Applied Horticulture*, vol. 15, no. 3, pp. 224–226, 2013.

[4] N. Shaari, "Lemba (Curculigo latifolia) leaf as a new materials for textiles," in *Proceedings of the 4th International Symposium on Environmentally Conscious Design and Inverse Manufacturing*, Tokyo, Japan, 2005.

[5] F. B. Ahmad and D. K. Holdsworth, "Medicinal plants of Sabah, Malaysia, part II. The muruts," *International Journal of Pharmacognosy*, vol. 32, no. 4, pp. 378–383, 1994.

[6] C. Wiart, *Medicinal Plant of Southeast Asia*, Pelanduk Publications, Serdang, Malaysia, 2000.

[7] H. Yamashita, S. Theerasilp, T. Aiuchi, K. Nakaya, Y. Nakamura, and Y. Kurihara, "Purification and complete amino acid sequence of a new type of sweet protein with taste-modifying activity, curculin," *The Journal of Biological Chemistry*, vol. 265, no. 26, pp. 15770–15775, 1990.

[8] R. Kant, "Sweet proteins-potential replacement for artificial low calorie sweeteners," *Nutrition Journal*, vol. 4, article 5, 2005.

[9] T. Masuda and N. Kitabatake, "Developments in biotechnological production of sweet proteins," *Journal of Bioscience and Bioengineering*, vol. 102, no. 5, pp. 375–389, 2006.

[10] Y. Nie, X. Dong, Y. He et al., "Medicinal plants of genus Curculigo: traditional uses and a phytochemical and ethnopharmacological review," *Journal of Ethnopharmacology*, vol. 147, no. 3, pp. 547–563, 2013.

[11] I. Grzegorczyk, A. Matkowski, and H. Wysokińska, "Antioxidant activity of extracts from in vitro cultures of Salvia officinalis L.," *Food Chemistry*, vol. 104, no. 2, pp. 536–541, 2007.

[12] R. Farzinebrahimi, R. M. Taha, K. Rashid, and J. S. Yaacob, "The effect of various media and hormones via suspension culture on secondary metabolic activities of (Cape Jasmine) Gardenia jasminoides ellis," *The Scientific World Journal*, vol. 2014, Article ID 407284, 7 pages, 2014.

[13] R. Farzinebrahimi, R. M. Taha, and M. Fadaie Nasab, "In vitro plant regeneration, antioxidant and antibacterial studies on broccoli, Brassica oleracea var. italica," *Pakistan Journal of Botany*, vol. 44, no. 6, pp. 2117–2122, 2012.

[14] A. Khorasani, W. Sani, K. Philip, R. M. Taha, and A. Rafat, "Antioxidant and antibacterial activities of ethanolic extracts of Asparagus officinalis cv. Mary Washington: Comparison of in vivo and in vitro grown plant bioactivities," *African Journal of Biotechnology*, vol. 9, no. 49, pp. 8460–8466, 2010.

[15] A. Rafat, P. Koshy, and M. Sekaran, "Antioxidant potential and content of phenolic compounds in ethanolic extracts of selected parts of Andrographis paniculata," *Journal Medicinal Plants Research*, vol. 4, no. 3, pp. 197–202, 2010.

[16] A. Bakrudeen, G. Subha Shanthi, T. Gouthaman, M. Kavitha, and M. Rao, "In vitro micropropagation of Catharanthus roseus—an anticancer medicinal plant," *Acta Botanica Hungarica*, vol. 53, no. 1-2, pp. 197–209, 2011.

[17] N. Babaei, N. A. P. Abdullah, G. Saleh, and T. L. Abdullah, "An efficient in vitro plantlet regeneration from shoot tip cultures of Curculigo latifolia, a medicinal plant," *The Scientific World Journal*, vol. 2014, Article ID 275028, 9 pages, 2014.

[18] S. V. Francis, S. K. Senapati, and G. R. Rout, "Rapid clonal propagation of Curculigo orchioides Gaertn., an endangered medicinal plant," *In Vitro Cellular & Developmental Biology—Plant*, vol. 43, no. 2, pp. 140–143, 2007.

[19] T. D. Thomas, "High-frequency, direct bulblet induction from rhizome explants of Curculigo orchioides Gaertn., an endangered medicinal herb," *In Vitro Cellular & Developmental Biology*, vol. 43, no. 5, pp. 442–448, 2007.

[20] B. B. Wala and Y. T. Jasrai, "Micropropagation of an endangered medicinal plant Curculigo orchioides Gaertn," *Plant Tissue Culture*, vol. 13, no. 1, pp. 13–19, 2003.

[21] C. L. Lim-Ho, *Tissue Culture of Curculigo latifolia Dry. ex W.T. Ait. (Hypoxidaceae)*, Botanic Gardens, Singapore, 1981.

[22] R. M. Taha, "Tissue culture studies of Citrus hystrix D.C. and Severinia buxifolia (poir) tenore," *Asia-Pacific Journal of Molecular Biology and Biotechnology*, vol. 1, pp. 36–42, 1993.

[23] T. Murashige and F. Skoog, "A revised medium for rapid growth and bio assays with tobacco tissue cultures," *Physiologia Plantarum*, vol. 15, no. 3, pp. 473–497, 1962.

[24] A. B. A. Ahmed, R. Pallela, A. S. Rao, M. V. Rao, and R. Mat Taha, "Optimized conditions for callus induction, plant regeneration and alkaloids accumulation in stem and shoot tip explants of Phyla nodiflora," *Spanish Journal of Agricultural Research*, vol. 9, no. 4, pp. 1262–1270, 2011.

[25] K. A. Gomez and A. A. Gomez, *Statistical Procedures for Agricultural Research with Emphasis on Rice*, 1976.

[26] P. Vinesi, M. Serafini, M. Nicoletti, L. Spanò, and P. Betto, "Plant regeneration and hypoxoside content in *Hypoxis obtusa*," *Journal of Natural Products*, vol. 53, no. 1, pp. 196–199, 1990.

[27] Y. M. Page and J. Van Staden, "*In vitro* propagation of *Hypoxis rooperi*," *Plant Cell, Tissue and Organ Culture*, vol. 3, no. 4, pp. 359–362, 1984.

[28] M. R. Appleton, G. D. Ascough, and J. Van Staden, "*In vitro* regeneration of *Hypoxis colchicifolia* plantlets," *South African Journal of Botany*, vol. 80, pp. 25–35, 2012.

[29] M. R. Appleton and J. van Staden, "Micropropagation of some South African *Hypoxis* species with medicinal and horticultural potential," *Acta Horticulturae*, vol. 420, pp. 75–77, 1995.

[30] B. E. Nsibande, *In vitro regeneration of four hypoxis species and transformation of Camelina sativa and Crambe abyssinica [M.S. thesis]*, The Swedish University of Agricultural Sciences. Sveriges lantbruksuniversitet, 2012.

[31] I. M. Mahomed and J. A. O. Ojewole, "Hypoglycemic effect of *Hypoxis hemerocallidea* corm (*African potato*) aqueous extract in rats," *Methods and Findings in Experimental and Clinical Pharmacology*, vol. 25, no. 8, pp. 617–619, 2003.

[32] K. S. Nagesh and C. Shanthamma, "Antibacterial activity of *Curculigo orchioides* rhizome extract on pathogenic bacteria," *African Journal of Microbiology Research*, vol. 3, no. 1, pp. 005–009, 2009.

[33] A. Al-Mariri and M. Safi, "*In vitro* antibacterial activity of several plant extracts and oils against some gram-negative bacteria," *Iranian Journal of Medical Sciences*, vol. 39, no. 1, pp. 36–43, 2014.

[34] N. Sarac and A. Ugur, "The *in vitro* antimicrobial activities of the essential oils of some *Lamiaceae* species from Turkey," *Journal of Medicinal Food*, vol. 12, no. 4, pp. 902–907, 2009.

6

The Effects of *Chunghyul-Dan* (A Korean Medicine Herbal Complex) on Cardiovascular and Cerebrovascular Diseases: A Narrative Review

Woo-Sang Jung, Seungwon Kwon, Seung-Yeon Cho, Seong-Uk Park, Sang-Kwan Moon, Jung-Mi Park, Chang-Nam Ko, and Ki-Ho Cho

Department of Cardiology and Neurology, College of Korean Medicine, Kyung Hee University, Seoul 02447, Republic of Korea

Correspondence should be addressed to Seungwon Kwon; kkokkottung@hanmail.net

Academic Editor: Yong C. Boo

Chunghyul-dan (CHD) is a herbal complex containing 80% ethanol extract and is composed of *Scutellariae Radix*, *Coptidis Rhizoma*, *Phellodendri Cortex*, *Gardeniae Fructus*, and *Rhei Rhizoma*. We have published several experimental and clinical research articles on CHD. It has shown antilipidemic, antihypertensive, antiatherosclerotic, and inhibitory effects on ischemic stroke recurrence with clinical safety in the previous studies. The antilipidemic effect of CHD results from 3-hydroxy-3-methylglutaryl-coenzyme A (HMG-CoA) reductase and pancreatic lipase-inhibitory activity. The antihypertensive effect likely results from the inhibitory effect on endogenous catecholamine(s) release and harmonization of all components showing the antihypertensive effects. Furthermore, anti-inflammatory and antioxidant effects on endothelial cells are implicated to dictate the antiatherosclerotic effects of CHD. It also showed neuroprotective effects on cerebrovascular and parkinsonian models. These effects of CHD could be helpful for the prevention of the recurrence of ischemic stroke. Therefore, we suggest that CHD could be a promising medication for treating and preventing cerebrovascular and cardiovascular diseases. However, to validate and better understand these findings, well-designed clinical studies are required.

1. Introduction: Background, History, and Development

Chunghyul-dan (CHD) is a capsulated herbal complex, which contains an 80% ethanol extract (300 mg per capsule) composed of *Scutellariae Radix*, *Coptidis Rhizoma*, *Phellodendri Cortex*, *Gardeniae Fructus*, and *Rhei Rhizoma* (Table 1). It is also known as Daehwang-Hwang-Ryung-Haedok-Tang (Daio-orengedokuto in Japanese), which means Hwang-Ryung-Haedok-Tang (HRHT, Orengedokuto in Japanese) plus Daehwang (*Rhei Rhizoma*). In other words, CHD consists of HRHT and *Rhei Rhizoma*.

Various herbal medicines have been used to treat cardiovascular and cerebrovascular diseases such as atherosclerosis, angina, and stroke in Korean medicine clinics. HRHT, which consists of *Scutellariae Radix*, *Coptidis Rhizoma*, *Phellodendri Cortex*, and *Gardeniae Fructus*, is one of the most famous

herbal medicines for treating cardiovascular and cerebrovascular diseases. The first record of the medicinal properties of the HRHT was documented in the Chinese medicine classic, "Oe-Dae-Bi-Yo (published in 752)." Traditionally, it has been used to treat pathological inflammation in gastrointestinal and cardiovascular and cerebrovascular diseases.

The modern clinical and experimental studies have also shown various evidences for the effect of HRHT on cardiovascular and cerebrovascular diseases. For instance, HRHT enhanced cerebral blood flow, decreased blood pressure, and exerted anti-inflammatory and vasodilatory effects [1]. Clinically, HRHT showed effects on abdominal obesity [2] and on the accessory symptoms of hypertension [3]. It could be suggested that these clinical effects are based on anti-inflammatory [4], antilipidemic [5], and antiplatelet effects [6] of HRHT. Furthermore, each herb in the HRHT is known to have neuroprotective, antioxidant, and antihypertensive

TABLE 1: Composition of *Chunghyul-dan*.

Constituent herbs	Scientific name (country of origin)	Weight (g)
Scutellariae Radix	*Scutellaria baicalensis* Georgi (Korea)	0.28
Coptidis Rhizoma	*Coptis japonica* Makino (Korea)	0.28
Phellodendri Cortex	*Phellodendron amurense* Ruprecht (Korea)	0.28
Gardeniae Fructus	*Gardenia jasminoides* Ellis (Korea)	0.28
Rhei Rhizoma	*Rheum palmatum* L. (China)	0.07
Total		1.2

effects [7–11]. Based on this, it was suggested that HRHT could have effects on cardiovascular disease and cerebrovascular disease.

To enhance the above-mentioned effects of HRHT, we combined HRHT and *Rhei Rhizoma*. The resulting combination medication was named as *Chunghyul-dan* (CHD), which means "purification of blood." A previous meta-analysis [12] suggested that *Rhei Rhizoma*-based herbal preparations have significant effects on the improvement of the clinical efficacy rates, the Barthel Index, National Institutes of Health Stroke Scale, Glasgow Coma Scale, and neurological deficit scores when compared with controls using only western medicine. *Rhei Rhizoma* has been used to remove blood stasis (oehyul in Korean and oketsu in Japanese). Clinically, *Rhei Rhizoma* has been used to treat severe gastrointestinal disorders including constipation or ileus, severe inflammation such as appendicitis or pneumonia, hypertension, and cerebrovascular diseases. Furthermore, *Rhei Rhizoma* has shown neuroprotective effects on experimental ischemic stroke [13] and antilipidemic effects [14].

The process of CHD development is as follows. Herbs were extracted with 80% ethanol in boiling water for 2 hours. The extracts were filtered, evaporated with a rotary vacuum evaporator, and freeze-dried. To standardize the quality of CHD, berberine in *Coptidis Rhizoma* and *Phellodendri Cortex*, baicalin in *Scutellariae Radix*, geniposide in *Gardeniae Fructus*, and sennoside A in *Rhei Rhizoma* were quantitatively assayed according to the standardized methods [15]. To enhance dry weight yields (%) of extract, CHD was extracted with 80% ethanol instead of water. In previous studies, extracted yield of each herb with 80% ethanol was higher than extracted yields with water [16, 17]. Furthermore, we used capsulated form to improve drug compliance.

Since 2002, we have reported extensive experimental and clinical research articles related to CHD. It has shown antilipidemic, antihypertensive, antiatherosclerotic, and enhancing effects on vascular endothelial cells. Furthermore, CHD shows inhibitory effect on recurrence of ischemic stroke (small vessel occlusion type). From here onwards, this review introduces and provides the effects of CHD on cardiovascular and cerebrovascular diseases.

2. CHD in Dyslipidemia

Dyslipidemia is defined as an abnormal amount of cholesterol and fat in the blood. It is known as a moderate risk factor for cardiovascular and cerebrovascular diseases such as

hypertension [18], coronary artery disease [19], and ischemic stroke [20]. The conventional therapies for dyslipidemia are statins (3-hydroxy-3-methylglutaryl-coenzyme A [HMG-CoA] reductase inhibitors), fibric acid derivatives, and bile acid sequestrants. Among these, statins are the most preferred therapeutic option. Although statins are an effective medication for dyslipidemia, they have severe adverse effects such as myopathy, rhabdomyolysis, and hepatic dysfunction [21, 22]. Therefore, new types of effective and safer antilipidemic agents need to be explored.

Chung et al. [23] investigated the effects of CHD on serum lipids in patients with hyperlipidemia (see Table 2). CHD (1800 mg/day for 8 weeks) was administered to 34 patients (10 males and 24 females) with serum levels of total cholesterol, LDL cholesterol, and triglycerides higher than 200 mg/dL, 130 mg/dL, and 200 mg/dL, respectively. Follow-up lipid profile check was performed after 4 weeks (34 patients) and 8 weeks (15 patients). Four weeks later, total cholesterol and LDL cholesterol levels showed significant decrease (-8.3% ($p < 0.05$) and -7.4% ($p < 0.05$), resp.). Eight weeks later, total cholesterol and triglyceride levels showed significant decrease (-7.7% ($p < 0.05$) and -21.1% ($p < 0.05$), resp.). No serious adverse effect was observed during the follow-up. Kim et al. [24] investigated the antilipidemic effect of CHD and compared it with atorvastatin. Study design was a case-control, open-label study. The subjects were divided into 2 groups, CHD group (further subdivided into two groups based on dosage; i.e., CHD 1 group received 600 mg/day CHD and CHD 2 group received 1200 mg/day CHD) and atorvastatin group (receiving 10 mg/day atorvastatin), to investigate and identify the dose-dependent effect of CHD on hyperlipidemia. Although atorvastatin was more powerful than 600 mg or 1200 mg CHD in lowering lipid levels, both CHD 1 and CHD 2 groups showed a statistically significant lipid-lowering effect (total cholesterol ($p < 0.05$), from 268.1 ± 30.2 mg/dL to 248.6 ± 29.2 mg/dL). There was no adverse effect such as hepatic or renal toxicity during CHD treatment. However, there was no significant difference between CHD 1 and CHD 2 groups in lowering lipids. Cho et al. [25] conducted a case-control, open-label study for evaluating the therapeutic effects of CHD on hypercholesterolemia. The subjects of this study were hyperlipidemia patients whose total serum cholesterol was more than 240 mg/dL. Subjects were divided into two groups, namely, CHD group and atorvastatin group that were treated (8 weeks) with CHD (600 mg/day, $n = 21$) and atorvastatin (10 mg/day, $n = 12$), respectively. After 8 weeks, CHD showed significant

TABLE 2: The efficacy of *Chunghyul-dan* in cardiovascular and cerebrovascular diseases in clinical studies [23–25, 32, 44, 56–58].

Disease	Author (year)	Subjects and Design	Intervention	Results
Dyslipidemia	Chung et al. [23]	34 hyperlipidemia patients Before and after study	1800 mg/day CHD for 8 weeks	After 4 weeks, total cholesterol: −8.3% ($p < 0.05$), LDL cholesterol: −7.4% ($p < 0.05$ After 8 weeks, total cholesterol: −7.7% ($p < 0.05$), triglyceride: −21.1% ($p < 0.05$)
	Kim et al. [24]	62 hyperlipidemia patients Case-control, open-label study	CHD1: 600 mg/day CHD2: 1200 mg/day Atorvastatin: 10 mg/day atorvastatin for 8 weeks	After 8 weeks, in CHD 1 and 2, total cholesterol: 268.1 ± 30.2 mg/dL → 248.6 ± 29.2 mg/dL ($p < 0.05$) There was no significant difference between CHD 1 and 2 group Atorvastatin was superior to 600 mg or 1200 mg CHD
	Cho et al. [56]	33 hyperlipidemia patients Case-control, open-label study	CHD: 600 mg/day CHD Atorvastatin: 10 mg/day atorvastatin for 8 weeks	After 8 weeks, in CHD group, total cholesterol: 269.5 ± 21.3 mg/dL → 246.9 ± 23.7 mg/dL ($p < 0.01$), LDL cholesterol: 171.2 ± 29.8 mg/dL → 155.4 ± 26.5 mg/dL ($p < 0.05$) CHD was superior to historical controls used diet therapy or placebo Atorvastatin was superior to 600 mg CHD
Hypertension	Yun et al. [32]	28 stroke patients with stage 1 hypertension Randomized controlled, open-label study	CHD: 1200 mg/day CHD Control: No treatment for 2 weeks	After 2 weeks, in CHD group SBP: 141.37 ± 8.96 mmHg → 132.28 ± 9.46 mmHg ($p = 0.03$, vs control, $p = 0.036$) In control group, SBP: 138.71 ± 11.36 mmHg → 132.27 ± 8.93 mmHg ($p > 0.05$)
Atherosclerosis (Arterial stiffness)	Park et al. [44]	35 subjects with increased baPWV (>1400 cm/sec) Randomized controlled, open-label study	CHD: 1800 mg/day CHD Control: No treatment for 8 weeks	After 8 weeks, in CHD group baPWV: 1736.0 ± 271.1 cm/sec → 1599.0 ± 301.9 cm/sec ($p = 0.032$) In control group, baPWV: 1668.3 ± 116.2 cm/sec → 1653.3 ± 184.1 cm/sec ($p = 0.774$)
Stroke prevention (SVO type)	Cho et al. [25]	31 asymptomatic ischemic stroke patients Observational study	600 mg/day CHD for 1 year	Complete follow-up patients ($n = 21$): no stroke recurrence Lost follow-up/dropped-out patients ($n = 10$): 2 patients suffered recurrence
	Cho et al. [57]	158 ischemic stroke patients Observational study	600 mg/day CHD for 1 year	Complete follow-up patients ($n = 73$): 3 patients (4.1%) experienced stroke recurrence Lost follow-up/dropped-out patients ($n = 85$): Among 85, 54 patients included in the final analysis → 8 patients (9.4%) had stroke recurrence. OR of CHD for stroke recurrence (vs lost to follow up): 0.12 times
	Cho et al. [58]	356 ischemic stroke patients Case-control, open-label study	CHD: 600 mg/day CHD Antiplatelet: Antiplatelet agent therapy for 2 years	In CHD group, recurrence occurred in 3 subjects (2.0%). In Antiplatelet group, recurrence occurred in 17 subjects (8.2%) OR of CHD for stroke recurrence(vs Antiplatelet group): 0.208 times

CHD: *Chunghyul-dan*; LDL: low-density lipoprotein; SBP: systolic blood pressure; baPWV: brachial-ankle pulse wave velocity; SVO: small vessel occlusion.

lipid-lowering effect (total cholesterol ($p < 0.01$), from 269.5 ± 21.3 mg/dL to 246.9 ± 23.7 mg/dL; LDL cholesterol ($p < 0.05$), from 171.2 ± 29.8 mg/dL to 155.4 ± 26.5 mg/dL). Although the antilipidemic effect of CHD was less than atorvastatin, it was higher than historical controls from previous studies using diet therapy or placebo. During CHD treatment, there was no adverse effect on hepatic or renal toxicity.

CHD has also shown antilipidemic effect in previous experimental studies. It inhibits HMG-CoA reductase and pancreatic lipase. Kim et al. [1] assessed the HMG-CoA reductase and pancreatic lipase-inhibitory effects of CHD in hyperlipidemic model rats treated with Triton WR-1339. They showed that CHD decreased total serum cholesterol and LDL cholesterol levels in the hyperlipidemic model rats. It potently inhibited HMG-CoA reductase and pancreatic lipase, simultaneously. Therefore, they suggested that the antilipidemic effect of CHD could originate from the inhibition of pancreatic lipase and HMG-CoA reductase. Another experimental study [17] also showed that *Rhei Rhizoma*, which is a component of CHD, exerted inhibitory effects on pancreatic lipase. Flavonoid extracts from *Scutellariae Radix* such as wogonin showed antilipidemic and body weight reducing effect in mice [26, 27]. Furthermore, alkaloids from *Coptidis Rhizoma* [28, 29] and crocin isolated from *Gardeniae Fructus* [30] also revealed antihyperglycemia and antihyperlipidemia effect in experimental studies.

Therefore, we suggest that CHD could be a safe-effective medication for controlling dyslipidemia. Although the effect of CHD on dyslipidemia is lower than that of statins, it did not show any adverse effects such as myopathy or hepatic dysfunction. The mechanism of the effect of CHD on dyslipidemia can be implicated to results from its pancreatic lipase-inhibitory effects. CHD can be an alternative medication for controlling dyslipidemia in the patients with adverse effects of statins. Further studies, such as examining whether statin with CHD therapy is superior to statin only therapy, are needed to ascertain the effect of CHD on dyslipidemia and clinical use.

3. CHD in Hypertension

Hypertension is one of the risk factors for atherosclerotic diseases such as stroke and coronary artery disease. In a previous clinical study, HRHT (a component of CHD) exhibited therapeutic effects on abdominal obesity [2] and the accessory symptoms of hypertension [3].

We conducted a preliminary study to determine an optimal dose for antihypertensive effect of CHD [31]. In this study, 1200 mg/day CHD (twice a day, p.o., 600 mg/each time) showed short-term antihypertensive effect on stroke patients with stage 1 hypertension (systolic blood pressure 140–159 mmHg and diastolic blood pressure 90–99 mmHg).

Based on the preliminary study, Yun et al. [32] evaluated the antihypertensive efficacy of CHD on stroke in patients with stage 1 hypertension using 24-hour ambulatory blood pressure monitoring (24ABPM). Forty stroke patients with stage 1 hypertension were enrolled for the study. They were randomly assigned into two groups: CHD group and control

group. Subjects in CHD group ($n = 15$) were treated with CHD (1200 mg/day) for 2 weeks, whereas control group ($n = 13$) did not receive CHD. Systolic blood pressure (SBP) of CHD group decreased from 141.37 ± 8.96 mmHg to 132.28 ± 9.46 mmHg after 2-week CHD administration ($p = 0.03$). However, SBP of control group did not show statistically significant decrease (from 138.71 ± 11.36 mmHg to 132.27 ± 8.93 mmHg). After 2 weeks of treatment, there was a significant difference in SBP between the CHD and the control groups ($p = 0.036$, Mann-Whitney U test). However, diastolic blood pressure and pulse rate in both groups had no significant change after treatment.

The antihypertensive effect of CHD can be explained by the findings of the following studies. HRHT and SamHwang-SaShim-Tang (SHSST, Sanoushasin-to in Japanese) exert an inhibitory effect on releasing endogenous catecholamines in experimental studies [33, 34]. Another study suggested that SHSST attenuated the increase in systemic and pulmonary arterial blood pressure induced by U46619 in rats. It downregulated the expression of phosphodiesterase type 5 (PDE5), Rho-kinase (ROCK) II, and cyclooxygenase-2 (COX-2) and upregulated the expression of soluble guanylyl cyclase (sGC) alpha(1) and sGCbeta(1) in U46619 treated primary pulmonary smooth muscle cells [35]. Berberine, a main compound of *Coptidis Rhizoma*, has shown inhibitory effects on endoplasmic reticulum stress in the carotid arteries of spontaneously hypertensive rats [36]. Furthermore, *Scutellariae Radix* showed inhibitory effect on adenylate cyclase activity in experimental studies [33, 34]. In addition, crocetin (a carotenoid from *Gardeniae Fructus*) also showed protective effect against hypertension and cerebral thrombogenesis in stroke-prone spontaneously hypertensive rats [9]. Furthermore, *Rhei Rhizoma* has a depressive effect on noradrenergic and dopaminergic nerve activities [33, 34] that also may be a mechanism of antihypertensive effects of CHD.

Based on these findings, we suggest that CHD can be used as an antihypertensive agent for stage I hypertension. However, further evaluation with a larger sample size and long-term follow-up is warranted.

4. CHD in Endothelial Dysfunction and Atherosclerosis

The effect of CHD on atherosclerosis, especially in endothelial cell dysfunction, has been reported. Endothelial cell dysfunctions are responsible for cardiovascular diseases such as the focal localization of atherosclerotic plaque [37]. Deregulation of endothelial cell function is closely associated with the incidence of atherosclerosis. Therefore, we investigated the effect of CHD on vascular endothelial cell dysfunction. CHD exhibited antiapoptotic effects and acted as a cell-cycle-progression and cell-migration-promoting agent in a previous study [38]. Molecular studies showed that CHD activates nitric oxide synthase (NOS) mRNA, which plays an important role in the protection against atherosclerosis. It suppresses vascular cell adhesion molecule-1 (VCAM-1) mRNA, which is expressed in human endothelial cells on sites predisposed to atherosclerotic lesions [39]. Another study [40] implicated CHD in controlling a variety of inflammation related activities by regulating MCP-1 and VCAM-1 gene expression in endothelial cell. Based on this, we suggest that antiatherosclerotic effect of CHD stems from antiapoptotic, anti-inflammatory, and antioxidant effects in human vascular endothelial cells.

The effects of components of CHD on atherosclerosis have also been reported. Wogonin, an active component of *Scutellariae Radix*, revealed inhibitory effect on monocyte chemotactic protein-1 gene expression in human endothelial cells [41]. Berberine, a natural extract from *Coptidis Rhizoma*, also revealed antiatherosclerotic effect via suppression of adhesion molecule expression including vascular cell adhesion molecule-1 (VCAM-1) and intercellular adhesion molecule-1 (ICAM-1) [42] and activation of AMP-activated protein kinase (AMPK) [43].

To ascertain the clinical antiatherosclerotic effects of CHD, we investigated the effect of CHD on increased arterial stiffness using brachial-ankle pulse wave velocity (baPWV) [44]. Arterial stiffness is a contributor to the progression of atherosclerosis [45], as the increased cycle stress on the arterial walls can affect the progression. Pulse wave velocity (PWV) is a surrogate marker for atherosclerosis and is a valuable index of arterial stiffness [46]. Subjects (35) with increased baPWV (>1400 cm/sec) were enrolled for this study. All subjects were randomized and divided into 2 groups; the CHD group ($n = 20$) received 1800 mg CHD for 8 weeks and the control group ($n = 15$) was without CHD medication. After 8 weeks, baPWV was significantly decreased in the CHD group (from 1736.0 ± 271.1 cm/sec to 1599.0 ± 301.9 cm/sec, $p = 0.032$), while there was no significant change in the control (from 1668.3 ± 116.2 cm/sec to 1653.3 ± 184.1 cm/sec, $p = 0.774$). There was no clinical adverse effect.

Arterial stiffness is closely associated with atherosclerosis [46] and there is a correlation of PWV and intima-media thickness (IMT) [47]. Based on the above findings, it is suggested that CHD may prevent the progression of atherosclerosis. The mechanism of CHD mediated antiatherosclerotic effects could be the antiapoptotic and NOS activation effects on endothelial cells.

5. The Neuroprotective Effect of CHD in Brain Ischemia and Cerebrovascular and Neurodegenerative Diseases

Traditionally, HRHT and *Rhei Rhizoma* have been the most famous herbal preparations for stroke and ischemic brain pathology in East Asia. As mentioned above, HRHT enhances cerebral blood flow, decreases blood pressure, and exerts anti-inflammatory and vasodilatory effects [1]. Furthermore, *Rhei Rhizoma*-based herbal medicines have significant effects on the improvement of stroke as compared with controls using only western medicine in a meta-analysis [12]. Therefore, we hypothesized that CHD could also exert neuroprotective effect on brain ischemia and neurodegenerative disease.

Previous experimental studies suggested that components of CHD such as *Rhei Rhizoma* [48] and *Scutellariae Radix* [49] revealed neuroprotective and prophylactic effects on the brain ischemia of rats. Berberine, the major pharmacological active constituent of *Coptidis Rhizoma*, is also suggested to regulate neuronal apoptosis in cerebral ischemia [8]. Geniposide, a pharmacologically active component purified from *Gardeniae Fructus*, is also suggested as a suppressor of neuroinflammation through inhibiting receptor for advanced glycation end products- (RAGE-) dependent signaling pathway in Alzheimer model [50, 51].

In an experimental study [52], CHD decreased the lipopolysaccharide- (LPS-) induced expression of mRNAs encoding inducible NO synthase, tumor necrosis factor- (TNF-) alpha, interleukin-1beta, cyclooxygenase-2, and prostaglandin E2 in rat brain microglia. Furthermore, CHD significantly decreased LPS-induced phosphorylation of the ERK1/2 and p38 signaling proteins. These results suggest that CHD exerts neuroprotective effect by reducing the release of various proinflammatory molecules from activated microglia.

An experimental study using rat model of focal ischemia-reperfusion investigated the effect of CHD on ischemic brain damage [53]. CHD was administered just before reperfusion and then 2 hours after reperfusion to evaluate its neuroprotective effect. After CHD treatment, cerebral infarct volume indicated significant reduction (100, 200, and 400 mg/kg; $p < 0.05$). It also lowered microglial activation and neutrophil infiltration ($p < 0.05$). Brain-derived neurotrophic factor- (BDNF-) positive cells were significantly increased after CHD treatment ($p < 0.05$). It is thus likely that the neuroprotective mechanisms of CHD result from inhibition of microglial activation, reduction of neutrophil infiltration, and enhancement of BDNF expression. Subsequently, another study [54] showed that CHD treatment markedly decreased the cytotoxicity in 42-hour hypoxia condition and H/R condition ($p < 0.01$ and $p < 0.05$, resp.). It also significantly decreased Bax expression ($p < 0.01$) and slightly decreased Bcl-2 expression. Based on these findings, it is likely that CHD shows neuroprotective effect in N2a cells subjected to H/R by increasing the expression of the proapoptotic protein Bax.

As CHD inhibited microglial activation, the neuroprotective effects of CHD on Parkinson's disease (PD) models were also investigated [55]. In an *in vivo* study, CHD (50 mg/kg, 5 days) reduced dopaminergic neuronal damage in the substantia nigra pars compacta (SNpc) and striatum and ameliorated bradykinesia. In an *in vitro* study, CHD exhibited significant protective effects in PC12 cells by inhibiting intracellular reactive oxygen species (ROS) generation and by regulatory effects on the heme oxygenase-1 and gp91 phagocytic oxidase. Furthermore, CHD protected dopaminergic neurons in a primary mesencephalic culture against 1-methyl-4-phenylpyridinium (MPP+) neurotoxicity. These results indicated that CHD could protect neuronal cell death in PD model by inhibition of ROS generation and associated mitochondrial dysfunction.

Based on these findings, it is likely that the anti-inflammatory and antioxidant properties of CHD on brain provide the neuroprotective effect. Therefore, CHD may be used as an alternative agent for brain ischemia as well as neurodegenerative diseases in the near future. However, further clinical studies using perfusion CT to evaluate the effect of CHD in clinical set-up are required.

6. CHD in Prevention of Small Vessel Occlusion (SVO) Type Ischemic Stroke

As mentioned earlier, CHD has antilipidemic [17, 23–25], antihypertensive [31, 32], anti-inflammatory [52, 53], and antioxidative [54] effects and can improve endothelial cells [38–41]. It was predicted that CHD could improve and prevent the progress of microangiopathy, which is strongly associated with small vessel disease type ischemic stroke. Clinical studies were conducted to evaluate the effectiveness of CHD on the prevention of small vessel occlusion type ischemic stroke.

First, the inhibitory effect of CHD on stroke occurrence in subjects with asymptomatic SVO type ischemic stroke was investigated through observational study. For this study [56], patients who had spotty lesions (3 mm in diameter or larger) in area supplied by deep perforating artery, showing high intensity in T2 weighted (TR = 3000, TE = 80) and FLAIR images and low intensity in the T1 weighted (TR = 450, TE = 10) image were included. According to the inclusion criteria, 31 patients were recruited. 600 mg/day CHD was administered to all subjects for 1 year. Stroke occurrence and adverse effects were monitored for 1 year. Follow-up brain MRI was performed to detect new ischemic lesions 1 year after the treatment. Ten subjects dropped out and only 21 subjects completed the follow-up. Among the 21 subjects who completed follow-up, no subject experienced clinical symptoms characterized by typical stroke and no new lesions were detected in the follow-up MRI. However, among the 10 drop-out patients, 2 patients experienced ischemic stroke. The CHD administration period for drop-out patients was 2.3 ± 1.8 months.

To further understand these results, the inhibitory effect of CHD on stroke recurrence in subjects with SVO type ischemic stroke (including asymptomatic and symptomatic stroke) was investigated [57]. Seventy-three patients with SVO type ischemic stroke were treated with 600 mg/day CHD for 1 year. Among them, three patients (4.1%) experienced new ischemic stroke (symptomatic stroke = 2; asymptomatic stroke = 1).

An expansion study with a 2-year follow-up was conducted in multicenters [58]. There were 2 groups in this study: the CHD group (n = 148) with 600 mg/day CHD for 2 years and the control group (n = 208) with antiplatelet agents. New brain lesions occurred in only 3 subjects (2.0%) of the CHD group, whereas 17 subjects (8.2%) experienced stroke recurrence in the control. The OR of the CHD group for stroke recurrence was 0.232 times that of the control. Furthermore, the OR of the CHD group decreased to 0.208 when adjusted for other relevant risk factors (age, sex, antiplatelet gage medication, smoking, previous stroke, hypertension, diabetes mellitus, and hyperlipidemia). Although it was not a randomized controlled study, we suggest that the inhibitory rate of CHD on stroke recurrence is much higher than that of antiplatelet agents.

A conclusion about the effect of CHD on prevention of SVO type stroke recurrence cannot be reached due to lack of randomized controlled studies. However, from the limited data available, recurrence rate of SVO stroke in the CHD therapy group (2.0%) was lower than conventional antiplatelet therapy (6.1~12.8%) using aspirin, clopidogrel, cilostazol, triflusal, or dipyridamole [59–65]. The most common adverse effect of antiplatelet agent therapy is bleeding, which can be fatal. For instance, the overall incidence rate of hemorrhagic events was 5.58 per 1000 person-years for aspirin users and 3.60 per 1000 person-years for those without aspirin use, and the incidence rate ratio (IRR) was 1.55 (95% CI, 1.48–1.63) [66]. However, there were no serious adverse events such as bleeding during CHD treatment. Based on this, we suggest that CHD may be a safe and effective agent for prevention of SVO type ischemic stroke. We are now conducting long-term follow-up study for the effect of CHD on SVO type stroke patients to improve our understanding.

7. Safety and Adverse Effect

To examine the safety of CHD, a retrospective cohort review study was performed [67]. Among 656 subjects with CHD treatment, there were clinical adverse effects in 13 subjects (2.0%), 8 with gastrointestinal symptoms such as indigestion, headache, insomnia, chest discomforts, general fatigue, and thirst appearing in 1 subject, respectively. This apparent frequency of adverse effects was much lower than the safety of previous medications such as statins [68, 69]. There were no serious adverse effects such as hepatic or renal dysfunction. Furthermore, other studies on effects of CHD on dyslipidemia [23–25], hypertension [32], and arterial stiffness [44] did not show any other adverse effects. Therefore, it may be suggested that CHD is a safe medication.

8. Summary and Future Considerations

CHD has antilipidemic, antihypertensive, antiatherosclerotic, antioxidant, and neuroprotective effects, which could exert an inhibitory effect on microangiopathy resulting in prevention of ischemic stroke. Furthermore, several clinical trials have proven its status as a safe alternative medication. To confirm the effect of CHD, well-designed and large sized clinical studies are required to assess the potential of CHD and validate these findings.

Competing Interests

The authors declare that they have no competing interests.

References

[1] Y.-S. Kim, E.-A. Jung, J.-E. Shin et al., "Daio-Orengedokuto inhibits HMG-CoA reductase and pancreatic lipase," *Biological and Pharmaceutical Bulletin*, vol. 25, no. 11, pp. 1442–1445, 2002.

[2] S. Kwon, W. Jung, A. R. Byun, S. Moon, K. Cho, and K. Shin, "Administration of Hwang-Ryun-Haedok-tang, a herbal complex, for patients with abdominal obesity: a case series," *Explore*, vol. 11, no. 5, pp. 401–406, 2015.

[3] K. Arakawa, T. Saruta, K. Abe et al., "Improvement of accessory symptoms of hypertension by TSUMURA Orengedokuto Extract, a four herbal drugs containing Kampo-Medicine Granules for ethical use: a double-blind, placebo-controlled study," *Phytomedicine*, vol. 13, no. 1-2, pp. 1–10, 2006.

[4] N. Oshima, Y. Narukawa, N. Hada, and F. Kiuchi, "Quantitative analysis of anti-inflammatory activity of orengedokuto: importance of combination of flavonoids in inhibition of PGE2 production in mouse macrophage-like cell line J774.1," *Journal of Natural Medicines*, vol. 67, no. 2, pp. 281–288, 2013.

[5] N. Ikarashi, M. Tajima, K. Suzuki et al., "Inhibition of preadipocyte differentiation and lipid accumulation by Orengedokuto treatment of 3T3-L1 cultures," *Phytotherapy Research*, vol. 26, no. 1, pp. 91–100, 2012.

[6] Y. Kimura, M. Shimizu, S. Kohara, F. Yoshii, H. Sato, and Y. Shinohara, "Antiplatelet effects of a Kampo medicine, Orengedokuto," *Journal of Stroke and Cerebrovascular Diseases*, vol. 15, no. 6, pp. 277–282, 2006.

[7] Y. S. Hwang, C. Y. Shin, Y. Huh, and J. H. Ryu, "Hwangryun-Hae-Dok-tang (Huanglian-Jie-Du-Tang) extract and its constituents reduce ischemia-reperfusion brain injury and neutrophil infiltration in rats," *Life Sciences*, vol. 71, no. 18, pp. 2105–2117, 2002.

[8] Q. Zhang, Z. Qian, L. Pan, H. Li, and H. Zhu, "Hypoxia-inducible factor 1 mediates the anti-apoptosis of berberine in neurons during hypoxia/ischemia," *Acta Physiologica Hungarica*, vol. 99, no. 3, pp. 311–323, 2012.

[9] S. Higashino, Y. Sasaki, J. C. Giddings et al., "Crocetin, a carotenoid from *Gardenia jasminoides* Ellis, protects against hypertension and cerebral thrombogenesis in stroke-prone spontaneously hypertensive rats," *Phytotherapy Research*, vol. 28, no. 9, pp. 1315–1319, 2014.

[10] R. H. Hughes, V. A. Silva, I. Ahmed, D. I. Shreiber, and B. Morrison III, "Neuroprotection by genipin against reactive oxygen and reactive nitrogen species-mediated injury in organotypic hippocampal slice cultures," *Brain Research*, vol. 1543, pp. 308–314, 2014.

[11] H. Y. Chow, J. C. C. Wang, and K. K. Cheng, "Cardiovascular effects of *Gardenia florida* L. (Gardeniae fructus) extract," *The American Journal of Chinese Medicine*, vol. 4, no. 1, pp. 47–51, 1976.

[12] L. Lu, H.-Q. Li, D.-L. Fu, G.-Q. Zheng, and J.-P. Fan, "Rhubarb root and rhizome-based Chinese herbal prescriptions for acute ischemic stroke: a systematic review and meta-analysis," *Complementary Therapies in Medicine*, vol. 22, no. 6, pp. 1060–1070, 2014.

[13] A.-J. Liu, L. Song, Y. Li et al., "Active compounds of rhubarb root and rhizome in animal model experiments of focal cerebral ischemia," *Evidence-Based Complementary and Alternative Medicine*, vol. 2015, Article ID 210546, 13 pages, 2015.

[14] Z.-W. Wang, M. Guo, D. Ma, and R.-Q. Wang, "Effects of Rhubarbs from different regions on blood lipid and antioxidation of hyperlipidemia rats," *Zhongguo Ying Yong Sheng Li Xue Za Zhi*, vol. 31, no. 3, pp. 278–281, 2015.

[15] J. Hayakawa, N. Noda, S. Yamada, E. Mikami, and K. Uno, "Studies on physical chemical quality evaluation of crude drugs preparations. III. Analysis of gardenia fruits and its preparations," *Yakugaku Zasshi*, vol. 105, pp. 996–1000, 1986.

[16] J. C. Jang, K. S. Lee, Y. S. Kim et al., "Purgative activities of whangryunhaedoktang and chunghyuldanm," *Natural Product Science*, vol. 9, pp. 64–67, 2003.

[17] H. K. Yang, Y. S. Kim, H. S. Bae et al., "Rhei rhizoma and chunghyuldan inhibit pancreatic lipase," *Natural Product Sciences*, vol. 9, no. 1, pp. 38–43, 2003.

[18] M. J. Martin, W. S. Browner, S. B. Hulley, L. H. Kuller, and D. Wentworth, "Serum cholesterol, blood pressure, and mortality: implications from a cohort of 361 662 men," *The Lancet*, vol. 328, no. 8513, pp. 933–936, 1986.

[19] J. Stamler, D. Wentworth, and J. D. Neaton, "Is relationship between serum cholesterol and risk of premature death from coronary heart disease continuous and graded?. Findings in 356,222 primary screenees of the Multiple Risk Factor Intervention Trial (MRFIT)," *The Journal of the American Medical Association*, vol. 256, no. 20, pp. 2823–2828, 1986.

[20] B. J. Ansell, "Cholesterol, stroke risk, and stroke prevention," *Current Atherosclerosis Reports*, vol. 2, no. 2, pp. 92–96, 2000.

[21] W. Insull, S. Kafonek, D. Goldner, and F. Zieve, "Comparison of efficacy and safety of atorvastatin (10 mg) with simvastatin (10 mg) at six weeks," *American Journal of Cardiology*, vol. 87, no. 5, pp. 554–559, 2001.

[22] D. Black, M. Davidson, M. Koren et al., "Cost effectiveness of treatment to National Cholesterol Education Panel (NCEP) targets with HMG-CoA reductase inhibitors. Trial design," *PharmacoEconomics*, vol. 12, no. 2, pp. 278–285, 1997.

[23] K. H. Chung, Y. S. Choi, L. D. Kim et al., "Effects of chunghyuldan on serum lipids in patients with hyperlipidemia," *Korean Journal of Oriental Internal Medicine*, vol. 24, no. 3, pp. 543–550, 2003.

[24] T. K. Kim, W. S. Jung, S. W. Park, K. H. Cho, and Y. S. Kim, "Comparison of efficacy and safety between chunghyuldan (HH-333) and atorvastatin (Lipitor®)," *Korean Journal of Oriental Internal Medicine*, vol. 24, no. 4, pp. 837–845, 2003.

[25] K. H. Cho, H. S. Kang, W. S. Jung, S. U. Park, and S. K. Moon, "Efficacy and safety of Chunghyul-dan (Qingwie-dan) in patients with hypercholesterolemia," *The American Journal of Chinese Medicine*, vol. 33, no. 2, pp. 241–248, 2005.

[26] E.-J. Bak, J. Kim, Y. H. Choi et al., "Wogonin ameliorates hyperglycemia and dyslipidemia via PPARα activation in db/db mice," *Clinical Nutrition*, vol. 33, no. 1, pp. 156–163, 2014.

[27] K. H. Song, S. H. Lee, B.-Y. Kim, A. Y. Park, and J. Y. Kim, "Extracts of scutellaria baicalensis reduced body weight and blood triglyceride in db/db mice," *Phytotherapy Research*, vol. 27, no. 2, pp. 244–250, 2013.

[28] H. Ma, Y. Hu, Z. Zou, M. Feng, X. Ye, and X. Li, "Antihyperglycemia and antihyperlipidemia effect of protoberberine alkaloids from rhizoma coptidis in HepG2 cell and diabetic KK-Ay mice," *Drug Development Research*, 2016.

[29] S. Kou, B. Han, Y. Wang et al., "Synergetic cholesterol-lowering effects of main alkaloids from *Rhizoma Coptidis* in HepG2 cells and hypercholesterolemia hamsters," *Life Sciences*, vol. 151, pp. 50–60, 2016.

[30] I.-A. Lee, J. H. Lee, N.-I. Baek, and D.-H. Kim, "Antihyperlipidemic effect of crocin isolated from the fructus of Gardenia jasminoides and its metabolite crocetin," *Biological and Pharmaceutical Bulletin*, vol. 28, no. 11, pp. 2106–2110, 2005.

[31] S. P. Yun, L. D. Kim, S. H. Lee et al., "Effects of Chunghyul-dan on stage 1 hypertensive patients with stroke-preliminary study for optimal dose," *Korean Journal of Oriental Internal Medicine*, pp. 74–81, 2004.

[32] S. P. Yun, W. S. Jung, S. U. Park et al., "Anti-hypertensive effect of *Chunghyul-dan* (*Qingxue-dan*) on stroke patients with essential hypertension," *American Journal of Chinese Medicine*, vol. 33, no. 3, pp. 357–364, 2005.

[33] F. Sanae, Y. Komatsu, S. Amagaya, K. Chisaki, and H. Hayashi, "Effects of 9 Kampo medicines clinically used in hypertension on hemodynamic changes induced by theophylline in rats," *Biological and Pharmaceutical Bulletin*, vol. 23, no. 6, pp. 762–765, 2000.

[34] F. Sanae, Y. Komatsu, K. Chisaki, T. Kido, A. Ishige, and H. Hayashi, "Effects of Sano-shashin-to and the constituent herbal medicines on theophylline-induced increase in arterial blood pressure of rats," *Biological and Pharmaceutical Bulletin*, vol. 24, no. 10, pp. 1137–1141, 2001.

[35] H.-H. Tsai, I.-J. Chen, and Y.-C. Lo, "Effects of San-Huang-Xie-Xin-Tang on U46619-induced increase in pulmonary arterial blood pressure," *Journal of Ethnopharmacology*, vol. 117, no. 3, pp. 457–462, 2008.

[36] L. Liu, J. Liu, Z. Huang et al., "Berberine improves endothelial function by inhibiting endoplasmic reticulum stress in the carotid arteries of spontaneously hypertensive rats," *Biochemical and Biophysical Research Communications*, vol. 458, no. 4, Article ID 33419, pp. 796–801, 2015.

[37] P. F. Davies, "Flow-mediated endothelial mechanotransduction," *Physiological Reviews*, vol. 75, no. 3, pp. 519–560, 1995.

[38] K.-H. Cho, W.-S. Jung, S.-U. Park et al., "Daio-Orengedokudo works as a cell-proliferating compound in endothelial cells," *Canadian Journal of Physiology and Pharmacology*, vol. 82, no. 6, pp. 380–386, 2004.

[39] S.-U. Park, W.-S. Jung, S.-K. Moon et al., "Chunghyuldan activates NOS mRNA expression and suppresses VCAM-1 mRNA expression in human endothelial cells," *Canadian Journal of Physiology and Pharmacology*, vol. 83, no. 12, pp. 1101–1108, 2005.

[40] W. S. Jung, J. Cho, K. In et al., "Chunghyul-dan acts as an Anti-Inflammatory agent in endothelial cells by regulating gene expression," *Animal Cells and Systems*, vol. 14, no. 4, pp. 275–282, 2010.

[41] Y.-L. Chang, J.-J. Shen, B.-S. Wung, J.-J. Cheng, and D. L. Wang, "Chinese herbal remedy wogonin inhibits monocyte chemotactic protein-1 gene expression in human endothelial cells," *Molecular Pharmacology*, vol. 60, no. 3, pp. 507–513, 2001.

[42] Z. Huang, X. Cai, S. Li et al., "Berberine-attenuated monocyte adhesion to endothelial cells induced by oxidized low-density lipoprotein via inhibition of adhesion molecule expression," *Molecular Medicine Reports*, vol. 7, no. 2, pp. 461–465, 2013.

[43] Q. Wang, M. Zhang, B. Liang, N. Shirwany, Y. Zhu, and M.-H. Zou, "Activation of AMP-activated protein kinase is required for berberine-induced reduction of atherosclerosis in mice: the role of uncoupling protein 2," *PLoS ONE*, vol. 6, no. 9, Article ID e25436, 2011.

[44] S. U. Park, W. S. Jung, S. K. Moon et al., "Chunghyul-Dan (Qingxie-dan) improves arterial stiffness in patients with increased baPWV," *The American Journal of Chinese Medicine*, vol. 34, no. 4, pp. 553–563, 2006.

[45] J. Y.-J. Shyy and S. Chien, "Role of integrins in endothelial mechanosensing of shear stress," *Circulation Research*, vol. 91, no. 9, pp. 769–775, 2002.

[46] N. M. van Popele, D. E. Grobbee, M. L. Bots et al., "Association between arterial stiffness and atherosclerosis: the Rotterdam Study," *Stroke*, vol. 32, no. 2, pp. 454–460, 2001.

[47] H. Taniwaki, T. Kawagishi, M. Emoto et al., "Correlation between the intima-media thickness of the carotid artery and aortic pulse-wave velocity in patients with type 2 diabetes. Vessel wall properties in type 2 diabetes," *Diabetes Care*, vol. 22, no. 11, pp. 1851–1857, 1999.

[48] D. K. Ahn, D. H. Won, and J. H. Kim, "Neuroprotective effects of the Rhei Rhizoma on the Rats' transient forebrain ischemia caused by 4-vessel-occlusion," *Korean Journal of Herbology*, vol. 14, no. 1, pp. 111–120, 1999.

[49] B. C. Lee, K. H. Leem, Y. O. Kim et al., "Neuroprotective effects of scutellariae radix on the brain ischemia induced by four-vessel occlusion in rats," *Korean Journal of Herbology*, vol. 14, no. 2, pp. 89–96, 1999.

[50] C. Lv, L. Wang, X. Liu et al., "Geniposide attenuates oligomeric $A\beta_{1-42}$-induced inflammatory response by targeting RAGE-dependent signaling in BV2 cells," *Current Alzheimer Research*, vol. 11, no. 5, pp. 430–440, 2014.

[51] C. Lv, L. Wang, X. Liu et al., "Multi-faced neuroprotective effects of geniposide depending on the RAGE-mediated signaling in an Alzheimer mouse model," *Neuropharmacology*, vol. 89, pp. 175–184, 2015.

[52] K. N. Nam, H.-J. Jung, M.-H. Kim et al., "Chunghyuldan attenuates brain microglial inflammatory response," *Canadian Journal of Physiology and Pharmacology*, vol. 87, no. 6, pp. 448–454, 2009.

[53] K.-H. Cho, J. K. Oh, Y. S. Jang et al., "Combination drug therapy using edaravone and Daio-Orengedoku-to after transient focal ischemia in rats," *Methods and Findings in Experimental and Clinical Pharmacology*, vol. 30, no. 6, pp. 443–450, 2008.

[54] C.-N. Ko, I.-S. Park, S.-U. Park et al., "Neuroprotective effect of Chunghyuldan (Qing Xue Dan) on hypoxia-reoxygenation induced damage of neuroblastoma 2a cell lines," *Chinese Journal of Integrative Medicine*, vol. 19, no. 12, pp. 940–944, 2013.

[55] H. G. Kim, M. S. Ju, D.-H. Kim et al., "Protective effects of Chunghyuldan against ROS-mediated neuronal cell death in models of Parkinson's disease," *Basic & Clinical Pharmacology & Toxicology*, vol. 107, no. 6, pp. 958–964, 2010.

[56] K. H. Cho, N. G. Ji, W. S. Jung et al., "Chunghyul-dan for the prevention of stroke progression in silent brain infarction," *The Journal of Korean Oriental Medicine*, vol. 26, no. 2, pp. 77–84, 2005.

[57] K. H. Cho, N. G. Jee, W. S. Jung et al., "A preliminary study on the inhibitory effect of chunghyul-dan on stroke recurrence in patients with small vessel disease," *The Journal of Korean Oriental Medicine*, vol. 28, no. 1, pp. 224–236, 2007.

[58] K. Cho, K. Noh, W. Jung et al., "A preliminary study on the inhibitory effect of Chunghyul-dan on stroke recurrence in patients with small vessel disease," *Neurological Research*, vol. 30, no. 6, pp. 655–658, 2008.

[59] ESPS Group, "European stroke prevention study," *Stroke*, vol. 21, no. 8, pp. 1122–1130, 1990.

[60] B. Farrell, J. Godwin, S. Richards, and C. Warlow, "The United Kingdom transient ischaemic attack (UK-TIA) aspirin trial: Final results," *Journal of Neurology, Neurosurgery & Psychiatry*, vol. 54, no. 12, pp. 1044–1054, 1991.

[61] The SALT Collaborative Group, "Swedish Aspirin Low-dose Trial (SALT) of 75 mg aspirin as secondary prophylaxis after cerebrovascular ischaemic events," *The Lancet*, vol. 338, no. 8779, pp. 1345–1349, 1991.

[62] H. C. Diener, L. Cunha, C. Forbes, J. Sivenius, P. Smets, and A. Lowenthal, "European Stroke Prevention Study 2. Dipyridamole and acetylsalicylic acid in the secondary prevention of stroke," *Journal of the Neurological Sciences*, vol. 143, no. 1-2, pp. 1–13, 1996.

[63] P. H.-C. Diener, P. J. Bogousslavsky, P. L. M. Brass et al., "Aspirin and clopidogrel compared with clopidogrel alone after

recent ischaemic stroke or transient ischaemic attack in high-risk patients (MATCH): randomised, double-blind, placebo-controlled trial," *The Lancet*, vol. 364, no. 9431, pp. 331–337, 2004.

[64] Y. Shinohara, Y. Katayama, S. Uchiyama et al., "Cilostazol for prevention of secondary stroke (CSPS 2): an aspirin-controlled, double-blind, randomised non-inferiority trial," *The Lancet Neurology*, vol. 9, no. 10, pp. 959–968, 2010.

[65] J. Matías-Guiu, J. M. Ferro, J. Alvarez-Sabín et al., "Comparison of triflusal and aspirin for prevention of vascular events in patients after cerebral infarction: the TACIP study: a randomized, double-blind, multicenter trial," *Stroke*, vol. 34, no. 4, pp. 840–848, 2003.

[66] G. De Berardis, G. Lucisano, A. D'Ettorre et al., "Association of aspirin use with major bleeding in patients with and without diabetes," *The Journal of the American Medical Association*, vol. 307, no. 21, pp. 2286–2294, 2012.

[67] K. H. Cho, W. S. Jung, S. U. Park, S. K. Moon, Y. S. Kim, and H. S. Hae, "Clinical assessment on the safety of chunghyul-dan (Qingwie-dan)," *The Journal of Korean Oriental Medicine*, vol. 24, no. 3, pp. 45–50, 2003.

[68] M. Davidson, J. McKenney, E. Stein et al., "Comparison of one-year efficacy and safety of atorvastatin versus lovastatin in primary hypercholesterolemia," *The American Journal of Cardiology*, vol. 79, no. 11, pp. 1475–1481, 1997.

[69] S. Bertolini, G. B. Bon, L. M. Campbell et al., "Efficacy and safety of atorvastatin compared to pravastatin in patients with hypercholesterolemia," *Atherosclerosis*, vol. 130, no. 1-2, pp. 191–197, 1997.

7

Composition Analysis and Inhibitory Effect of *Sterculia lychnophora* against Biofilm Formation by *Streptococcus mutans*

Yang Yang,[1] Bok-Im Park,[2] Eun-Hee Hwang,[1] and Yong-Ouk You[2]

[1]Department of Food and Nutrition, School of Human Environmental Sciences, Wonkwang University,
Iksan 570-749, Republic of Korea
[2]Department of Oral Biochemistry, School of Dentistry, Wonkwang University, Iksan 570-749, Republic of Korea

Correspondence should be addressed to Eun-Hee Hwang; ehhwang@wku.ac.kr and Yong-Ouk You; hope7788@wku.ac.kr

Academic Editor: Xiangqian Liu

Pangdahai is a traditional Chinese drug, specifically described in the Chinese Pharmacopoeia as the seeds of *Sterculia lychnophora* Hance. Here, we separated *S. lychnophora* husk and kernel, analyzed the nutrient contents, and investigated the inhibitory effects of *S. lychnophora* ethanol extracts on cariogenic properties of *Streptococcus mutans*, important bacteria in dental caries and plaque formation. Ethanol extracts of *S. lychnophora* showed dose-dependent antibacterial activity against *S. mutans* with significant inhibition at concentrations higher than 0.01 mg/mL compared with the control group ($p < 0.05$). Furthermore, biofilm formation was decreased by *S. lychnophora* at concentrations > 0.03 mg/mL, while bacterial viability was decreased dose-dependently at high concentrations (0.04, 0.08, 0.16, and 0.32 mg/mL). Preliminary phytochemical analysis of the ethanol extract revealed a strong presence of alkaloid, phenolics, glycosides, and peptides while the presence of steroids, terpenoids, flavonoids, and organic acids was low. The *S. lychnophora* husk had higher moisture and ash content than the kernel, while the protein and fat content of the husk were lower ($p < 0.05$) than those of the kernel. These results indicate that *S. lychnophora* may have antibacterial effects against *S. mutans*, which are likely related to the alkaloid, phenolics, glycosides, and peptides, the major components of *S. lychnophora*.

1. Introduction

The Chinese traditional medicine Pangdahai consists of the dried mature seeds of *Sterculia lychnophora* Hance, a deciduous tree that belongs to the Sterculiaceae family. The trees grow mainly in tropical zones including Vietnam, India, Malaysia, Thailand, Indonesia, Gwangdong, and the Hainan Island in China [1]. The immature seed has an oval shape and looks similar to an olive while the mature seed has a length and approximate width of 2–2.5 and 1.2–1.7 cm, respectively, and weighs about 2 g (Figure 1). The outer layer of the seed is very thin and brittle, and when soaked in water its exposed interior is yellowish brown with a spongy mucus rich consistency [2].

In the dictionary of traditional Chinese medicine, *S. lych-nophora* is odorless, has a viscous consistency when chewed at length, is cool or cold in nature, and has a slightly sweet or bittersweet taste. It has been used to treat the pharyngitis, constipation, and tussis in most cases [3, 4]. In China, *S. lychnophora* is commonly boiled or soaked in hot water and consumed as beverage for the treatment of sore throat or bloating. Recent report has shown neuroprotective effect [4]. However, anticariogenic effect or antibacterial activity of *S. lychnophora* is not well known. The main constituents are bassorin in the outer seed layer as well as galactose and pentose (mainly arabinose), 15.06% and 24.7%, respectively, in the peel [5].

Dental caries constitutes the most common chronic ecological disease in dentistry and is known as tooth decay or cavities. It is an infectious disease in which the hard tissues of the teeth such as the enamel, dentin, and cementum are gradually and irreversibly destroyed [6, 7]. Dental caries is caused by some types of oral *Streptococci* including the Gram-positive *Streptococcus mutans*, which is the most important

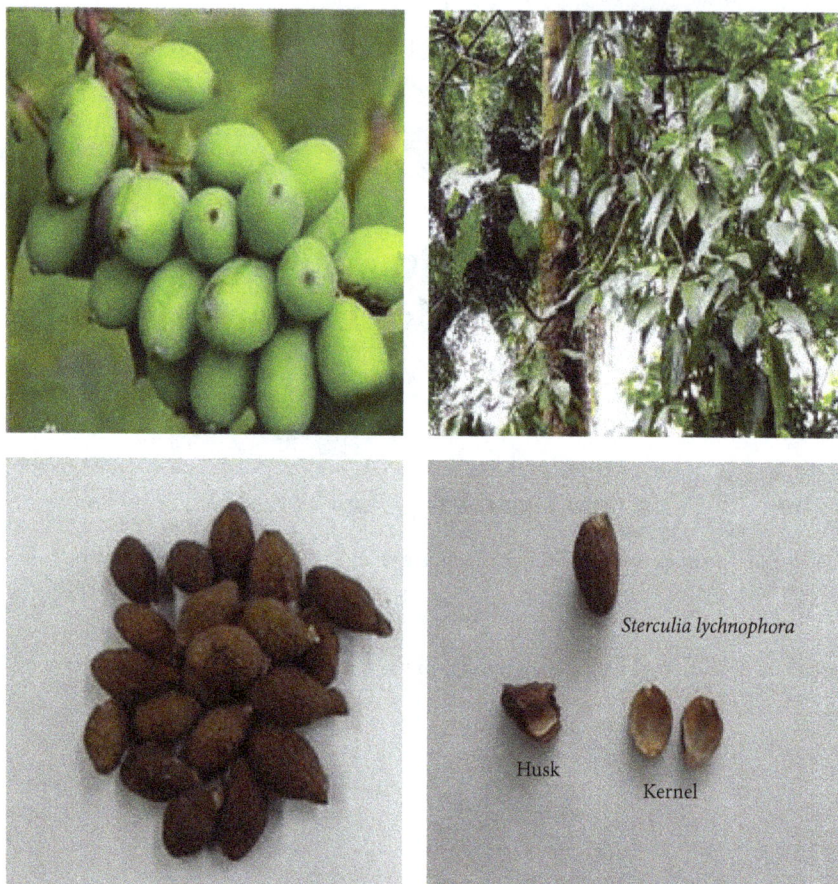

FIGURE 1: Photographs of *Sterculia lychnophora* Hance plant parts.

cariogenic bacteria and primary causative agent of this disease [8, 9]. *S. mutans* metabolizes the carbohydrates contained in consumed foods and produces organic acids, which initiate tooth enamel decay. Although fluoride compounds have been used to inhibit the formation of dental caries, high levels are cytotoxic [10]. Therefore, the development of new and safe agents that protect against the formation of dental caries is important. Natural products are good candidates for drug discovery including anticariogenic cariogenic agents. In the present study, we show *S. lychnophora* inhibits the growth as well as acid production and biofilm formation of *S. mutans*. This is the first report of anticariogenic effect of *S. lychnophora*. Furthermore, we analyzed the composition of phytochemicals and nutrient components of *S. lychnophora*.

2. Materials and Methods

2.1. Materials. Brain heart infusion (BHI) broth was purchased from Difco Laboratories (Detroit, MI, USA). Glucose and dimethyl sulfoxide (DMSO) were obtained from Sigma-Aldrich Co. (St. Louis, MO, USA). *Streptococcus mutans* ATCC 25175 was purchased from the American Type Culture Collection (ATCC, Rockville, MD, USA).

2.2. Plant Material and Extraction. Pangdahai was obtained from the Oriental Drug Store Dae Hak Yak Kuk (Iksan,

South Korea) and was authenticated by Young-Hoi Kim at the College of Environmental and Bioresource Sciences, Chonbuk National University (Jeonju, South Korea). A voucher specimen (number 18-03-12) has been deposited at the Herbarium of the Department of Oral Biochemistry in Wonkwang University. The husk and kernels of the *S. lychnophora* plant material were separated prior to use. The ethanol extract was prepared using 300 g of plant material, which was placed in a 3000 mL flask and macerated with 3000 mL of 70% ethanol for 72 h at room temperature. The ethanol extract samples were then dried, weighed, and stored at −20°C and the yield was 10.68 g (3.56%). The ethanol extract was dissolved in DMSO to obtain the desired stock solution for the experiments. The final concentration of DMSO was adjusted to 0.1% (v/v) in the culture systems, which did not interfere with the test while control groups were treated with medium containing 0.1% DMSO.

2.3. Inhibition of Growth and Acid Production. Bacterial growth inhibition was determined using a modification of methods described previously [11]. The cell growth evaluation was performed at 37°C in tubes with 0.95 mL of BHI broth containing varying concentrations of *S. lychnophora* extracts. The tubes were inoculated with 0.05 mL of an overnight culture of *S. mutans* grown in BHI broth at a final density of 5×10^5 colony-forming units (CFU)/mL and incubated at

37°C. After a 24 h incubation, the minimum inhibitory concentration (MIC), defined as the lowest concentration that inhibited the visible growth of *S. mutans* following overnight incubation, was determined by measuring the optical density (OD) of the growth media at 550 nm using an enzyme-linked immunosorbent assay (ELISA) plate reader (Molecular Devices Co., Sunnyvale, CA, USA). In addition, the pH of the culture media was determined using a pH meter (HANNA Instrument, Philippines). The measurements were performed in triplicate for each concentration of the test extracts and sodium fluoride (NaF, 1%) was used as a positive control.

2.4. Biofilm Assay. The biofilm assay used in this study was based on a method described previously [12]. *S. lychnophora* extract was added to BHI broth containing 1% glucose in 35 mm polystyrene dishes or 24-well plates (Nunc, Copenhagen, Denmark). The culture media were then inoculated with a seed culture of methicillin-resistant *S. mutans* at a final density of 5×10^5 CFU/mL. After culturing for 48 h at 37°C, the supernatant was removed completely, and the dishes, wells, or wells containing the composite resin teeth were rinsed with distilled water. The amount of biofilm formed in the wells was measured by staining with 0.1% safranin, followed by treatment with 30% acetic acid to release the bound safranin from the stained cells, and the absorbance of the solution was measured at 530 nm. The biofilm formed on the surface of the resin teeth was also stained with 0.1% safranin and photographed.

2.5. Scanning Electron Microscopy (SEM). The biofilm formed on the 35 mm polystyrene dishes was also examined using scanning electron microscopy (SEM) using a modification of a previously described method [13]. The biofilm formed on the dishes was rinsed with distilled water and fixed with 2.5% glutaraldehyde in 0.1 M sodium cacodylate buffer (pH 7.2) at 4°C for 24 h. After sequential dehydration with graded concentrations of ethanol (60, 70, 80, 90, 95, and 100%), the samples were freeze-dried, sputter-coated with gold (108A sputter coater, Cressington Scientific Instruments Inc., Watford, England, UK), and observed using a scanning electron microscope (JSM-6360 SEM, JEOL, Tokyo, Japan).

2.6. Confocal Laser Scanning Microscopy. The bactericidal effect of the *S. lychnophora* extracts was determined using confocal laser scanning microscopy. The *S. mutans* culture (in BHI) was diluted with additional BHI medium to a density of approximately 1×10^7 CFU/mL and then treated with high concentrations (8–64 mg/mL) of *S. lychnophora* extracts at 37°C under aerobic conditions. After a 30 min incubation, the bacteria were washed with PBS and stained using a LIVE/DEAD BacLight Bacterial Viability Kit (Molecular Probes, Eugene, OR, USA) according to the manufacturer's instructions, for 15 min. Stained bacteria were observed using a confocal laser scanning microscope (LSM 510, Zeiss, Germany). This method is based on two nucleic acid stains: green fluorescent SYTO 9 and red fluorescent propidium iodide stains, which differ in their ability to penetrate healthy bacterial cell and label live bacteria and those with damaged membranes, respectively.

2.7. Phytochemical Screening. The ethanol extracts of *S. lychnophora* were analyzed using phytochemical test [14]. The alkaloids, phenolics, glycosides, peptides, flavonoids, steroids, and organic acids were determined using Mayer's reagent, ferric chloride reagent, Molisch test, Biuret reagent, Mg-HCl reagent, Liebermann-Burchard reagent, and silver nitrate reagent, respectively.

2.8. Analytical Assays. The proximate components (moisture, protein, fat, carbohydrate, and ash) and mineral contents of the *S. lychnophora* extracts were analyzed using the Association of Official Analytical Chemists (AOAC) methods [15]. The following analyses were performed for the proximate nutrient determination. Moisture loss was determined after exposing the extract samples to a temperature of 110°C for 5 h in a forced draft oven. Total nitrogen was determined using the Kjeldahl method with a semiautomatic nitrogen analyzer. The ash content was determined by extracting ether soluble material from the extract samples with petroleum ether in a Soxhlet extractor for 8 h. Then, 2 g of the sample was charred and ashed to a constant weight at 550°C for 5 h in a muffled furnace. The carbohydrate content was calculated using the fresh weight-derived data, according to the following equation:

$$g/100\,g \text{ carbohydrate} = 100\,g/100\,g$$
$$- (g/100\,g \text{ moisture} + g/100\,g \text{ protein} \qquad (1)$$
$$+ g/100\,g \text{ fat} + g/100\,g \text{ ash}).$$

2.9. Mineral Content Analysis. The *S. lychnophora* extract contents of Ca, Fe, Na, K, Mg, and Zn were analyzed using an atomic absorption spectrophotometer while the P content was determined using a spectrophotometer.

2.10. Dietary Fiber Analysis. The *S. lychnophora* husk and kernel extracts were separately analyzed for their insoluble dietary fiber (IDF), soluble dietary fiber (SDF), and total dietary fiber (TDF) using the relevant AOAC methods [15].

2.11. Statistical Analysis. All the experiments were performed in triplicate and the data were analyzed using the Statistical Package for the Social Sciences (SPSS) version 18.0 program. The data are expressed as the mean ± standard error (SE). The differences between the means of the experimental and control groups were evaluated using Student's *t*-test and *p* values < 0.05 were considered statistically significant.

3. Results

3.1. Inhibition of Bacterial Growth and Acid Production. The ethanol extract of *S. lychnophora* showed significant dose-dependent antibacterial activity against *S. mutans* at concentrations of 0.01, 0.02, 0.03, and 0.04 mg/mL (Figure 2). Furthermore, compared to the control group, the inhibitory effects observed in the extract-treated groups were significant at concentrations higher than 0.01 mg/mL ($p < 0.05$) while the 0.1% NaF positive control exhibited antibacterial activity as well. A comparison of the extract-treated and control

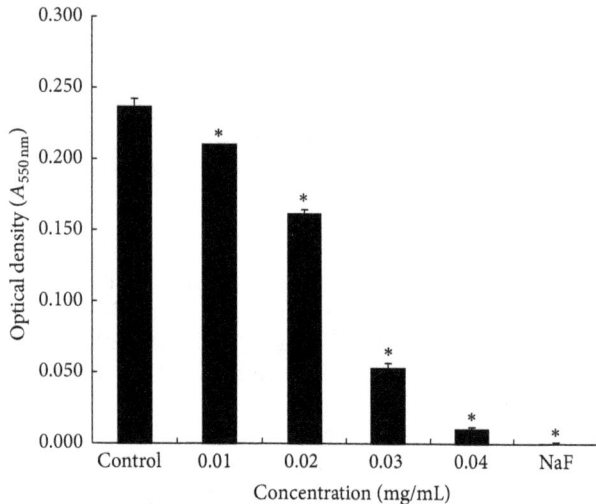

FIGURE 2: Optical density of S. mutans culture supernatants following treatment with varying concentrations of ethanol extracts of S. lychnophora. *$p < 0.05$ when compared with the control group after incubation.

TABLE 1: The pH of S. mutans incubated with ethanol extract of S. lychnophora.

Conc. (mg/mL)	pH (before incubation)	pH (after incubation)
Control	7.24 ± 0.06	5.37 ± 0.01
0.01	7.26 ± 0.06	$5.42 \pm 0.02^*$
0.02	7.25 ± 0.00	$5.62 \pm 0.02^*$
0.03	7.25 ± 0.00	$6.55 \pm 0.03^*$
0.04	7.25 ± 0.00	$7.23 \pm 0.02^*$
0.1% NaF	7.30 ± 0.06	$7.29 \pm 0.00^*$

*$p < 0.05$ when compared with the control group after incubation.

groups at the concentrations tested (0.01, 0.02, 0.03, and 0.04 mg/mL) revealed antibacterial effects of 11.02, 31.78, 77.54, and 95.76%, respectively.

The inhibitory effects of S. lychnophora ethanol extract against acid production by S. mutans, determined by the effects of the extract on pH, are shown in Table 1. The pH was significantly decreased in the untreated control group (pH 5.37 ± 0.01) but this effect was significantly inhibited in the positive control group (0.1% NaF, pH 7.29 ± 0.00). S. lychnophora extract (0.01–0.04 mg/mL) showed significant inhibition. These results indicate that the ethanol extract of S. lychnophora may inhibit organic acid production by S. mutans.

3.2. Inhibitory Effect of S. lychnophora on Biofilm Formation. The inhibitory effects of the extract of S. lychnophora on the biofilm formation by S. mutans evaluated using safranin staining are shown in Figure 3. The extract of S. lychnophora (0.01–0.04 mg/mL) inhibited the formation of S. mutans biofilm, which was also inhibited by the positive control (0.1% NaF). Furthermore, the S. lychnophora extract induced significant dose-dependent changes in the color intensity (OD) of the stained biofilm.

TABLE 2: Phytochemical screening of the ethanol extract from S. lychnophora.

Plant constituent	Contents
Alkaloid	+++
Phenolics	+++
Glycosides	+++
Peptides	+++
Steroids, terpenoids	+
Flavonoids	+
Organic acids	+

+++: strong; ++: moderate; +: weak; −: absent.

The SEM photographs (Figure 4) illustrate the results obtained using safranin staining. S. mutans attached and aggregated to the surface of the polystyrene 35 mm dishes and formed the visible biofilm in the control group. However, the biofilm formation was decreased in the presence of S. lychnophora at concentrations higher than 0.03 mg/mL and in the presence of the positive control (0.1% NaF).

In addition, we observed biofilm formation on the surface of the resin teeth following safranin staining (Figure 5). The extract of S. lychnophora (0.01–0.04 mg/mL) inhibited the formation of biofilm on the surface of resin teeth, and the inhibition was particularly potent at concentrations higher than 0.03 mg/mL.

3.3. Bactericidal Effect of S. lychnophora against S. mutans. The bactericidal effect of S. lychnophora is showed in Figure 6. The bactericidal effect of S. lychnophora was determined by staining the cultured bacteria with LIVE/DEAD BacLight Bacterial Viability Kit followed by confocal laser scanning microscopy. Bacterial viability decreased at high concentrations (0.04, 0.08, 0.16, and 0.32 mg/mL) of S. lychnophora extract, dose-dependently. This result suggests that high concentration of S. lychnophora extract may be bactericidal against S. mutans.

3.4. Phytochemical Screening. The results of the phytochemical tests for the ethanol extract are shown in Table 2. The preliminary phytochemical analysis is performed on the ethanol extracts. The ethanol extract revealed a strong presence of alkaloid, phenolics, glycosides, and peptides while the presence of steroids, terpenoids, flavonoids, and organic acids was low.

3.5. Proximate Composition. The results of the proximate composition analysis of S. lychnophora extracts are shown in Table 3. Moisture ($11.97\% \pm 0.19$) and ash ($5.38\% \pm 0.10$) of husk were higher than moisture ($7.83\% \pm 0.05$) and ash ($2.65\% \pm 0.03$) of kernel. Protein ($3.12\% \pm 0.07$) and fat ($0.02\% \pm 0.01$) of husk were lower than protein ($17.24\% \pm 0.23$) and fat ($6.47\% \pm 0.25$) of kernel. No significant difference was found in the levels of carbohydrate between the husk ($79.54\% \pm 0.21$) and kernel ($65.79\% \pm 0.17$).

3.6. Minerals Analysis. The results of the mineral content analysis of S. lychnophora extracts are shown in Table 4. The

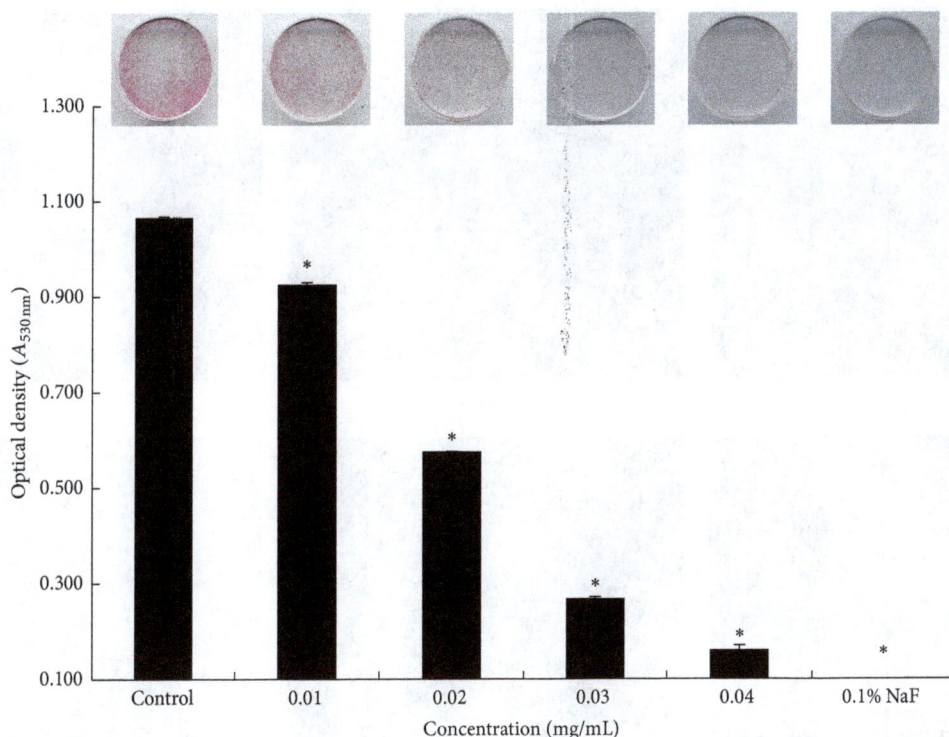

FIGURE 3: Safranin staining of S. mutans biofilm formation. Control, 0.01, 0.02, 0.03, and 0.04 mg/mL ethanol extract of S. lychnophora and positive control 0.1% sodium fluoride (NaF). $^*p < 0.05$ when compared with the control group after incubation.

TABLE 3: The proximate composition of S. lychnophora.

	Husk (%)	Kernel (%)
Moisture	$11.97 \pm 0.19^*$	$7.83 \pm 0.05^*$
Protein	$3.12 \pm 0.07^*$	$17.24 \pm 0.23^*$
Fat	$0.02 \pm 0.01^*$	$6.47 \pm 0.25^*$
Ash	$5.38 \pm 0.10^*$	$2.65 \pm 0.03^*$
Carbohydrate	79.54 ± 0.21	65.79 ± 0.17

$^*p < 0.05$ when compared with the husk and kernel.

TABLE 4: Mineral contents of S. lychnophora.

	Husk (mg/100 g)	Kernel (mg/100 g)
Calcium	$367.64 \pm 6.39^*$	$85.84 \pm 3.07^*$
Copper	$0.89 \pm 0.01^*$	$1.81 \pm 0.08^*$
Iron	$6.57 \pm 0.47^*$	$4.15 \pm 0.11^*$
Magnesium	$405.41 \pm 15.68^*$	$218.94 \pm 5.46^*$
Phosphorus	$11.5 \pm 0.01^*$	$76.81 \pm 6.49^*$
Potassium	$1734.76 \pm 33.75^*$	$1111.32 \pm 4.77^*$
Sodium	2.9 ± 0.05	2.46 ± 0.25

$^*p < 0.05$ when compared with the husk and kernel.

TABLE 5: Content of dietary fiber in husk and kernel of S. lychnophora.

	Husk (mg/100 g)	Kernel (mg/100 g)
Insoluble dietary fiber (IDF)	$58.08 \pm 0.06^*$	$1.31 \pm 0.01^*$
Soluble dietary fiber (SDF)	$14.05 \pm 0.23^*$	$0.42 \pm 0.02^*$
Total dietary fiber (TDF)	$72.13 \pm 0.29^*$	$1.73 \pm 0.03^*$

$^*p < 0.05$ when compared with the husk and kernel.

difference was found in the levels of Na between the husk and kernel.

3.7. Dietary Fiber Analysis. Table 5 shows the IDF, SDF, and TDF of the S. lychnophora husk and kernel. The IDF, SDF, and TDF of husk are higher than those of kernel significantly.

4. Discussion

There have been numerous research studies on the prevention and treatment of dental caries, which is one of the most frequently contracted and chronic dental diseases in humans. It is known that this disease affects 85.7% of people on average. Dental caries, once contracted, is not self-limiting and, therefore, cannot be cured without treatment [16]. Furthermore, if left untreated dental caries may develop into pulpitis, which can cause severe pain and eventually result in the necessary extraction of teeth [16].

S. mutans is commonly found in the dental plaque of humans and is the most cariogenic bacteria against the tooth

husk showed Ca, Fe, Mg, and K contents that were significantly higher ($p < 0.05$) than those of the kernel. The husk had copper levels of 0.89 ± 0.01 mg/100 g and phosphorus contents of 11.50 ± 0.01 mg/100 g, which were both significantly lower ($p < 0.05$) than those of kernel. No significant

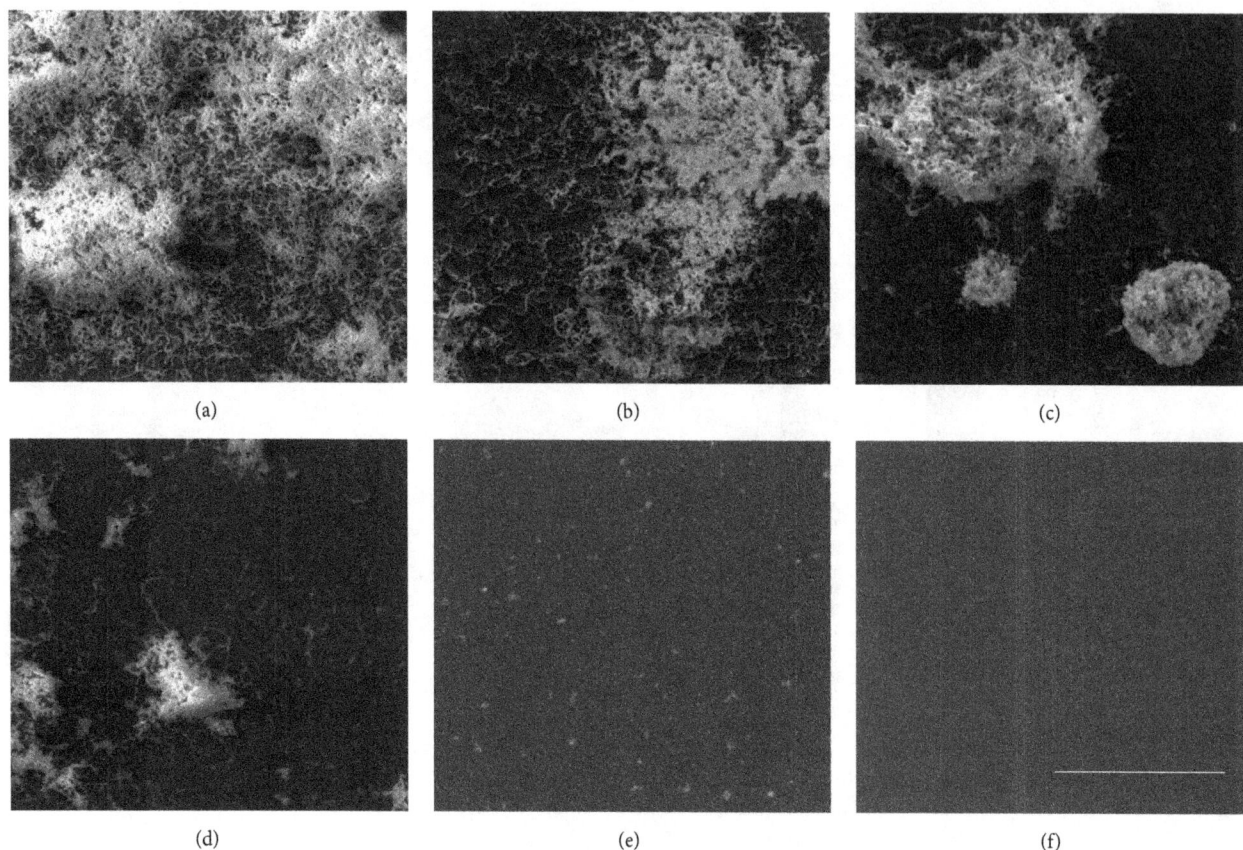

FIGURE 4: Scanning electron microscopy of S. mutans biofilms grown in the presence of ethanol extract of S. lychnophora: (a) control, (b) 0.01, (c) 0.02, (d) 0.03, and (e) 0.04 mg/mL extract and (f) positive control (0.1% NaF), scale bar = 10 μm.

enamel. It metabolizes dietary sugars and produces organic acids such as propionic, butyric, lactic, and formic acids as metabolic products, which can lower the pH of dental plaque and demineralize the tooth enamel and thereby initiate dental caries [17, 18].

Adhesion and colonization of S. mutans on the acquired enamel pellicle coated tooth surface are the initial step of the formation of dental plaque, which is a type of biofilm. The biofilm formation enhances bacterial resistance to both the host defense system and antimicrobials. Several natural substances have been developed for the treatment and prevention of dental diseases. The methanol extracts from leaves of green perilla and mugwort [19] as well as white ginseng [20] were reported to have excellent antibiotic effect against S. mutans. However, it was reported that ethanol extracts of S. lychnophora have more outstanding antibiotic effects than these substances. The methanol extracts of Aralia continentalis [21] as well as Dianthus superbus [22] were reported to have effects at 2 mg/mL and 4 mg/mL, respectively, against S. mutans. In addition, the ethanol extracts of S. lychnophora have a superior antibiotic effect to these substances as well. We aimed to provide scientific evidence of how S. lychnophora extracts can reduce the growth of germs that cause dental caries.

In this study, we prepared the ethanol extract of S. lychnophora and investigated its potential effects against the cariogenic properties of S. mutans. The extract of S. lychnophora inhibited the growth of S. mutans. It is commonly known as the main bacteria responsible for the formation of dental plaque and dental caries [7]. The ethanol extract of S. lychnophora inhibited the decrease in pH induced by S. mutans. These results suggest that the ethanol extract of S. lychnophora may inhibit organic acid production by S. mutans. Furthermore, the ethanol extract of S. lychnophora inhibited biofilm formation by S. mutans at concentrations ranging from 0.01 to 0.04 mg/mL and the SEM data on the biofilm formation corroborated the safranin staining data. The extract of S. lychnophora (0.01-0.04 mg/mL) also inhibited the biofilm formation on the resin tooth surface. In the present study, we have used 0.1% NaF as a positive control. It exhibited antibacterial activity and inhibited the decrease of pH and biofilm formation of S. mutans as S. lychnophora. However, previous reports have shown that fluoride compounds have cytotoxicity when fluoride compound was used at concentrations higher than 80 ppm [23]. Fluoride compounds have been investigated to inhibit the dental caries, but dental caries still remains the major cause of tooth loss. Therefore, it is necessary to develop new agents

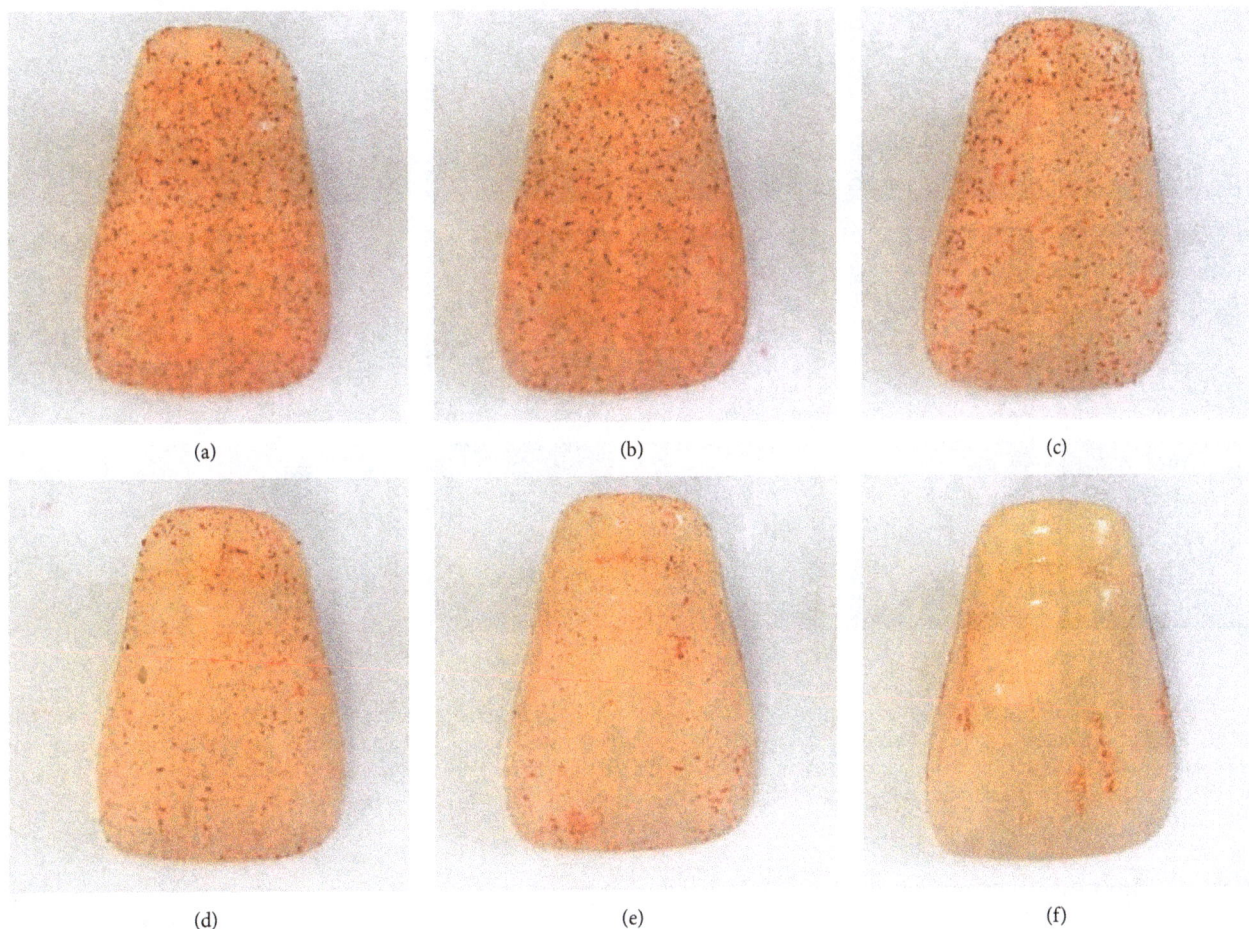

FIGURE 5: *S. mutans* biofilms on resin tooth surface following incubation with ethanol extract of *S. lychnophora*: (a) control, (b) 0.01, (c) 0.02, (d) 0.03, and (e) 0.04 mg/mL extract and (f) positive control, 0.1% sodium fluoride (NaF).

having better effect against dental caries. In this experiment, we found a strong presence of alkaloid, phenolics, glycosides, and peptides and a low presence of steroids, flavonoids, and organic acids. These compounds may have been responsible for the anticariogenic activity observed in the present study [24, 25].

The *S. lychnophora* ethanol extract showed levels of alkaloid, phenolics, glycosides, and peptides that were greater than those reported for the ethanol extract of *Aralia continentalis* [21]. In the results of the ethanol extract of *Aralia continentalis*, it had the strong presence of flavonoids and organic acids, moderate presence of phenolics and steroids, and the weak presence of alkaloids.

Then, we investigated the proximate composition of the *S. lychnophora* husk and kernel. The husk had moisture and ash contents that were significantly higher ($p < 0.05$) than those of the kernel as well as protein levels and fat contents that were significantly lower ($p < 0.05$) than those of kernel. According to the study by Li and Chen [26], the levels of Fe and P were 183.0 and 2786.0 mg/kg in *S. lychnophora* from China, and P was 2017.0 mg/kg in samples from Cambodia, which was more than that observed in our study. The levels of

Ca, Mg, and Na at 1210.0, 3323.0, and 8.1 mg/kg, respectively, were higher in our study. The IDF level of the husk was higher than that in the peel of persimmon (15.71%), jujube (16.88%), citron (7.32%), cereal, and potato samples (7.36%) [27, 28]. The dried soymilk residue contained about 16% of SDF, which is higher than that of the husk of *S. lychnophora* [29]. The ISF level of the kernel was lower than that of the pulp of persimmon (1.95%), jujube (1.95%), and citron (2.61%) [27].

In conclusion, we demonstrated that the ethanol extract of *S. lychnophora* may inhibit acid production and biofilm formation, which may be due to the organic acids and glycosides, which are the major components of the extract of *S. lychnophora*. Therefore, we provided scientific evidence of the potential efficacy of the ethanol extract of *S. lychnophora* in the treatment of dental caries and a basis for its continued ethnomedicinal application and future development as a standard treatment.

Competing Interests

The authors declare that they have no competing interests.

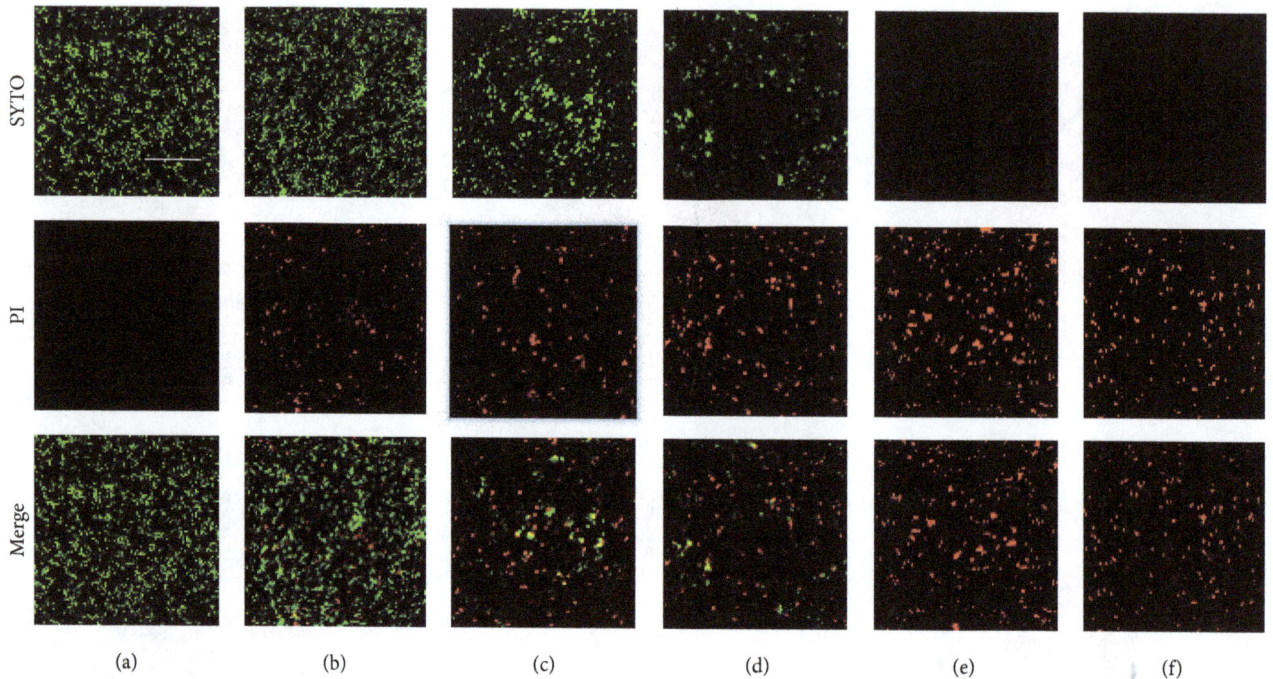

FIGURE 6: Bactericidal effect of *S. lychnophora* cultured *S. mutans* treated with *S. lychnophora* and stained with LIVE/DEAD BacLight Bacterial Viability Kit. Stained bacteria were observed using confocal laser scanning microscopy. Treatment with *S. lychnophora* decreased green-labeled living bacteria (SYTO 9 stain) and increased red-labeled dead bacteria (PI stain) dose-dependently. (a) Control, (b) 0.04, (c) 0.08, (d) 0.16, and (e) 0.32 mg/mL extract and (f) positive control sodium fluoride 0.1% (NaF), scale bar = 50 μm, objective lens (×100).

Acknowledgments

This research was supported by Basic Science Research Program through the National Research Foundation of Korea (NRF) funded by the Ministry of Education, Science and Technology (no. 2013R1A1A4A03011203).

References

[1] K. I. Suh and G. Y. Jeong, *An Easy Herbal Medicine*, Daegu Hanny University Publishing, Seoul, Republic of Korea, 2007.

[2] Z. Zhao, "An illustrated Chinese materia medica in Hong Kong," in *Herbal Medicine*, Z. Zhao, Ed., School of Chinese Medicine, Hong Kong Baptist University Publishing, Hong Kong, 2004.

[3] H. Carl-Herman, *A Materia Medical for Chinese Medicine: Plants, Minerals and Animal Products*, Elsevier Publishing, 2009 (German).

[4] R.-F. Wang, X.-W. Wu, and D. Geng, "Two cerebrosides isolated from the seeds of *Sterculia lychnophora* and their neuroprotective effect," *Molecules*, vol. 18, no. 1, pp. 1181–1187, 2013.

[5] Jiangsu New Medical College, *The Dictionary of Traditional Chinese Medicine*, Science and Technology Publishing, Shanghai, China, 1979.

[6] X.-Y. Wang, Q. Zhang, and Z. Chen, "A possible role of LIM mineralization protein 1 in tertiary dentinogenesis of dental caries treatment," *Medical Hypotheses*, vol. 69, no. 3, pp. 584–586, 2007.

[7] K.-H. Lee, B.-S. Kim, K.-S. Keum et al., "Essential oil of *Curcuma longa* inhibits *Streptococcus mutans* biofilm formation," *Journal of Food Science*, vol. 76, no. 9, pp. 226–230, 2011.

[8] M. A. Salam, N. Matsumoto, K. Matin et al., "Establishment of an animal model using recombinant NOD. B10. D2 mice to study initial adhesion of oral streptococci," *Clinical and Diagnostic Laboratory Immunology*, vol. 11, no. 2, pp. 379–386, 2004.

[9] S.-I. Jeong, B.-S. Kim, K.-S. Keum et al., "Kaurenoic acid from *Aralia continentalis* inhibits biofilm formation of *Streptococcus mutans*," *Evidence-Based Complementary and Alternative Medicine*, vol. 2013, Article ID 160592, 9 pages, 2013.

[10] S. Y. Kang, S. Y. An, M. W. Lee et al., "Effect of *Aconitum koreanum* extract on the growth, acid production, adhesion and insoluble glucan synthesis of *Streptococcus Mutans*," *Korean Journal of Oriental Physiology and Pathology*, vol. 29, no. 1, pp. 27–32, 2015.

[11] B.-K. Choi, K.-Y. Kim, Y.-J. Yoo, S.-J. Oh, J.-H. Choi, and C.-Y. Kim, "In vitro antimicrobial activity of a chitooligosaccharide mixture against *Actinobacillus actinomycetemcomitans* and *Streptococcus mutans*," *International Journal of Antimicrobial Agents*, vol. 18, no. 6, pp. 553–557, 2001.

[12] E. O'Neill, H. Humphreys, and J. P. O'Gara, "Carriage of both the fnbA and fnbB genes and growth at 37° C promote FnBP-mediated biofilm development in meticillin-resistant *Staphylococcus aureus* clinical isolates," *Journal of Medical Microbiology*, vol. 58, no. 4, pp. 399–402, 2009.

[13] K. Nakamiya, S. Hashimoto, H. Ito, J. S. Edmonds, A. Yasuhara, and M. Morita, "Microbial treatment of bis (2-ethylhexyl) phthalate in polyvinyl chloride with isolated bacteria," *Journal of Bioscience and Bioengineering*, vol. 99, no. 2, pp. 115–119, 2005.

[14] W. S. Woo, *Experimental Methods for Phytochemistry*, Seoul National University Press, Seoul, Republic of Korea, 2001.

[15] V. A. Arlington, *Official Methods of Analysis of AOAC*, Association of Official Analytical Chemists, 17th edition, 2001.

[16] J. M. Awika, L. W. Rooney, X. Wu, R. L. Prior, and L. Cisneros-Zevallos, "Screening methods to measure antioxidant activity of Sorghum (*Sorghum bicolor*) and Sorghum products," *Journal of Agricultural and Food Chemistry*, vol. 51, no. 23, pp. 6657–6662, 2003.

[17] J. Cohen-Berneron, D. Steinberg, J. D. Featherstone, and O. Feuerstein, "Sustained effects of blue light on *Streptococcus mutans* in regrown biofilm," *Lasers in Medical Science*, vol. 31, no. 3, pp. 445–452, 2016.

[18] M. Lu, "Analysis of pathogenic bacteria and drug resistance of oral infection," *Chinese Journal of Nosocomiology*, vol. 11, no. 3, pp. 144–152, 2010.

[19] M. J. Lee, *Anti-microbial activities, anti-cariogenic effect against oral microbes and growth—inhibitory effect on oral tumor cell by extracts of Perilla and Mugwort [M.S. thesis]*, Keimyung University, Daegu, Republic of Korea, 2006.

[20] M. S. Han, *A study on ginseng dentifrice used of extruded ginseng extracts [M.S. thesis]*, Kongju National University, Gongju, South Korea, 2008.

[21] D.-H. Lee, B.-R. Seo, H.-Y. Kim et al., "Inhibitory effect of *Aralia continentalis* on the cariogenic properties of *Streptococcus mutans*," *Journal of Ethnopharmacology*, vol. 137, no. 2, pp. 979–984, 2011.

[22] H. H. Yu, D. K. Kim, J. K. Kim, and Y. O. You, "Effects of *Dianthus superbus* on activity of *Streptococcus mutans*," *Korean Journal of Oriental Physiology and Pathology*, vol. 24, no. 3, pp. 854–858, 2010.

[23] J. H. Jeng, C. C. Hsieh, W. H. Lan et al., "Cytotoxicity of sodium fluoride on human oral mucosal fibroblasts and its mechanisms," *Cell Biology and Toxicology*, vol. 14, no. 6, pp. 383–389, 1998.

[24] Y.-O. You, N.-Y. Choi, S.-Y. Kang, and K.-J. Kim, "Antibacterial activity of *Rhus javanica* against methicillin-resistant *Staphylococcus aureus*," *Evidence-Based Complementary and Alternative Medicine*, vol. 2013, Article ID 549207, 8 pages, 2013.

[25] N.-Y. Choi, S.-Y. Kang, and K.-J. Kim, "*Artemisia princeps* inhibits biofilm formation and virulence-factor expression of antibiotic-resistant bacteria," *BioMed Research International*, vol. 2015, Article ID 239519, 7 pages, 2015.

[26] W. K. Li and J. M. Chen, "The comparison studies on the trace elements in home and abroad *Sterculia lychnophora*," *Spectroscopy and Spectral Analysis*, vol. 13, no. 3, pp. 45–47, 1993.

[27] M. Y. Kang, Y. H. Jeong, and J. B. Eun, "Identification and determination of dietary fibers in citron, jujube and persimmon," *Korean Journal of Food Preservation*, vol. 10, no. 3, pp. 60–64, 2003.

[28] N.-G. Asp, C.-G. Johansson, H. Hallmer, and M. Siljeström, "Rapid enzymatic assay of insoluble and soluble dietary fiber," *Journal of Agricultural and Food Chemistry*, vol. 31, no. 3, pp. 476–482, 1983.

[29] M. N. Kweon, H. S. Ryu, and S. I. Mun, "Evaluation of tofu containing dried soymilk residue (DSR)," *International Journal of Food Sciences and Nutrition*, vol. 22, no. 3, pp. 262–265, 1993.

8

Effect of *Dangguibohyul-Tang,* a Mixed Extract of *Astragalus membranaceus* and *Angelica sinensis,* on Allergic and Inflammatory Skin Reaction Compared with Single Extracts of *Astragalus membranaceus* or *Angelica sinensis*

You Yeon Choi,[1] Mi Hye Kim,[1] Jongki Hong,[2] Kyuseok Kim,[3] and Woong Mo Yang[1]

[1]Department of Convergence Korean Medical Science, College of Korean Medicine, Kyung Hee University, Seoul 02447, Republic of Korea
[2]College of Pharmacy, Kyung Hee University, Seoul 02447, Republic of Korea
[3]Department of Ophthalmology, Otorhinolaryngology and Dermatology of Korean Medicine, College of Korean Medicine, Kyung Hee University, Seoul 02447, Republic of Korea

Correspondence should be addressed to Kyuseok Kim; kmdkskim@khu.ac.kr and Woong Mo Yang; wmyang@khu.ac.kr

Academic Editor: Ying-Ju Lin

Dangguibohyul-tang (DBT), herbal formula composed of *Astragalus membranaceus* (AM) and *Angelica sinensis* (AS) at a ratio of 5 : 1, has been used for the treatment of various skin diseases in traditional medicine. We investigated the effect of DBT on allergic and inflammatory skin reaction in atopic dermatitis-like model compared to the single extract of AM or AS. DBT treatment showed the remission of clinical symptoms, including decreased skin thickness and scratching behavior, the total serum IgE level, and the number of mast cells compared to DNCB group as well as the single extract of AM- or AS-treated group. Levels of cytokines (IL-4, IL-6, IFN-γ, TNF-α, and IL-1β) and inflammatory mediators (NF-κB, phospho-IκBα, and phospho-MAPKs) were significantly decreased in AM, AS, and DBT groups. These results demonstrated that AM, AS, and DBT may have the therapeutic property on atopic dermatitis by inhibition of allergic and inflammatory mediators and DBT formula; a mixed extract of AM and AS based on the herb pairs theory especially might be more effective on antiallergic reaction as compared with the single extract of AM or AS.

1. Introduction

Atopic dermatitis (AD) is one of the most common chronic and recurrent inflammatory skin diseases which affect environmental, genetic, immunologic, and biochemical factors [1]. The pathogenesis of AD has been known to be caused by T helper (Th) 1/2 dysregulation and skin barrier disorder [2, 3]. In addition, mast cells (MCs) in allergic diseases including AD have shown playing a crucial role in the secretion of histamine, leukotrienes, prostaglandin D2, proteolytic enzymes, and several cytokines including interleukin- (IL-) 1β, IL-4, IL-6, tumor necrosis factor- (TNF-) α, and interferon- (IFN-) γ [4].

In conventional medicine, most clinicians mainly focus on the regulation of T cell inflammation with corticosteroids, antihistamines, or immunosuppressive agents [5]. However, long-term uses of these agents can induce serious side effects such as facial edema, skin atrophy, striae distensae, and perioral dermatitis [6]. Therefore, a wide variety of plant-derived medicines with fewer side effects have been investigated as potential alternatives for allergic skin diseases instead of conventional therapy [7, 8].

Many studies have reported that natural products and their compounds inhibit the development of allergic skin diseases. *Dangguibohyul-tang* (DBT; herbal decoction), which combines simply with two herbs, *Astragalus membranaceus* (AM) and *Angelica sinensis* (AS), is widely used herbal formulas for the treatment of hematopoietic function, menopausal symptoms, and immune responses [9–11]. A recent pharmacological study indicated that DBT reduces inflammatory

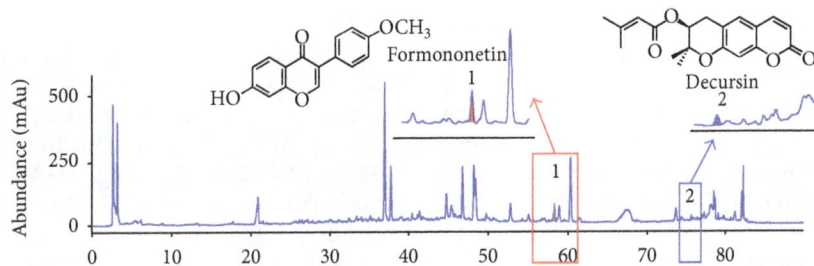

FIGURE 1: HPLC chromatogram of the DBT by HPLC analysis. The amounts of formononetin and decursin in the DBT extracts were determined as marker chemicals.

symptoms in AD-like mice [12]. Also, Dang-Gui-Yin-Zi, a similar herbal formula containing AM and AS, is commonly used for treating atopic dermatitis in clinical practice [13]. Additionally, the weight ratio of 5 : 1 for AM to AS in accord with the ancient preparation showed the best properties of DBT to achieve the maximum activity [14–16]. However, until now, there was no study to assess the antiallergic and anti-inflammatory effect of multiformulas DBT prepared from AM and AS compared with the single extract of AM or AS from the perspective of herb pairs [17].

Based on these backgrounds, we investigated the efficacy and the mechanism of DBT (the weight ratio of 5 : 1 for AM to AS) on allergic and inflammatory skin reaction compared to the single extract of AM or AS via AD-like mouse model.

2. Materials and Methods

2.1. Preparation of Sample. AM and AS were prepared same as previous reports [18, 19]. Briefly, each of the AM and AS crude materials was extracted with 300 mL of 70% ethanol for 24 h. The extracts were filtered, concentrated, lyophilized, and stored at −80°C. The yield of AM dried extract was approximately 25.0% (w/w, dry weight 7.5 g) and the extract of AS yielded 37.3% (w/w) for dry weight 11.2 g. Each voucher specimen (# AM001 and # AS070) was deposited in the herbarium of the college of pharmacy's laboratory. DBT mixture amounts of AM and AS were weighed according to a ratio of 5 to 1 and then mixed well in a vortex. A voucher specimen of DBT (# DBD E70) was deposited at our laboratory.

2.2. Standardization of DBT. DBT was identified by formononetin and decursin using reverse-phase high-performance liquid chromatography (HPLC). 50 mg DBT was mixed with 1 mL methanol, sonicated for 30 min, and filtered through a 0.2 μm filter membrane. HPLC was performed by an Agilent 1100 series instrument and chromatographic separation was achieved on a SHISEIDO CAPCELL PAK C18 column (250 mm × 4.6 mm, 5 μm). Gradient elution was carried out with A : B (water : acetonitrile) as follows: 0 min, 99 : 1; 10 min, 99 : 1; 70 min, 50 : 50; 80 min, 0 : 100; 90 min, 0 : 100. The flow rate was 1.0 mL/min and the detection wavelength was 230 nm. The column temperature was maintained at 40°C. AM and AS were, respectively, characterized based on the content of formononetin and decursin (Figure 1).

2.3. Animal Treatment. Six-week-old female BALB/c mice were supplied by Raon Bio (Yongin, Republic of Korea). The mice were maintained in climate-controlled quarters with a 12 h light/12 h dark cycle (at 22–24°C, 55–60% humidity) and provided with access to a standard laboratory diet and water *ad libitum*. After 1 week of adaptation, the mice were randomly divided into six groups of 5 animals each: (1) vehicle: vehicle application, (2) DNCB: 2,4-dinitrochlorobenzene application with vehicle application as a negative control group, (3) DEX: dexamethasone (10 μM/100 μL/day, Sigma Aldrich, MO, USA) treatment with DNCB application as a positive control group, (4) AM: AM (100 mg/mL, 100 μL/day) treatment with DNCB application, (5) AS: AS (20 mg/mL, 100 μL/day) treatment with DNCB application, and (6) DBT: DBT (120 mg/mL, 100 μL/day) treatment with DNCB application.

In brief, the dorsal hair of mice was removed by an electronic hair clipper for sensitive skin. After 24 h, 100 μL of 1% DNCB solution (acetone : olive oil = 4 : 1, v/v solution) was applied on the back skin once a day for 3 d. After 4 days of sensitization, 100 μL of 0.5% DNCB solution was treated on the back during 10 days. 4 h before DNCB application, DEX, AM, AS, and DBT dissolved in phosphate-buffered saline (PBS) were topically applied to the dorsal skin. Before sample treatment, 100 μL of 4% sodium dodecyl sulfate (SDS) was applied to the lesions in order to remove cuticle and to help the absorption of sample [20]. At the end of experiment, serum was obtained by cardiac puncture and the dorsal skin was collected for molecular indicators. All procedures were performed in accordance with the guidelines of the Committee on Care and Use of Laboratory Animals of Kyung Hee University (KHUASP (SE)-14-030).

2.4. Histological Observation. To investigate the effects of DBT on DNCB-induced AD-like symptoms in mice, we evaluated the skin thickness. To evaluate skin thickening and mast cell infiltration, the dorsal skin samples (1 × 0.4 cm^2) were obtained at the end of the experiment (on day 19). The sample was fixed in 10% buffered formalin (Sigma Aldrich, MO, USA) for at least 24 h, progressively dehydrated in solution containing an increasing percentage of ethanol (70%, 80%, 95%, and 100%, v/v), embedded in paraffin under vacuum, and sectioned at 4 μm thickness. Deparaffinized skin sections were stained with hematoxylin and eosin (H&E) for skin thickening and toluidine blue for mast cell infiltration. Histopathological changes were examined using the Leica

Application Suite (LAS; Leica Microsystems, Buffalo Grove, IL). The magnification was ×100. The epidermal thickness was measured from the top layer (stratum corneum) to the bottom layer (stratum basale). The dermis thickness was measured in vertical distance between stratum basale layer and the subcutaneous tissues. Thickness was measured 3 times at regular intervals in one slide and obtained 15 results per group [21]. The number of mast cells was measured in the entire area of slides for each sample ($n = 5$).

2.5. Measurement of Scratching Behavior. The mice were monitored for 20 min using a digital-camera (model NEX-C3, Sony, Japan), 1 h after last DNCB sensitization. Scratching movement was determined by replaying the recorded video. One incident of scratching was defined as raising to lowering of a leg including a series of scratches at one time.

2.6. Measurement of Total Serum Immunoglobulin E (IgE) Levels and Cytokines. The collected blood was centrifuged for 30 min at 16,000 ×g, and serum sample was stored in −80°C until analysis. Serum concentrations of IgE were measured using mouse IgE ELISA kit (BD Pharmingen, CA, USA) according to the manufacturers' instructions. To measure cytokine on dorsal skin changes according to the topical application, the dorsal skin was removed from each mouse (100 mg, $n = 5$ per group) and homogenized. The dorsal skin was lysed using tissue protein extraction reagent (T-PER; Pierce, Rockford, IL, USA) containing a protease inhibitor cocktail (Roche, Indianapolis, IN, USA). The resulting lysate was centrifuged at 16,000 ×g for 30 min at 4°C and stored at −80°C until analysis. Protein concentrations were requantified under identical conditions using a protein assay reagent (Bio-Rad, Hercules, CA, USA).

2.7. Preparation of Protein Extraction in Dorsal Skin. Extraction of cytoplasmic and nuclear proteins was performed with standard protocols and our previous paper [22]. In brief, the cytoplasmic buffer (10 mM HEPES, pH 7.9, 10 mM KCl, 0.1 mM EDTA, 0.1 mM EGTA, 1 mM DTT, 0.15% Nonidet P-40, 50 mM β-glycerophosphate, 10 mM NaF, and 5 mM Na_3VO_4, containing the protease inhibitor cocktail) was used to analyze the phosphorylated IκBα in the cytoplasm and nuclear buffer (20 mM HEPES, pH 7.9, 400 mM NaCl, 1 mM EDTA, 1 mM EGTA, 1 mM DTT, 0.50% Nonidet P-40, 50 mM β-glycerophosphate, 10 mM NaF, and 5 mM Na_3VO_4, containing the protease inhibitor cocktail) was used to analyze the NF-κB protein levels in the nucleus. MAPKs (extracellular signal-regulated kinases; ERK1/2, p38 kinases, the c-Jun N-terminal kinases; JNK) were confirmed by total protein extracts using RIPA assay buffer containing protease inhibitor cocktail.

2.8. Detection of Inflammatory Protein Expression. Each denatured protein (30 μg; nuclear, cytoplasmic, and whole fraction) was loaded onto 15% polyacrylamide gels for electrophoresis. Then, the proteins were transferred to polyvinylidene fluoride (PVDF) membranes and incubated at room temperature for 1 h with 5% BSA (diluted in TBS-T; TBS buffer containing 0.1% Tween) to block nonspecific

binding. Primary antibodies reactive to mouse β-actin (Santa Cruz, USA), phosphorylated NF-κB (Santa Cruz, USA), phosphorylated IκBα (Santa Cruz, USA), ERK1/2 (Cell Signaling, USA), phosphorylated ERK1/2 (Cell Signaling, USA), p38 MAPK (Cell Signaling, USA), phosphorylated p38 MAPK (Cell Signaling, USA), JNK (Cell Signaling, USA), and phosphorylated JNK (Cell Signaling, USA) were used overnight (1 : 1,000 dilution; in TBS-T). The membrane was washed three times in TBS-T for 30 min, incubated with horseradish peroxidase-conjugated secondary antibodies (1 : 2,000 dilution; in TBS-T) for 2 h at room temperature (RT), washed three times in TBS-T for 30 min, and revealed with enhanced chemiluminescence (ECL). Immunoreactive bands were detected using an LAS-4000 mini system (Fujifilm Corporation, Tokyo, Kumamoto, Japan).

2.9. Statistical Analysis. All data are expressed as the mean ± standard deviation (SD). Significance was determined using one-way ANOVA with Duncan's multiple range test. In all analyses, $P < 0.05$ indicated statistical significance. GraphPad Prism 5 software (San Diego, CA, USA) was used for the statistical analysis.

3. Results

3.1. Amelioration of Hyperkeratosis and Hyperplasia. AD symptoms including dryness, erythema, and swelling were evidently seen in DNCB group. On the other hand, DBT-treated group significantly reduced AD symptoms (Figure 2(a)). As shown in microscopic analysis (Figure 2(b)), the dorsal skin of DNCB-treated mice (epidermis: 111.6 ± 15.5 μm, dermis: 505.3 ± 31.0 μm) was swollen and significantly thicker than those of the vehicle group (32.3 ± 6.3 μm, dermis: 178.3 ± 31.2 μm). Treatment with AM (epidermis: 43 ± 9.1 μm, dermis: 312.2 ± 51.0 μm), AS (epidermis: 65.8 ± 13.5 μm, dermis: 354.9 ± 49.3 μm), and DBT (epidermis: 39.1 ± 6.9 μm, dermis: 327.8 ± 38.2 μm) markedly attenuated DNCB-induced hyperkeratosis and hyperplasia. Particularly, the epidermis and dermis thickness of DBT-treated group were lower than those in AS-treated group.

3.2. Attenuation of Scratching Behavior. Intensive pruritus leads to extensive scratching as a hallmark of AD [23]. The distribution of the assessed level of scratching behavior was illustrated as the dot plot (Figure 3). The scratching behavior was markedly increased in DNCB-treated mice (179 ± 50) compared with the vehicle group (27 ± 5). This increased scratching behavior was significantly reduced by AM (50 ± 16), AS (63 ± 35), and DBT (40 ± 19) treatment. Consistently with histologic analysis, the reduction of pruritus by DBT treatment was greater than AS single treatment.

3.3. Inhibition of the Number of Mast Cells. The number of toluidine blue-stained mast cells of DNCB-treated mice (151 ± 15) was significantly increased compared with that of the vehicle group (44 ± 6). AM (56 ± 9), AS (70 ± 12), and DBT (45 ± 6) markedly lowered the number of mast cells in the skin of DNCB-treated mice (Figures 4(a) and 4(b)).

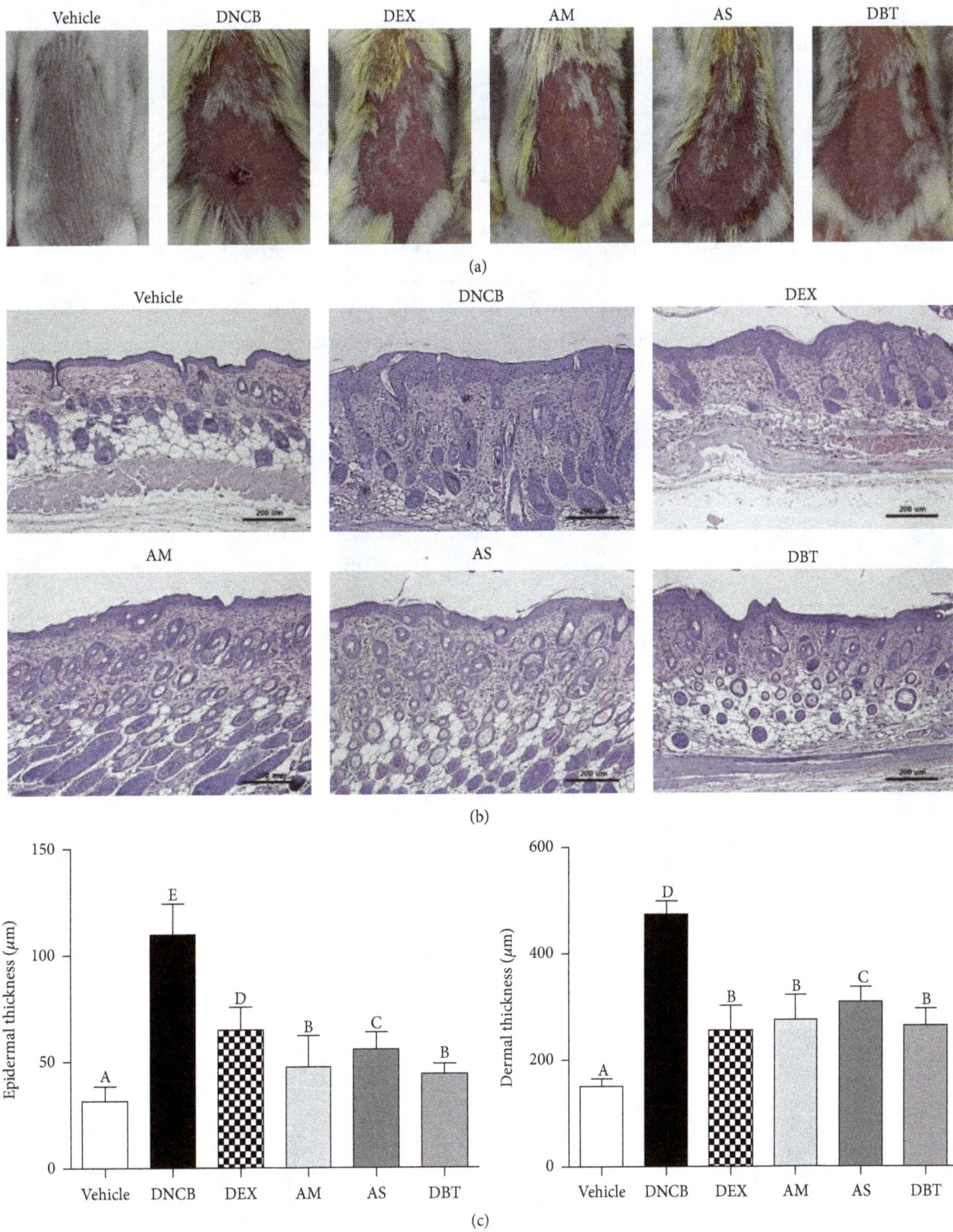

FIGURE 2: Effects of DBT on histological features of dorsal skin in DNCB-induced AD mice. (a) Representative mice of each treatment group on day 19. (b) Histological observation of the dorsal skin of each group by H&E staining. (c) The thickness of epidermis and dermis. Results are expressed as mean ± SD ($n = 5$). Magnifications are ×100 (scale bar: 200 μm).

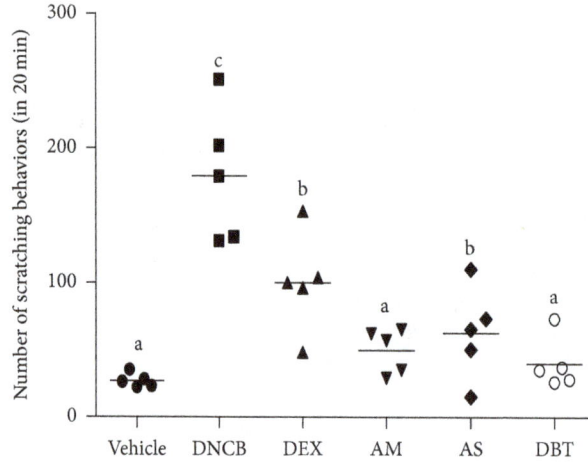

FIGURE 3: Effects of DBT on scratching behavior. The numbers of scratching behaviors are expressed as mean ± SD ($n = 5$).

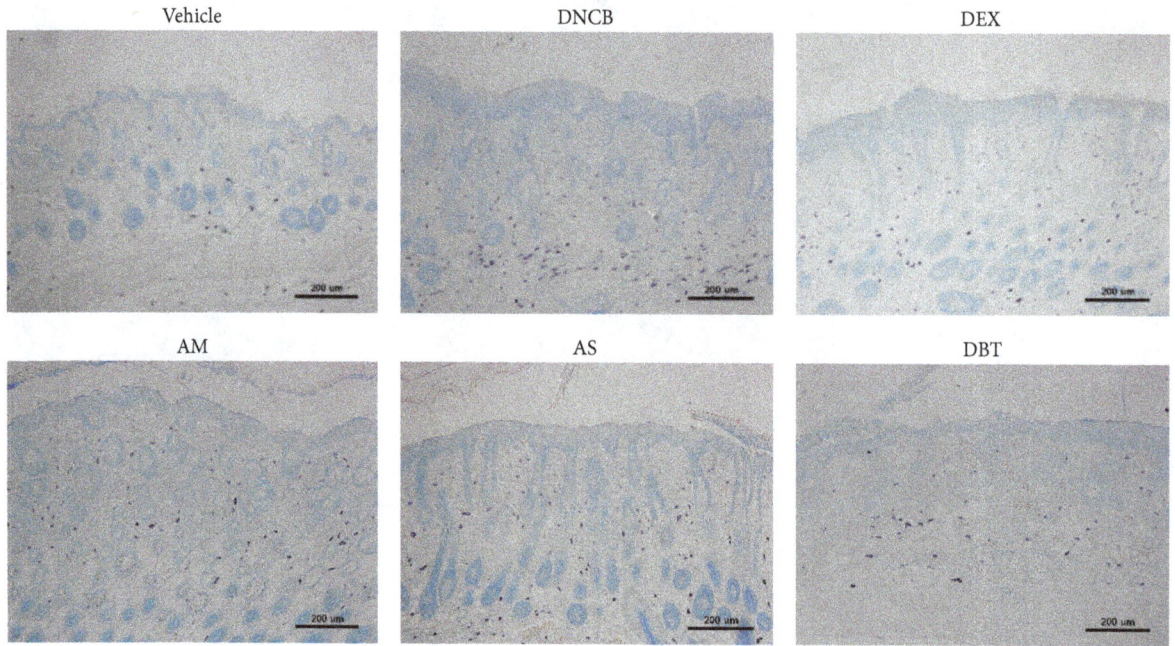

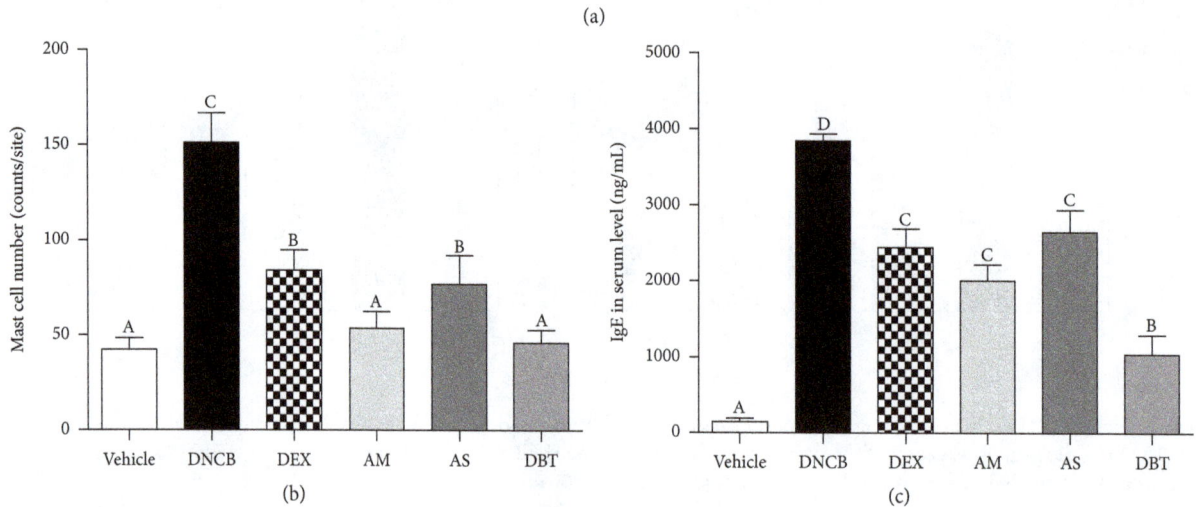

(a)

(b)

(c)

FIGURE 4: The number of mast cells and the level of IgE in DNCB-induced AD mice. (a, b) The number of mast cells observed by toluidine blue staining. Magnifications are ×100 (scale bar: 200 μm). (c) The level of IgE in serum. Results are expressed as mean ± SD ($n = 5$).

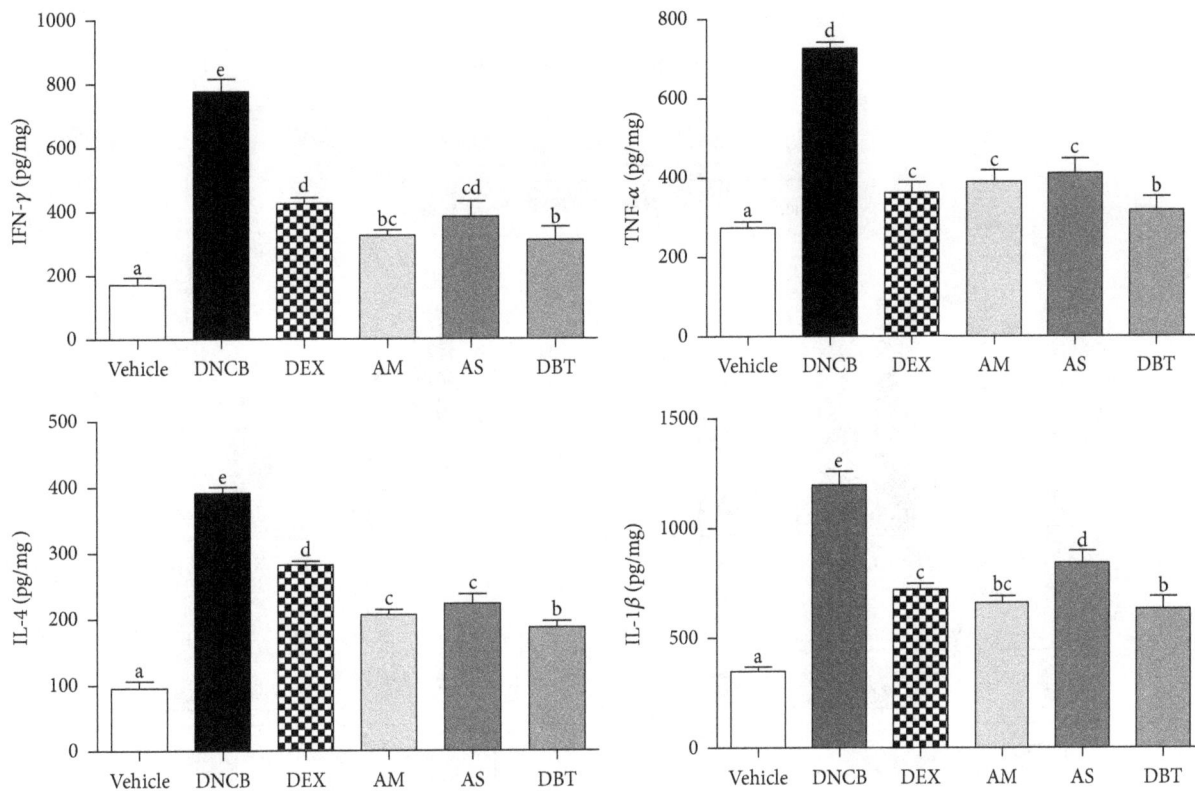

FIGURE 5: Effects of DBT on levels of Th2- and Th1-type cytokines. Values of cytokines are means ± standard error of the mean.

Compared with AS, DBT significantly decreased the number of mast cells.

3.4. Reduction of Serum IgE Level. We investigated whether DBT alters the serum level of IgE in DNCB-induced AD-like mice. We found that the level of IgE was markedly increased by DNCB application, compared to vehicle group. Treatment with AM, AS, DBT, and DEX group significantly reduced the IgE level of DNCB group (Figure 4(c)). DBT treatment showed more effective reduction in IgE level than the single extract of AM or AS.

3.5. Downregulation of Cytokines. Lesional skin of AD patients exhibits increased expression of Th2, Th1 cytokines and proinflammatory cytokines [24]. The cytokine levels in dorsal skin were significantly increased in DNCB (IL-4: 454.9%, IL-6: 1339.7%, IFN-γ: 524.6%, TNF-α: 247.8%, and IL-1β: 342.0%) compared to vehicle. Topical treatment of DEX, AM, AS, and DBT showed significantly lower levels of various cytokines compared with DNCB group (Figure 5). Particularly, the levels of IL-4 and TNF-α in DBT are significantly lower than in the single extract of AM or AS.

3.6. Inhibition of Inflammatory Mediators. Western blot analysis showed that DNCB challenge markedly upregulated the NF-κB (about 1.7-fold) and phosphorylation of IκBα (about 2.6-fold) compared to the vehicle group, whereas simultaneous treatment with DEX, AM, AS, and DBT attenuated

the DNCB-induced NF-κB activation and phosphorylation of IκBα (Figure 6(a)). Moreover, DBT significantly reduced NF-κB and phosphor-IκBα expressions as compared with the AM and AS groups. MAPKs phosphorylation was significantly upregulated by DNCB, including phosphorylation ERK, p38, and JNK pathways (Figure 6(b)). AM, AS, and DBT treatment inhibited the increased level of phosphorylation of ERK, p38, and JNK. The regulation of phospho-ERK and phospho-p38 levels in DBT was more effective than AS, whereas phospho-JNK level was even higher than that of AS.

4. Discussion

Hyperplasia is one of the main symptoms in AD [24]. In histological analysis, we confirmed that the dermis and epidermis were thickened in the DNCB-induced group compared to vehicle group. Our findings showed that thickening of the epidermis and dermis was significantly reduced in DBT, AS, and AM groups. These findings are in agreement with those of a previous study presenting that DBT significantly inhibited ear swelling compared with DNCB-sensitized mice [12]. Particularly, topical application of DBT markedly suppressed a skin thickening and hyperkeratosis of the epidermis as compared with the AS groups. Scratching behavior in DNCB-induced model could be a major feature in skin lesions as results of various immunological responses such as the elevation of serum IgE concentration and number of mast cells [1, 22]. Therefore, it is important to decrease the scratching behavior in controlling the skin lesions and

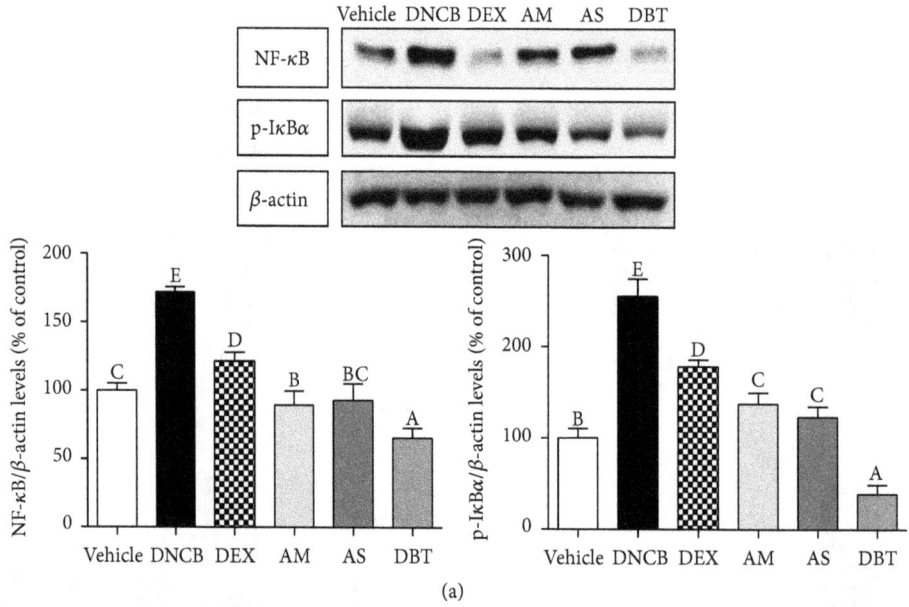

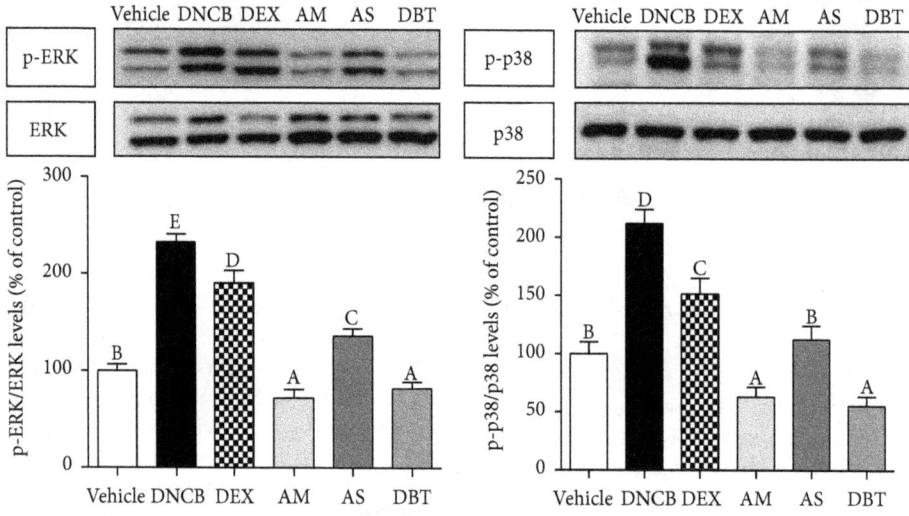

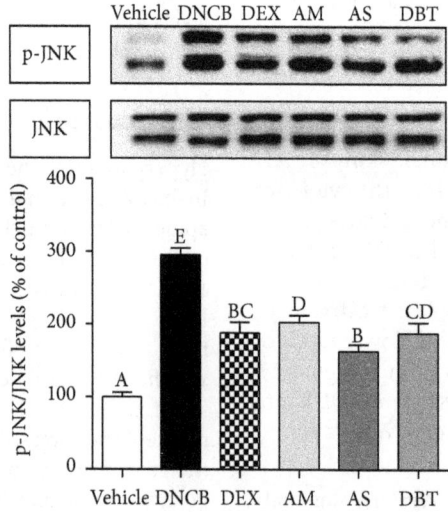

Figure 6: Effects of DBT on inflammatory mediators in DNCB-induced AD mice. (a) NF-κB and phosphor-IκBα levels (b) phosphor-MAPKs (ERK1/2, p38, and JNK) levels. Results are expressed as mean ± SD (n = 5).

various immunological reactions. DBT significantly inhibited the itching sign and decreased the elevation of serum IgE levels and degranulation of mast cells (MCs) compared to DNCB-induced group. These results are in close agreement with the findings of a similar previous study [12]. Particularly, DBT was more significantly effective on the inhibition of serum IgE levels compared to the single extract of AM or AS. These improvements could be partially attributed the antiallergic properties of DBT compared to the single extract of AM or AS in AD.

AD is involved in the dysregulation of Th type 1 and 2 cell-mediated immune responses [2]. Th2 cytokines, such as IL-4 and IL-6, promote B cell proliferation and cause IgE class switching in both acute and chronic AD [25]. On the other hand, Th1 cytokines, such as IFN-γ and IL-1β, are upregulated mainly in chronic stage [26]. Specifically, TNF-α regulates dermal-epidermal interactions in keratinocyte during inflammation, wound healing, and epidermal growth. Also, TNF-α stimulates IL-6 with enhancing the IL-4-induced IgE production [18, 22]. In close accordance with a previous study [12], topical application of DBT significantly inhibited the expression of AD-related pathogenic cytokines such as IL-4, IL-6, IFN-γ, TNF-α, and IL-1β regardless of Th1 and Th2 cytokines similarly to DEX group. Furthermore, DBT significantly suppressed DNCB-induced elevation of IL-4 and TNF-α compared to the single extract of AM or AS. Our comprehensive findings indicate that DBT may be more effective on suppressing an immune response by inhibiting both Th1- and Th2-type cytokine production as compared with the single extract of AM or AS in AD.

NF-κB signaling pathway, which is mediated by TNF-α, plays a critical role in the cellular immune and inflammatory response in epidermal keratinocytes [27]. In this study, we confirmed that activation of NF-κB results in skin thickening and that DBT reduced hyperplasia of epidermis in mice by suppressing expression of NF-κB. In addition, we have observed that the translocation of NF-κB to nucleus by DBT was inhibited as shown by a marked decrease of NF-κB in the nucleus and a decrease of phosphorylated IκBα in the cytoplasm.

Mitogen-activated protein kinase (MAPK) signaling is important in inflammatory skin diseases by controlling the activation, proliferation, degranulation, and migration of various immune cells. MAPK is divided into three groups: ERK controlling cell cycle progression, JNK regulating the cell proliferation and survival, and p38 MAPK relating to cell growth and differentiation, cell death, and inflammation [28]. Several studies have suggested that the development of MAPK inhibitors could be a therapeutic target for allergic diseases [29]. In the present study, DNCB challenge induced the increased activities of MAPK in consistency with the results of previous studies. Topical application of DBT inhibited the phosphorylation of ERK and p38 more than AS groups. These data suggest that inhibition of MAPK by DBT may contribute to its antiallergic and anti-inflammatory activities.

In conclusion, DBT with the weight ratio of 5 : 1 for AM to AS in accord with the ancient preparation not only prevented the degranulation of MCs and regulated the NF-κB signaling pathway, but also suppressed the phosphorylation of MAPK signaling molecules. Particularly, DBT formula could be more effective than AM or AS single treated groups on the antiallergic reactions by suppressing NF-κB signaling pathway and Th2-type cytokines mediating by TNF-α. These consecutive antiallergic and anti-inflammatory effects of DBT are believed to inhibit epidermal and dermal thickness and scratching behavior and to contribute significantly to the clinical efficacy in the management of AD.

Competing Interests

The authors have declared that there are no competing interests.

Authors' Contributions

You Yeon Choi participated in the data analysis and drafted this paper. Mi Hye Kim and Jongki Hong carried out the immunoassays and data analysis. Kyuseok Kim and Woong Mo Yang were the general supervisors for this research and participated in both the study design and critical revision of the paper and all agreed to accept equal responsibility for the accuracy of the content of the paper.

Acknowledgments

This work was supported by the National Research Foundation of Korea Grant funded by the Korean Government (NRF-2014R1A1A1005859).

References

[1] G. Yang, K. Lee, M.-H. Lee, S.-H. Kim, I.-H. Ham, and H.-Y. Choi, "Inhibitory effects of Chelidonium majus extract on atopic dermatitis-like skin lesions in NC/Nga mice," Journal of Ethnopharmacology, vol. 138, no. 2, pp. 398–403, 2011.

[2] D. Navi, J. Saegusa, and F. T. Liu, "Mast cells and immunological skin diseases," Clinical Reviews in Allergy & Immunology, vol. 33, no. 1-2, pp. 144–155, 2007.

[3] Y. Tomimori, Y. Tanaka, M. Goto, and Y. Fukuda, "Repeated topical challenge with chemical antigen elicits sustained dermatitis in NC/Nga mice in specific-pathogen-free condition," Journal of Investigative Dermatology, vol. 124, no. 1, pp. 119–124, 2005.

[4] B. S. Kim, J. K. Choi, H. J. Jung et al., "Effects of topical application of a recombinant staphylococcal enterotoxin A on DNCB and dust mite extract-induced atopic dermatitis-like lesions in a murine model," European Journal of Dermatology, vol. 24, no. 2, pp. 186–193, 2014.

[5] J. Del Rosso and S. F. Friedlander, "Corticosteroids: options in the era of steroid-sparing therapy," Journal of the American Academy of Dermatology, vol. 53, supplement 1, pp. S50–S58, 2005.

[6] M. Kawai, T. Hirano, S. Higa et al., "Flavonoids and related compounds as anti-allergic substances," Allergology International, vol. 56, no. 2, pp. 113–123, 2007.

[7] H. Kim, M. Kim, H. Kim, G. San Lee, W. G. An, and S. I. Cho, "Anti-inflammatory activities of Dictamnus dasycarpus Turcz., root bark on allergic contact dermatitis induced by dinitrofluorobenzene in mice," Journal of Ethnopharmacology, vol. 149, no. 2, pp. 471–477, 2013.

[8] K. Yamaura, M. Shimada, and K. Ueno, "Anthocyanins from bilberry (*Vaccinium myrtillus* L.) alleviate pruritus in a mouse model of chronic allergic contact dermatitis," *Pharmacognosy Research*, vol. 3, no. 3, pp. 173–177, 2011.

[9] K. Y. Z. Zheng, R. C. Y. Choi, H. Q. H. Xie et al., "The expression of erythropoietin triggered by danggui buxue tang, a Chinese herbal decoction prepared from radix Astragali and radix Angelicae Sinensis, is mediated by the hypoxia-inducible factor in cultured HEK293T cells," *Journal of Ethnopharmacology*, vol. 132, no. 1, pp. 259–267, 2010.

[10] M. Yang, G. C. F. Chan, R. Deng et al., "An herbal decoction of *Radix astragali* and *Radix angelicae* sinensis promotes hematopoiesis and thrombopoiesis," *Journal of Ethnopharmacology*, vol. 124, no. 1, pp. 87–97, 2009.

[11] Q. T. Gao, J. K. H. Cheung, J. Li et al., "A Chinese herbal decoction, Danggui Buxue Tang, activates extracellular signal-regulated kinase in cultured T-lymphocytes," *FEBS Letters*, vol. 581, no. 26, pp. 5087–5093, 2007.

[12] L.-W. Fang, C.-C. Cheng, T.-S. Hwang et al., "Danggui buxue tang inhibits 2,4-dinitrochlorobenzene: induced atopic dermatitis in mice," *Evidence-Based Complementary and Alternative Medicine*, vol. 2015, Article ID 672891, 10 pages, 2015.

[13] J. F. Lin, P. H. Liu, T. P. Huang et al., "Characteristics and prescription patterns of traditional Chinese medicine in atopic dermatitis patients: ten-year experiences at a Medical Center in Taiwan," *Complementary Therapies in Medicine*, vol. 22, no. 1, pp. 141–147, 2014.

[14] T. T. X. Dong, K. J. Zhao, Q. T. Gao et al., "Chemical and biological assessment of a Chinese herbal decoction containing *Radix astragali* and *Radix angelicae* sinensis: determination of drug ratio in having optimized properties," *Journal of Agricultural and Food Chemistry*, vol. 54, no. 7, pp. 2767–2774, 2006.

[15] Q. Gao, J. Li, J. K. H. Cheung et al., "Verification of the formulation and efficacy of Danggui Buxue Tang (a decoction of Radix Astragali and Radix Angelicae Sinensis): an exemplifying systematic approach to revealing the complexity of Chinese herbal medicine formulae," *Chinese Medicine*, vol. 2, article 12, 2007.

[16] Q. T. Gao, R. C. Y. Choi, A. W. H. Cheung et al., "Danggui buxue tang—a Chinese herbal decoction activates the phosphorylations of extracellular signal-regulated kinase and estrogen receptor α in cultured MCF-7 cells," *FEBS Letters*, vol. 581, no. 2, pp. 233–240, 2007.

[17] S. Wang, Y. Hu, W. Tan et al., "Compatibility art of traditional Chinese medicine: from the perspective of herb pairs," *Journal of Ethnopharmacology*, vol. 143, no. 2, pp. 412–423, 2012.

[18] J. H. Kim, M. H. Kim, G. Yang, Y. Huh, S. H. Kim, and W. M. Yang, "Effects of topical application of *Astragalus membranaceus* on allergic dermatitis," *Immunopharmacology and Immunotoxicology*, vol. 35, no. 1, pp. 151–156, 2012.

[19] M. H. Kim, Y. Y. Choi, I. H. Cho, J. Hong, S. H. Kim, and W. M. Yang, "*Angelica sinensis* induces hair regrowth via the inhibition of apoptosis signaling," *The American Journal of Chinese Medicine*, vol. 42, no. 4, pp. 1021–1034, 2014.

[20] Y.-Y. Sung, T. Yoon, J. Y. Jang, S.-J. Park, G.-H. Jeong, and H. K. Kim, "Inhibitory effects of Cinnamomum cassia extract on atopic dermatitis-like skin lesions induced by mite antigen in NC/Nga mice," *Journal of Ethnopharmacology*, vol. 133, no. 2, pp. 621–628, 2011.

[21] S. M. A. Hassan, A. J. Hussein, and A. K. Saeed, "Role of green tea in reducing epidermal thickness upon ultraviolet light-B injury in BALB/c mice," *Advances in Biology*, vol. 2015, Article ID 890632, 6 pages, 2015.

[22] Y. Y. Choi, M. H. Kim, J. Y. Lee, J. Hong, S.-H. Kim, and W. M. Yang, "Topical application of Kochia scoparia inhibits the development of contact dermatitis in mice," *Journal of Ethnopharmacology*, vol. 154, no. 2, pp. 380–385, 2014.

[23] K. Abe, K. Kobayashi, S. Yoshino, K. Taguchi, and H. Nojima, "Withdrawal of repeated morphine enhances histamine-induced scratching responses in mice," *Drug and Chemical Toxicology*, vol. 38, no. 2, pp. 167–173, 2014.

[24] L. S. Fonacier, S. C. Dreskin, and D. Y. Leung, "Allergic skin diseases," *Journal of Allergy and Clinical Immunology*, vol. 125, no. 2, supplement 2, pp. S138–S149, 2010.

[25] S.-L. Zhou, G.-H. Tan, F.-Y. Huang, H. Wang, Y.-Y. Lin, and S.-L. Chen, "Sanpao herbs inhibit development of atopic dermatitis in Balb/c mice," *Asian Pacific Journal of Allergy and Immunology*, vol. 32, no. 2, pp. 140–144, 2014.

[26] M. H. Kim, Y. Y. Choi, G. Yang, I.-H. Cho, D. Nam, and W. M. Yang, "Indirubin, a purple 3,2- bisindole, inhibited allergic contact dermatitis via regulating T helper (Th)-mediated immune system in DNCB-induced model," *Journal of Ethnopharmacology*, vol. 145, no. 1, pp. 214–219, 2013.

[27] J. Lee, YY. Choi, MH. Kim, JM. Han, JE. Lee, and EH. Kim, *Topical Application of Angelica sinensis Improves Pruritus and Skin Inflammation in Mice with Atopic Dermatitis-Like Symptoms. J Med Food*, doi, 10.1089/jmf.2015.3489, 2015.

[28] B. Kaminska, "MAPK signalling pathways as molecular targets for anti-inflammatory therapy—from molecular mechanisms to therapeutic benefits," *Biochimica et Biophysica Acta—Proteins and Proteomics*, vol. 1754, no. 1-2, pp. 253–262, 2005.

[29] S. R. Kim, K. S. Lee, S. J. Park, M. S. Jeon, and Y. C. Lee, "Inhibition of p38 MAPK reduces expression of vascular endothelial growth factor in allergic airway disease," *Journal of Clinical Immunology*, vol. 32, no. 3, pp. 574–586, 2012.

9

Inductive Effect of Palmatine on Apoptosis in RAW 264.7 Cells

Shintaro Ishikawa, Misako Tamaki, Yui Ogawa, Kiyomi Kaneki, Meng Zhang, Masataka Sunagawa, and Tadashi Hisamitsu

Department of Physiology, School of Medicine, Showa University, 1-5-8 Hatanodai, Shinagawa-ku, Tokyo 142-8555, Japan

Correspondence should be addressed to Shintaro Ishikawa; s-ishikawa@med.showa-u.ac.jp

Academic Editor: Yibin Feng

Osteoporosis is a serious public health problem characterized by low bone density and deterioration of the bone microarchitecture. Current treatment options target either osteoclast resorption or osteoblast formation. It has been reported that berberine, a close structural analog of palmatine, inhibited bone loss in an osteoporosis model. In this study, osseous metabolism was observed *in vitro* with osteoclast bone resorbing cells. We proved that mouse preosteoclastic cell line (RAW 264.7) has a higher sensitivity to palmatine than mouse osteoblastic cell line (MC3T3-E1); the cell survival rates significantly decreased at 40 μM palmatine. The NO_2^- level, a metabolic product of nitric monoxide (NO), and iNOS mRNA expression, an osteoclast with NO induced enzyme, also increased with higher dosage of palmatine. Furthermore, it was recognized that the cell viability decrease from palmatine was caused by apoptosis rather than necrosis. Additionally, osteoclast apoptosis from palmatine did not occur when iNOS was inhibited with N^G-nitro-L-arginine methyl ester hydrochloride (pan NOS inhibitor). These results indicate that palmatine plays an important role in osteoclast apoptosis via the NOS system. Hence, palmatine could be considered as a viable pharmaceutical candidate for osteoporosis bone resorption inhibitor.

1. Introduction

Osteoporosis is a serious public health problem characterized by low bone density and deterioration of the bone microarchitecture. It results in a loss of bone strength and fractures. Nevertheless, bone is an active tissue that continues to remodel via bone formation and resorption. These two counteracting processes are strongly connected and firmly regulated to maintain skeletal homeostasis [1]. In other words, osseous metabolism depends on dual cell processes, osteoclasts and osteoblasts, diffcrentiated bone resorbing cells derived from hematopoietic cells of monocyte-macrophage lineage, and bone forming cells of mesenchymal origin, respectively. Bone diseases frequently occur because of differentiation aberration or proliferation activity in the osteoclast and osteoblast. Current treatments for osteoporosis target either the osteoclast by inhibiting bone resorption (antiresorptive agents) or the osteoblast by stimulating bone formation (osteoanabolic agents).

Bone resorption of postmenopausal women progresses approximately two times faster than bone formation [2].

The possibility of suffering a fracture increases in women with decreased bone quantity, even if osteoporosis is in its early stages [3]. When bone quantity decreases (early stage), a physician may give advice on lifestyle improvement to the patient (e.g., diet and exercise). As osteoporosis progresses, pharmacotherapy, which inhibits bone resorption, will be an important treatment option. The first choice is usually bisphosphonate or raloxifene. An estrogenic pharmaceutical is chosen when patients have menopausal syndrome. However, careful medication selection will be crucial because of its possible side effects.

Palmatine is a quaternary protoberberine alkaloid. It is typically yellow in color and is an active constituent in a number of plants, such as *Rhizoma Coptidis* [4]. Alkaloids have been used in the treatment of jaundice, dysentery, hypertension, inflammation, and liver-related diseases [5]. It was previously reported that berberine, an isoquinoline alkaloid, which is a close structural analog of palmatine, inhibited bone loss in an osteoporosis model [6].

Our findings showed evidence that palmatine regulated osteoclast activity by secretion of cytokines of osteoblasts [7], but we did not discuss palmatine's influence on osteoclast-induced bone resorption. Because the effect of resorption could prevent osteoclast activity or directly inhibit osteoclasts, we investigated the influence of palmatine on osteoclast differentiation and function.

2. Materials and Methods

2.1. Reagents and Cell Culture. Palmatine chloride (Wako Pure Chemical Industries, Ltd., Tokyo, Japan) was used in the present study. Palmatine was dissolved in a culture medium in *in vitro* experiments. The culture medium used was Dulbecco's modified eagle medium (DMEM; Sigma-Aldrich Corporation, St. Louis, MO, USA) or alpha modified eagle minimum essential medium (α-MEM; Sigma-Aldrich Co.) supplemented with 10% heat-inactivated fetal calf serum (FCS; Nihon Bio-Supply Center, Tokyo, Japan) and a penicillin-streptomycin-neomycin (PSN) antibiotic mixture (5 mg each of penicillin and streptomycin and 10 mg of neomycin/mL, GIBCO 15640, Life Technologies, Inc.), sterilized with 0.2 μm pore filters, and stored at 4°C until its use. The mouse osteoblastic cell line MC3T3-E1 (DS Pharma Biomedical Co., Ltd., Osaka, Japan) was routinely cultured at 37°C in a humidified atmosphere of 5% CO_2 and maintained in α-MEM-FCS-PSN. The transformed murine monocytic cell line RAW 264.7 (DS Pharma Biomedical Co., Ltd.) was routinely cultured at 37°C in a humidified atmosphere of 5% CO_2 and maintained in DMEM-FCS-PSN. N^G-Nitro-L-arginine methyl ester hydrochloride (L-NAME) was obtained from Dojindo Laboratories, Kumamoto, Japan.

2.2. Cell Viability in Cytotoxicity CCK-8 Assays. Cell viability was measured using the cell counting kit-8 (CCK-8; Dojindo, Kumamoto, Japan) [8]. The cells were seeded in a 96-well flat-bottomed microplate (5×10^3 cells/well) and cultured in 100 μL of growth medium at 37°C and 5% CO_2 for 24 h or 5 days. The cell culture medium in each well was then replaced with 100 μL of cell growth medium containing palmatine at the following concentrations: 1, 5, 10, 40, and 100 μM [9, 10]. Additionally, L-NAME (10, 100, and 1000 μM) dissolved in PBS [11] was added. After incubation for 24 h or 5 days at 37°C, the cells were washed with PBS 3 times. Then, 10 μL of CCK-8 dye and 100 μL of α-MEM cell culture medium were added to each well, and cells were incubated for another 1 h at 37°C. Cell viability (%) was calculated using the following formula:

$$\text{Cell viability (\%)} = \frac{\left[OD_{\text{experimental sample}} - OD_{\text{blank}}\right]}{\left[OD_{\text{control}} - OD_{\text{blank}}\right]} \times 100\%.$$

(1)

$OD_{\text{experimental sample}}$ refers to the absorbance of a well with treated cells and CCK-8. OD_{blank} refers to the absorbance of a well with medium and CCK-8 but without cells. OD_{control} refers to the absorbance of a well with untreated cells and CCK-8 [7, 8]. The absorbance at 450 nm was measured by a microplate reader (Multiskan™ GO instrument; Thermo Fisher Scientific Inc., Waltham, MA, USA), and the results are presented as mean ± SD from triplicate wells.

2.3. Establishment of a Coculture System for Bone Resorption. It has been known that osteoblasts and osteoclasts interact in bone tissue [12]. Therefore, we observed the influence of palmatine for osteoblast and osteoclast crosstalk under a coculture in an *in vitro* system.

A novel coculture system was established using Transwell inserts (Corning Incorporated Number 3450, NY, USA) [12]. Osteoclast bone resorption activity was assessed using a bone resorption assay kit 24 (PG Research, Tokyo, Japan), under the same culture conditions as described above [13]. The bottom of the inserts was composed of polyester materials with a pore size of 0.4 μm, which only permits the passage of small, soluble factors. RAW 264.7 cells, a mouse preosteoclastic cell line, were embedded at a density of 5×10^5 cells/cm^2 in the lower compartment, bone resorption assay plate, of each insert. MC3T3-E1 cells, a monoclonal preosteoblastic cell line, were incubated at a density of 5×10^4 cells/cm^2 in the upper compartment of the inserts. After each cell was cultured for 24 h, the Transwell inserts with MC3T3-E1 cells were combined together in the bone resorption assay plate with RAW 264.7 cells. This coculture system was maintained in DMEM-FCS-PSN and supplemented with different concentrations of palmatine in 5% CO_2 at 37°C. After coculturing for 5 days, the sequential experiments were performed.

2.4. Quantification of Osteoclastic Activity: Biomimetic Calcium Phosphate Assay and Resorption Pit Assay. The cocultured cells were incubated on bone resorption assay plates and fluorescein-labeled CaP-coated 24-well plates without medium change under the light-shielded condition. After 5 days, 100 μL of the cell culture supernatant was transferred into a 96-well plate for fluorescence measurement, mixed with 50 μL of bone resorption assay buffer added to each well, and then mixed using a plate shaker. The fluorescence intensity, fluoresceinamine-labeled chondroitin sulfate, was measured using a fluorescence plate reader (Twinkle LB970, Berthold Japan, Tokyo, Japan) with excitation and emission wavelengths of 485 and 535 nm. The remaining plates were washed with PBS and treated with 5% sodium hypochlorite for 5 min. After washing the plates with tap water and drying them, five different regions in each well were photographed by microscopy (Olympus Co.) and the pit areas were measured with ImageJ software v. 1.48 (NIH, USA) [14].

2.5. Coculture for Tartrate-Resistant Acid Phosphatase (TRAP) Stain. RAW 264.7 cells and MC3T3-E1 cells were mixed at a rate of 5×10^4 cells and disseminated in the 24-well plate (IWAKI 3820-024; Asahi Glass Co., Ltd., Tokyo, Japan). This coculture system was maintained in DMEM-FCS-PSN and supplemented with different concentrations of palmatine in 5% CO_2 at 37°C. After coculturing for 5 days, the sequential experiments were performed. To confirm the generation of multinucleated osteoclast-like cells, the cultured RAW 264.7 cells were stained with TRAP (TRAP/ALP stain kit, Wako Pure), according to the manufacturer's instructions. TRAP-positive multinucleated (3 or more nuclei) osteoclasts were visualized by light microscopy and photographed. The number of mature osteoclasts, multinucleated RAW 264.7

cell, per a field (quadrangle of 2 mm × 2.5 mm) was counted to quantify the influence of palmatine [15, 16]. Each osteoclast formation assay was performed at least 3 times.

2.6. Apoptosis Detection. RAW 264.7 cells were plated in 24-well tissue culture plates at a cell density of 1×10^5 cells per well. After 24 h, the medium was replaced with medium containing the palmatine compounds. All treatments were performed in triplicate. The cells were treated for 24 h, after which they were harvested and the extent of apoptosis was assessed using the APOPercentage™ assay (Biocolor Ltd., Newtownabbey, Northern Ireland, UK) as previously described [17]. Briefly, the cells were removed by trypsinization, washed with PBS, and stained with APOPercentage dye for 30 min at 37°C. The dye uptake was quantified by the colorimetric method based on the manufacturer's instructions. The cells were lysed with the dye release reagent of attachment, and the absorbance was measured at 550 nm using a Multiskan GO instrument.

2.7. Detection of Supernatant Nitric Monoxide Level. The amount of nitrite/nitrate in the supernatant produced by RAW 264.7 cells was measured using an NO_2/NO_3 assay kit FX (NK08; Dojindo Laboratories, Kumamoto, Japan), based on manufacturer's instructions. The cells were seeded in a 24-well flat-bottomed microplate (1×10^5 cells/well) and cultured in 1000 μL of DMEM-FCS-PSN medium at 37°C and 5% CO_2 for 24 h. The cell culture medium in each well was then replaced with 1000 μL of cell growth medium containing palmatine at the following concentrations: 1, 5, 10, 40, and 100 μM [9, 10]. Then, L-NAME (10, 100, and 1000 μM), dissolved in PBS [11], was added. After incubation for 2 h, 4 h, or 5 days at 37°C, 80 μL of the supernatant was transferred to an empty 96-well plate, 2,3-diaminonaphthalene reagents of attachment were added to each well, and the plate was incubated. Fluorescence intensity was measured using a Twinkle LB970, with excitation and emission wavelengths of 355 and 450 nm.

2.8. PCR Primers and Reagent Kits. The reagents used for mRNA isolation (TaqMan Gene Expression Cells-to-CT™) and real-time reverse transcription-polymerase chain reaction (RT-PCR; TaqMan Gene Expression Assays) were purchased from Applied Biosystems (Foster City, CA, USA). Assays were conducted according to the manufacturer's instructions [18]. For RT-PCR comparison of gene expression, we selected *iNOS* (NOS2: TaqMan Gene Expression Assays; Assay ID: Mm00440502_m1). The 18S ribosomal RNA (Mm18s: TaqMan Gene Expression Assays; Assay ID: Mm03928990_g1) was used as a housekeeping gene to normalize RNA loading.

2.9. mRNA Isolation and Quantitative RT-PCR. After incubation for 2 h at 37°C, total RNA was isolated from RAW 264.7 cells using 50 μL of a lysis solution (P/N4383583). Each sample of total RNA was subjected to RT using a 20 × RT enzyme mix (P/N 4383585) and a 2 × RT buffer (P/N43833586) with a T100 thermal cycler (Bio-Rad Co., Hercules, CA, USA).

After RT reaction, the cDNA templates were amplified by PCR using TaqMan Gene Expression Assays, PCR primers, and RT master mix (P/N 4369016). Predesigned and validated gene-specific TaqMan Gene Expression Assays [17–19] were duplicated for quantitative RT-PCR, based on manufacturer's protocol. PCR assays were conducted as follows: 10 mins of denaturation at 95°C, 40 cycles of 15 s, denaturation at 95°C, and 1 min annealing and extension at 60°C. Samples were analyzed using an ABI Prism 7900HT Fast RT-PCR System (Applied Biosystems) [19, 20]. Relative quantification (RQ) studies [21] were prepared from collected data (threshold cycle numbers (Ct)) with ABI Prism 7900HT Sequence-Detection System (SDS) software v. 2.3 (Applied Biosystem).

2.10. Statistical Analysis. Data is expressed as means ± SD. All assays were repeated 3 times to ensure reproducibility. Statistical significance between the control and experimental groups was analyzed by one-way analysis of variance followed by Scheffé test. Probability (p) value < 0.05 was considered statistically significant.

3. Results

3.1. TRAP-Positive Cell Detection on Coculture. It is known that RAW 264.7 cells differentiate into osteoclastic cells over days in culture [22]. Therefore, RAW 264.7 cells' differentiation to osteoclast was examined by TRAP staining in culture of RAW 264.7 cells and MC3T3-E1 cells. As shown in Figure 1, RAW 264.7 cell fusion began and multinucleated giant cells developed in the control group on culture day 5. The multinuclear osteoclast per a field (quadrangle of 2 mm × 2.5 mm) decreased according to palmatine's dosage (Figure 1(m)).

3.2. Cell Viability for Palmatine with Cytotoxicity CCK-8 Assays. The proliferation of cells cultured with different palmatine concentrations was evaluated using the CCK-8 assay. Five days of palmatine treatment even at high dosage of 100 μM (Figure 2(a)) did not change the MC3T3-E1 cell survival rates. However, at concentration >5 μM (Figure 2(b)), RAW 264.7 cell survival rate significantly decreased.

Palmatine treatment of 24 h at concentration >40 μM (Figure 2(c)) significantly decreased the RAW 264.7 cell survival rate. Furthermore, the survival rate of the osteoclast-like differentiated mature RAW 264.7 cells, which were cocultured with MC3T3-E1, was not affected even by the high dosage of 100 μM palmatine (Figure 2(d)).

3.3. Apoptosis Detection with APOPercentage Assay. An apoptosis assay was carried out to confirm whether the cellular extinction by palmatine depends on necrosis or apoptosis. The pigmentary absorbance which was extracted from the apoptosis cell was measured. As shown in Figure 3, palmatine treatment for 24 h at concentration >10 μM significantly increased RAW 264.7 cell apoptosis rate.

3.4. Supernatant NO_2^- Level Detection. An experiment was performed to determine whether palmatine affected nitrous

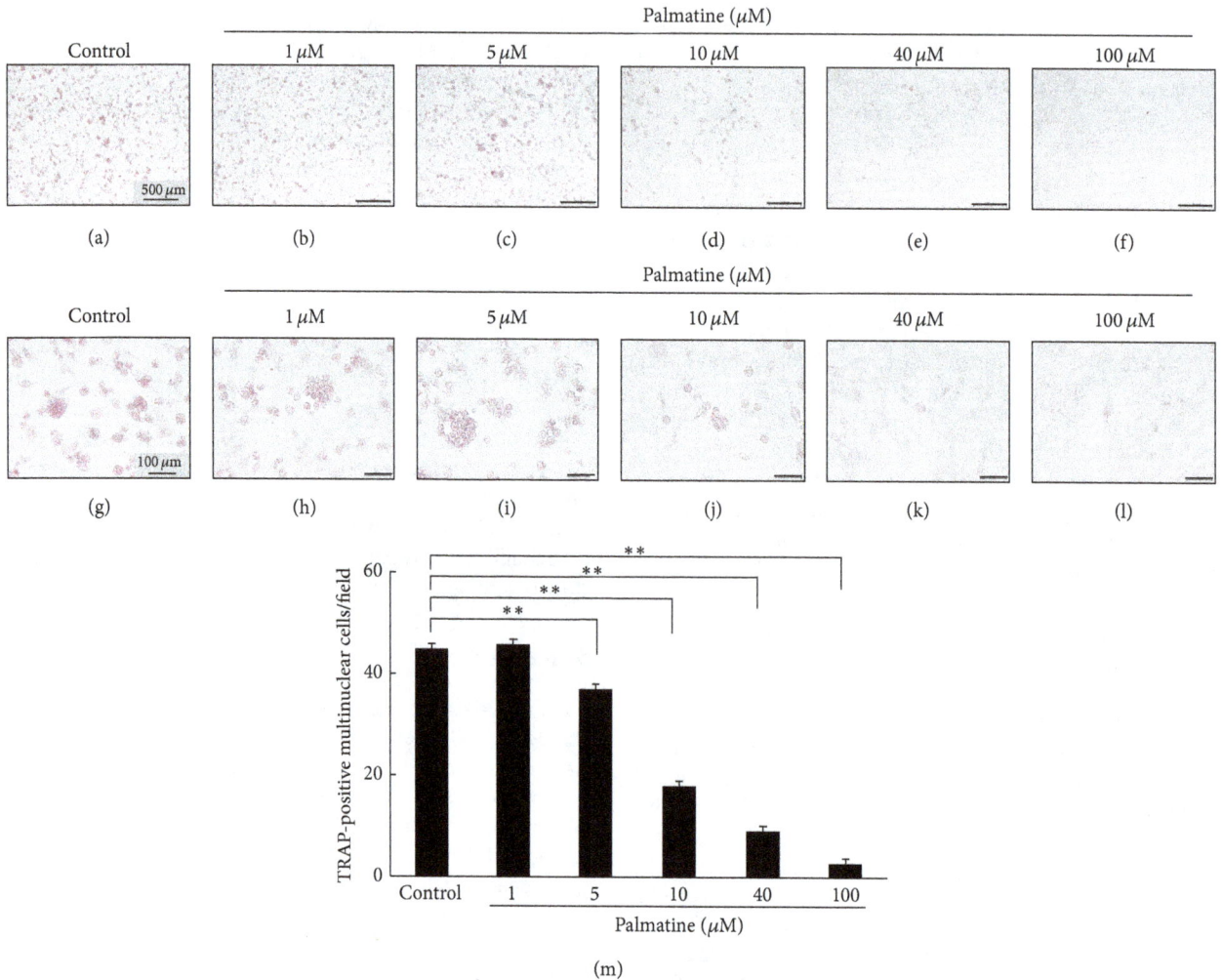

FIGURE 1: TRAP-positive cell detection with the coculture method. The differentiation to osteoclast of a RAW 264.7 cell was examined using TRAP staining in culture of a RAW 264.7 cell and an MC3T3-E1 cell for 5 days. Digital images were obtained using an optical microscope. RAW 264.7 cells, which were dyed using TRAP in the cell block section, show differentiation of a RAW 264.7 cell, cytogamy image. (a)–(f) ×100 magnification, (g)–(l) ×600 magnification. (m) The number of mature osteoclasts, multinucleated RAW 264.7 cell, per a field (quadrangle of 2 mm × 2.5 mm) was counted to quantify influence of palmatine. Asterisks indicate statistically significant differences ($^{**}p < 0.01$). Error bars denote ±SD.

acid ion (NO_2^-) production in RAW 264.7 cells using the NO_2/NO_3 assay kit FX. As shown in Figure 4, palmatine treatment of 2 h at high concentration 100 μM significantly increased the NO production in RAW 264.7 cells. Furthermore, a treatment of 4 h significantly increased the NO production in accordance with palmatine concentration.

3.5. iNOS mRNA Appearance in RAW 264.7 Cell. The next experiment examined whether addition of palmatine could change iNOS mRNA expression in RAW 264.7 cells using RT-PCR method. The proliferation of cells cultured with different palmatine dosages was examined using the CCK-8 assay. As shown in Figure 5, palmatine treatment of 2 h at concentration >10 μM significantly increased the iNOS mRNA expression in RAW 264.7 cells.

3.6. Cell Viability and Supernatant NO_2^- Level Detection for L-NAME Treatment. In order to assess whether NO affects the survival of RAW 264.7 cells, L-NAME was added. Firstly, to clarify the direct effect of L-NAME on the survival of RAW 264.7 cells, they were both cocultured for 5 days. Then the cell's condition of the controlled group and NO_2^- level were examined. The result was that the NO_2^- level decreased significantly, by 100 μM. The survival rate of the cells did not have significant difference in each of the concentrations. Therefore, the optimum concentration level of L-NAME, which has no cytotoxic effects and inhibits NO secretion, was set at 100 μM. L-NAME was dissolved in PBS and added to the culture medium (final concentration: 100 μM). The proliferation of cells cultured with different palmatine concentrations level was evaluated using the CCK-8 assay. As shown in Figure 6(c), L-NAME treatment of 24 h did not

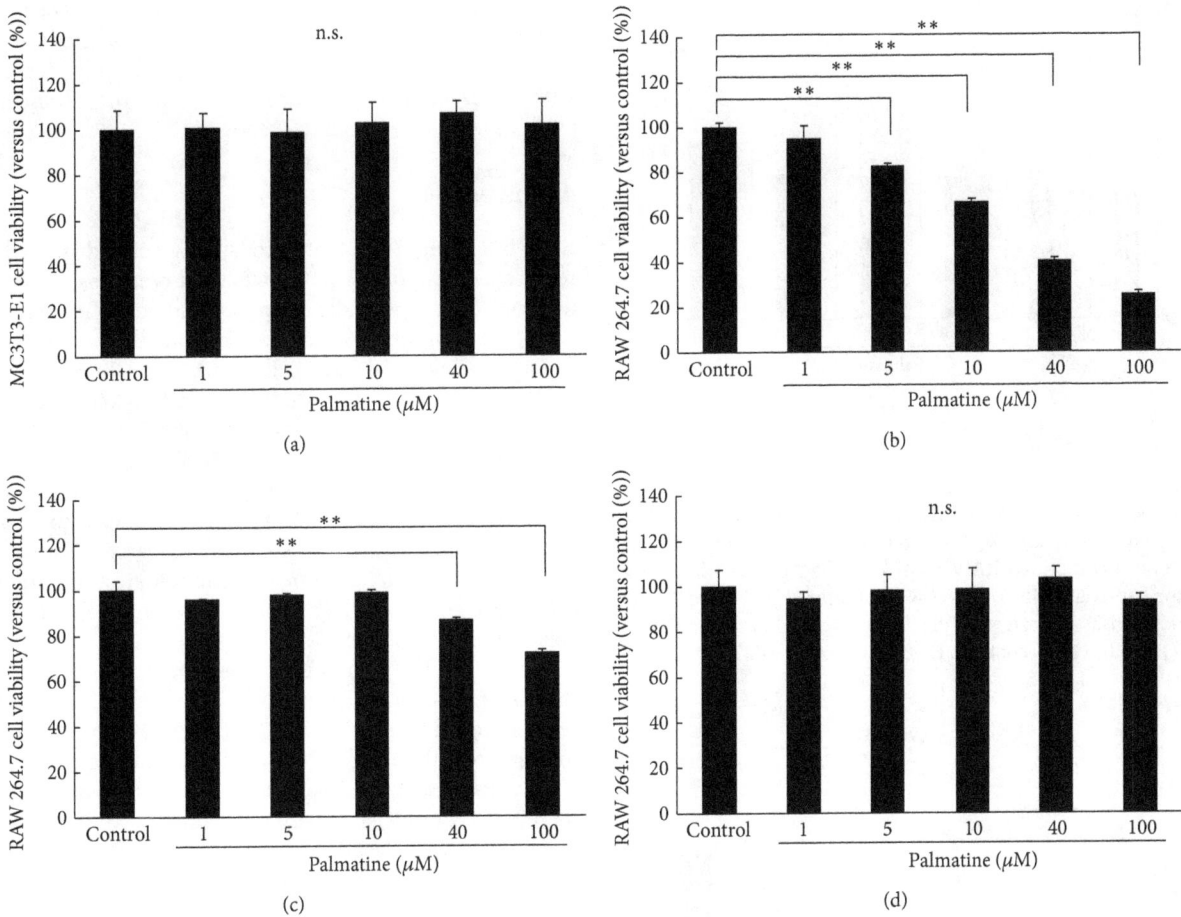

FIGURE 2: Cell viability for palmatine with cytotoxicity CCK-8 assays. The proliferation of cells cultured with different palmatine concentrations for 24 h or 5 days was evaluated using a CCK-8 assay. Seeded cells were incubated with or without palmatine for 24 h or 5 days. The cell viability was calculated using the following formula: cell viability (%) = $[OD_{experiment} - OD_{blank}]/[OD_{control} - OD_{blank}] \times 100\%$. The absorbance was measured at 450 nm. (a) The survival rate of MC3T3-E1 cells that were incubated in palmatine component medium for 5 days. (b) The survival rate of RAW 264.7 cells that were incubated in palmatine component medium for 5 days. (c) The survival rate of RAW 264.7 cells that were incubated in palmatine component medium for 24 h. (d) The survival rate of mature RAW 264.7 cells that were incubated in palmatine component medium for 5 days. Asterisks indicate statistically significant differences ($^{**}p < 0.01$, n.s., no significant difference). Error bars denote $\pm$ SD.

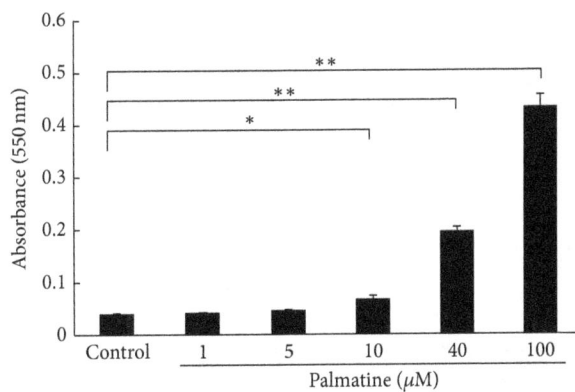

FIGURE 3: Apoptosis detection with an APOPercentage assay. The cell apoptotic rate was measured using an APOPercentage assay after the seeded cells were incubated with each palmatine concentration for 24 h. The absorbance at 550 nm was measured. Asterisks indicate statistically significant differences ($^{*}p < 0.05$, $^{**}p < 0.01$). Error bars denote $\pm$ SD.

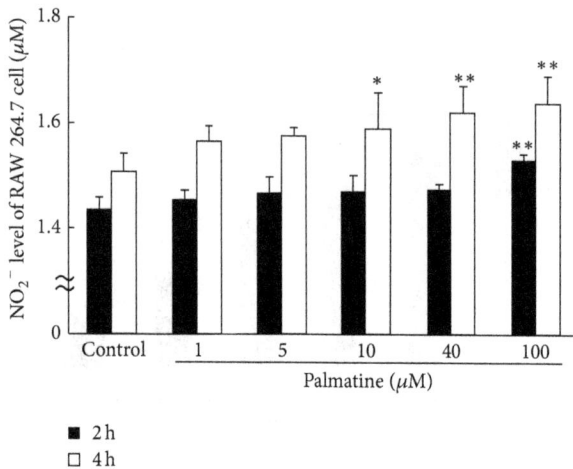

FIGURE 4: Supernatant NO_2^- level as a surrogate for NO. Nitrous acid ion (NO_2^-) production in RAW 264.7 cells was measured using the NO_2/NO_3 assay kit FX. The black bars show the supernatant NO_2^- level that cultured RAW 264.7 cells for 2 h. The white bars show the supernatant NO_2^- level which cultured RAW 264.7 cells for 4 h. Asterisks indicate statistically significant differences ($^*p < 0.05$, $^{**}p < 0.01$ versus control). Error bars denote $\pm$ SD.

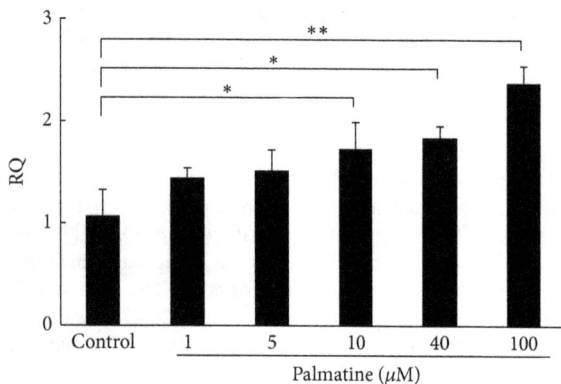

FIGURE 5: Relative quantity (RQ) of iNOS mRNA expression in RAW 264.7 cells. The experiment was conducted to examine whether addition of palmatine would change the iNOS mRNA expression in RAW 264.7 cells. After culture for 2 h, RAW 264.7 cells were collected and used for the measurement of iNOS mRNA expression by RT-PCR. Asterisks indicate statistically significant differences ($^*p < 0.05$, $^{**}p < 0.01$). Error bars denote $\pm$ SD.

change RAW 264.7 cell survival rates at any concentrations level.

3.7. Bone Resorption Evaluation on Coculture. Bone resorption ability of RAW 264.7 cells was examined using a bone resorption assay kit in the culture of RAW 264.7 and MC3T3-E1 cells. Bone resorption activity was evaluated by measuring the pit formation on a CaP-coated plate and the fluorescence intensity of the conditioned medium. The microscopic photographs (Figures 7(a)–7(l)) and the total pit

area (Figure 7(m)) indicated that the pit formation decreased with increasing palmatine dosage. The fluorescence intensity of the conditioned medium also significantly decreased with increasing palmatine dosage (Figure 7(n)). These assay evaluations showed a similar tendency.

4. Discussion

Bone is a living tissue that is constantly being degraded and replaced. Osteoporosis occurs when the creation of new bone does not keep up with the removal of old bone. In the current study, we examined the influence of palmatine on osteoclast function using RAW 264.7 cells and MC3T3-E1 cells *in vitro*.

The first part of this study was undertaken to examine the effects of palmatine on the differentiation on RAW 264.7 cells. Results of a coculture with MC3T3-E1, osteoblast-like cell, and RAW 264.7, osteoclast-like cell, and the osteoclast differentiation on TRAP staining were inhibited by palmatine dosage (Figure 1). The preliminary research showed that palmatine affected the bone immunological function in osteoblast and osteoclast. However, palmatine's effects on osteoclasts were not concluded.

Therefore, the second experiment in this study examined the direct influence of palmatine on osteoclast survival. Our results proved that RAW 264.7 cells have a higher sensitivity to palmatine than MC3T3-E1 cells. The survival rate significantly decreased as palmatine's dosage and exposure period increased (Figure 2). Furthermore, palmatine did not alter the cocultured, osteoclast differentiated mature RAW 264.7 cell. In other words, the result indicated that palmatine may be related to primary osteoclast differentiation or proapoptotic activity. Additionally, an apoptosis assay was carried out to confirm whether the cellular extinction from palmatine depends on necrosis or apoptosis. Apoptosis is a multistage process in which activity of caspase enzymes fluctuates, DNA becomes fragmented, and phosphatidyl serine is transferred to the exterior surface of the cell membrane [23]. Such transfer and exposure of phosphatidyl serine are linked to the onset of apoptosis. Necrotic cells are not involved in this transfer. Therefore, the degree of apoptosis was determined by this phosphatidyl serine transmembrane movement. We identified that the decrease in dosage of palmatine reduces RAW 264.7 cells and thereby induces apoptosis, rather than necrosis. Additionally, apoptosis increases according to the dosage of palmatine in a concentration-dependent manner (Figure 3). Further, it has been known that nitric oxide induces apoptosis in various cells lines. Simultaneously, activating the NO/cGMP signaling pathway, including NO, prevents apoptosis induced by diverse stimuli [24]. Even if higher density was applied to the MC3T3-E1 cells, apoptosis did not occur [7]. Thus, experimenting over a range of densities with palmatine may activate the NO/cGMP signal in the MC3T3-E1 cells.

The purpose of the third experiment was to find the factor that induced osteoclast apoptosis. Some researchers previously reported that NO was the important factor which induced osteoclast apoptosis [25–27]. The mechanism that NO induces apoptosis in a macrophage-like cell is related to the release of cytochrome c from mitochondria, increase in

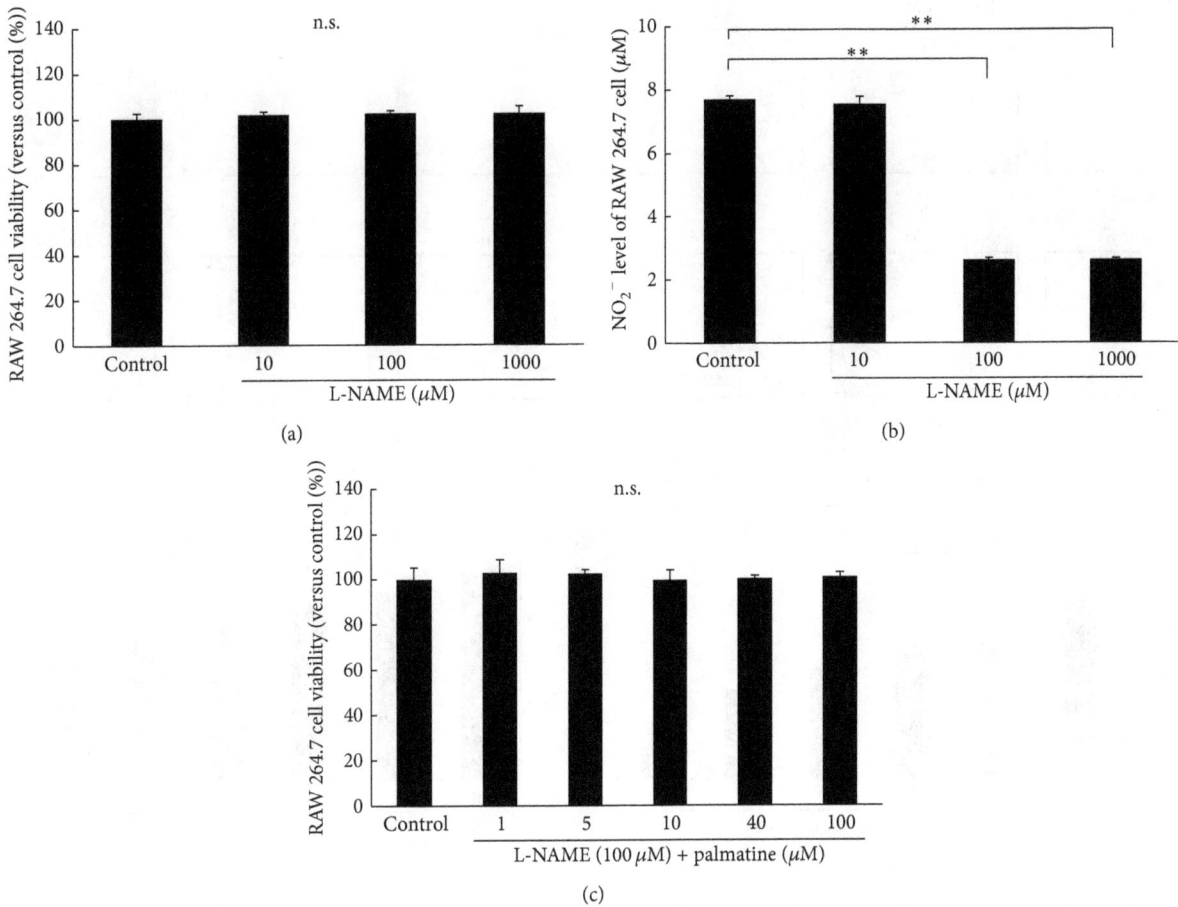

(a)

(b)

(c)

FIGURE 6: Cell viability and supernatant NO_2^- level detection for L-NAME treatment. NO release was inhibited by the addition of L-NAME to clarify whether NO affects the survival of RAW 264.7 cells. ((a) and (b)) The cell survival rate after culture and NO_2^- level were examined to clarify the direct influence of L-NAME on RAW 264.7 cells after 5 days in culture medium containing L-NAME. (c) The proliferation of cells cultured with different palmatine concentrations for 24 h was evaluated using a CCK-8 assay. The cell viability was calculated using the following formula: cell viability (%) = $[OD_{experiment} - OD_{blank}]/[OD_{control} - OD_{blank}] \times 100\%$. Absorbance was measured at 450 nm. Nitrous acid ion (NO_2^-) production in RAW 264.7 cells was measured using the NO_2/NO_3 assay kit FX. Asterisks indicate statistically significant differences ($^{**}p < 0.01$, n.s., no significant difference). Error bars denote ± SD.

the expression of the tumor suppressor p53, and accumulation of proapoptotic factors (e.g., the Bcl-2 family) [28]. Therefore, we investigated the relationship of palmatine and NO. The level of NO_2^-, a metabolic product of NO, was measured since half-life of NO is very short (3–6 s). NO in the culture supernatant increased as palmatine concentrations increased (Figure 4). Furthermore, the iNOS mRNA expression, which was an NO induced enzyme in osteoclast, also increased as palmatine concentrations increased (Figure 5). Additionally, osteoclast apoptosis from palmatine did not occur when iNOS was previously inhibited with L-NAME (pan NOS inhibitor/Figure 6). Furthermore, as palmatine dosage increased, bone resorption decreased (Figure 7). These results suggest that palmatine inhibits bone resorption and osteoclast formation, which supports our preliminary research [7]. It has also been reported that NO inhibits osteoclast differentiation [29] and bone resorption [30]. Hence, palmatine not only induces osteoclast apoptosis but also may inhibit osteoclast activities.

These results provide the first evidence that palmatine plays an important role in osteoclast apoptosis via the NOS system in osteoclasts. Thus, palmatine could be considered as a viable pharmaceutical candidate for osteoporosis bone resorption inhibitor. NO has been reported to be a mediator of bone turnover that has biphasic effects on regulating osteoblast survival and death [31]. NO may affect normal bone resorption by osteoclasts. Additionally, RAW 264.7 is a leukemic cell line. The apoptotic reactions of cancer cell lines to drug treatment may be different from normal monocytic cells. Therefore, we believe that palmatine's examination under varied conditions and on the nuclear intrinsic factor of normal osteoclasts would be necessary, as long as the role of NO on osteoclast activity is yet to be determined.

Competing Interests

The authors declare that they have no competing interests.

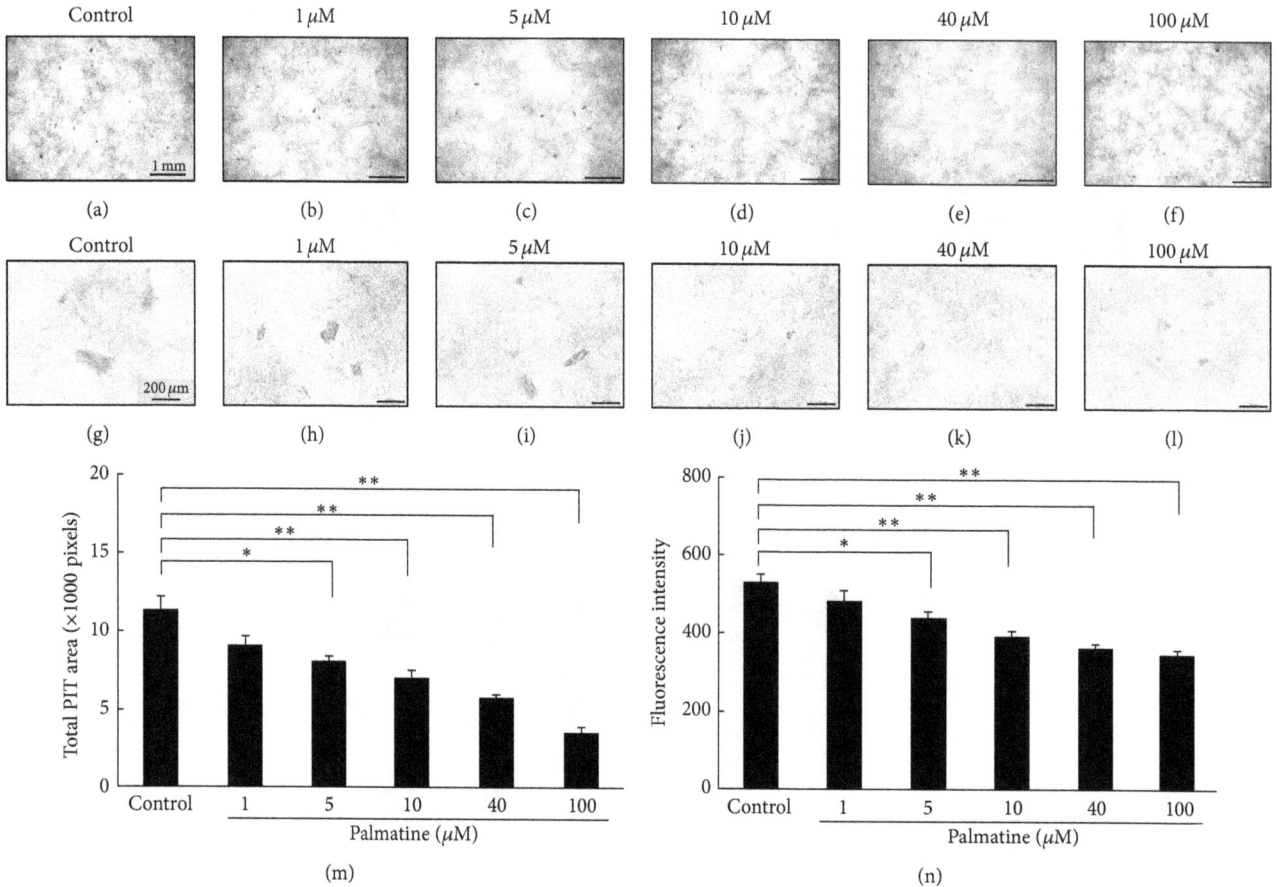

FIGURE 7: Bone resorption evaluation with a CaP-coated plate. Bone resorption ability of a RAW 264.7 cell examined using a bone resorption assay kit in culture of a RAW 264.7 cell and an MC3T3-E1 cell for 5 days. The bone resorption activity was evaluated by measuring the pit formation on a CaP-coated plate and the fluorescence intensity of the conditioned medium. (a)–(l) Digital images of pit formation on a CaP-coated plate were obtained using an optical microscope. The brown pit shows the locus where a mature RAW 264.7 cell (differentiation like osteoclast) dissolved a calcium plate. (a)–(f): ×40 magnification, (g)–(l): ×400 magnification. (m) The total pit area on a CaP-coated plate. (n) The fluorescence intensity of bone resorption dependence in the conditioned medium. Asterisks indicate statistically significant differences ($^*p < 0.05$, $^{**}p < 0.01$). Error bars denote ± SD.

Authors' Contributions

Shintaro Ishikawa and Tadashi Hisamitsu created the study design and helped draft the paper. Misako Tamaki, Yui Ogawa, Kiyomi Kaneki, Meng Zhang, Masataka Sunagawa, and Shintaro Ishikawa were responsible for data acquisition. Shintaro Ishikawa performed all statistical analysis and interpretation of the data. All authors have read and approved the paper.

References

[1] R. Tamma and A. Zallone, "Osteoblast and osteoclast crosstalks: from OAF to Ephrin," *Inflammation & Allergy-Drug Targets*, vol. 11, no. 3, pp. 196–200, 2012.

[2] M. S. Nanes and C. B. Kallen, "Osteoporosis," *Seminars in Nuclear Medicine*, vol. 44, no. 6, pp. 439–450, 2014.

[3] E. S. Siris, Y.-T. Chen, T. A. Abbott et al., "Bone mineral density thresholds for pharmacological intervention to prevent fractures," *Archives of Internal Medicine*, vol. 164, no. 10, pp. 1108–1112, 2004.

[4] H. A. Jung, B.-S. Min, T. Yokozawa, J.-H. Lee, Y. S. Kim, and J. S. Choi, "Anti-Alzheimer and antioxidant activities of coptidis rhizoma alkaloids," *Biological and Pharmaceutical Bulletin*, vol. 32, no. 8, pp. 1433–1438, 2009.

[5] L. Zhang, J. Li, F. Ma et al., "Synthesis and cytotoxicity evaluation of 13-n-alkyl berberine and palmatine analogues as anticancer agents," *Molecules*, vol. 17, no. 10, pp. 11294–11302, 2012.

[6] H. Chen, S. Emura, H. Isono, and S. Shoumura, "Effects of traditional Chinese medicine on bone loss in SAMP6: a murine model for senile osteoporosis," *Biological & Pharmaceutical Bulletin*, vol. 28, no. 5, pp. 865–869, 2005.

[7] S. Ishikawa, Y. Ogawa, M. Tamaki et al., "Influence of palmatine on bone metabolism in ovariectomized mice and cytokine secretion of osteoblasts," *In Vivo*, vol. 29, no. 6, pp. 671–677, 2015.

[8] C. Zhihong, L. Yezhen, G. Zhiyuan et al., "Comparison of the cytogenotoxicity induced by five different dental alloys using

four in vitro assays," *Dental Materials Journal*, vol. 30, no. 6, pp. 861–868, 2011.

[9] D. Dhingra and A. Bhankher, "Behavioral and biochemical evidences for antidepressant-like activity of palmatine in mice subjected to chronic unpredictable mild stress," *Pharmacological Reports*, vol. 66, no. 1, pp. 1–9, 2014.

[10] H. Ali and S. Dixit, "Extraction optimization of *Tinospora cordifolia* and assessment of the anticancer activity of its alkaloid palmatine," *The Scientific World Journal*, vol. 2013, Article ID 376216, 10 pages, 2013.

[11] K. Shibata, Y. Yoshimura, T. Kikuiri et al., "Effect of the release from mechanical stress on osteoclastogenesis in RAW264.7 cells," *International Journal of Molecular Medicine*, vol. 28, no. 1, pp. 73–79, 2011.

[12] X. Zhang, J. Li, Z. Wan et al., "Osteoblasts subjected to mechanical strain inhibit osteoclastic differentiation and bone resorption in a Co-culture system," *Annals of Biomedical Engineering*, vol. 41, no. 10, pp. 2056–2066, 2013.

[13] C.-H. Kuo, K.-F. Chen, S.-H. Chou et al., "Lung tumor-associated dendritic cell-derived resistin promoted cancer progression by increasing wolf-hirschhorn syndrome candidate 1/twist pathway," *Carcinogenesis*, vol. 34, no. 11, pp. 2600–2609, 2013.

[14] T. Hayakawa, Y. Yoshimura, T. Kikuiri et al., "Optimal compressive force accelerates osteoclastogenesis in RAW264.7 cells," *Molecular Medicine Reports*, vol. 12, no. 4, pp. 5879–5885, 2015.

[15] R. Sanuki, C. Shionome, A. Kuwabara et al., "Compressive force induces osteoclast differentiation via prostaglandin E_2 production in MC3T3-E1 cells," *Connective Tissue Research*, vol. 51, no. 2, pp. 150–158, 2010.

[16] Y. Wang, B. Wang, L. Fu, A. Lan, and Y. Zhou, "Effect of fetal bovine serum on osteoclast formation in vitro," *Journal of Hard Tissue Biology*, vol. 23, no. 3, pp. 303–308, 2014.

[17] F. K. Keter, S. Kanyanda, S. S. L. Lyantagaye, J. Darkwa, D. J. G. Rees, and M. Meyer, "In vitro evaluation of dichloro-bis(pyrazole)palladium(II) and dichloro-bis(pyrazole)platinum(II) complexes as anticancer agents," *Cancer Chemotherapy and Pharmacology*, vol. 63, no. 1, pp. 127–138, 2008.

[18] E. Swartzman, M. Shannon, P. Lieu et al., "Expanding applications of protein analysis using proximity ligation and qPCR," *Methods*, vol. 50, no. 4, pp. S23–S26, 2010.

[19] C. C. Barbacioru, Y. Wang, R. D. Canales et al., "Effect of various normalization methods on Applied Biosystems expression array system data," *BMC Bioinformatics*, vol. 7, article 533, 2006.

[20] A. Martínez, M. Sánchez-Lopez, J. Varadé et al., "Role of the MHC2TA gene in autoimmune diseases," *Annals of the Rheumatic Diseases*, vol. 66, no. 3, pp. 325–329, 2007.

[21] J. P. Kósa, A. Kis, K. Bácsi et al., "The protective role of bone morphogenetic protein-8 in the glucocorticoid-induced apoptosis on bone cells," *Bone*, vol. 48, no. 5, pp. 1052–1057, 2011.

[22] T. Miyazaki, S. Miyauchi, T. Anada, H. Imaizumi, and O. Suzuki, "Evaluation of osteoclastic resorption activity using calcium phosphate coating combined with labeled polyanion," *Analytical Biochemistry*, vol. 410, no. 1, pp. 7–12, 2011.

[23] M. Suzanne and H. Steller, "Shaping organisms with apoptosis," *Cell Death and Differentiation*, vol. 20, no. 5, pp. 669–675, 2013.

[24] Y. Yoshioka, A. Yamamuro, and S. Maeda, "Nitric oxide/cGMP signaling pathway protects RAW264 cells against nitric oxide-induced apoptosis by inhibiting the activation of p38 mitogen-activated protein kinase," *Journal of Pharmacological Sciences*, vol. 101, no. 2, pp. 126–134, 2006.

[25] M. Suetsugu, A. Takeshita, K. Matsumoto, A. Takahashi, C. Sasuga, and T. Yasui, "Synergistic enhancement by transforming growth factor-β1 of nitric oxide-induced apoptosis in macrophage-like cell line RAW264.7 cells," *The Journal of Meikai Dental Medicine*, vol. 38, no. 2, pp. 166–181, 2009 (Japanese).

[26] S.-K. Lin, S.-H. Kok, L.-D. Lin et al., "Nitric oxide promotes the progression of periapical lesion via inducing macrophage and osteoblast apoptosis," *Oral Microbiology and Immunology*, vol. 22, no. 1, pp. 24–29, 2007.

[27] G. Oktem, S. Uslu, S. H. Vatansever, H. Aktug, M. E. Yurtseven, and A. Uysal, "Evaluation of the relationship between inducible nitric oxide synthase (iNOS) activity and effects of melatonin in experimental osteoporosis in the rat," *Surgical and Radiologic Anatomy*, vol. 28, no. 2, pp. 157–162, 2006.

[28] L. Boscá, M. Zeini, P. G. Través, and S. Hortelano, "Nitric oxide and cell viability in inflammatory cells: a role for NO in macrophage function and fate," *Toxicology*, vol. 208, no. 2, pp. 249–258, 2005.

[29] Y. Sun, X. Chen, Z. Chen et al., "Neuropeptide FF attenuates RANKL-induced differentiation of macrophage-like cells into osteoclast-like cells," *Archives of Oral Biology*, vol. 60, no. 2, pp. 282–292, 2015.

[30] P. H. Stern and J. Diamond, "Sodium nitroprusside increases cyclic GMP in fetal rat bone cells and inhibits resorption of fetal rat limb bones," *Research Communications in Chemical Pathology and Pharmacology*, vol. 75, no. 1, pp. 19–28, 1992.

[31] R. Mentaverri, S. Kamel, A. Wattel et al., "Regulation of bone resorption and osteoclast survival by nitric oxide: possible involvement of NMDA-receptor," *Journal of Cellular Biochemistry*, vol. 88, no. 6, pp. 1145–1156, 2003.

10

Cardioprotective Effect of Electroacupuncture Pretreatment on Myocardial Ischemia/Reperfusion Injury via Antiapoptotic Signaling

Sheng-feng Lu,[1] Yan Huang,[1,2] Ning Wang,[1] Wei-xing Shen,[1] Shu-ping Fu,[1] Qian Li,[1] Mei-ling Yu,[1] Wan-xin Liu,[3] Xia Chen,[1] Xin-yue Jing,[1] and Bing-mei Zhu[1,4]

[1]*Key Laboratory of Acupuncture and Medicine Research of Ministry of Education, Nanjing University of Chinese Medicine, Nanjing 210023, China*
[2]*Key Laboratory of Acupuncture and Immunological Effects, Shanghai University of Traditional Chinese Medicine, Shanghai 200030, China*
[3]*School of Veterinary Medicine, University of Pennsylvania, 3800 Spruce Street, Philadelphia, PA 19104, USA*
[4]*Jiangxi University of Traditional Chinese Medicine, Nanchang 330004, China*

Correspondence should be addressed to Bing-mei Zhu; zhubm64@hotmail.com

Academic Editor: Ching-Liang Hsieh

Objectives. Our previous study has used RNA-seq technology to show that apoptotic molecules were involved in the myocardial protection of electroacupuncture pretreatment (EAP) on the ischemia/reperfusion (I/R) animal model. Therefore, this study was designed to investigate how EAP protects myocardium against myocardial I/R injury through antiapoptotic mechanism. *Methods.* By using rats with myocardial I/R, we ligated the left anterior descending artery (LAD) for 30 minutes followed by 4 hr of reperfusion after EAP at the Neiguan (PC6) acupoint for 12 days; we employed arrhythmia scores, serum myocardial enzymes, and cardiac troponin T (cTnT) to evaluate the cardioprotective effect. Heart tissues were harvested for western blot analyses for the expressions of pro- and antiapoptotic signaling molecules. *Results.* Our preliminary findings showed that EAP increased the survival of the animals along with declined arrhythmia scores and decreased CK, LDH, CK-Mb, and cTnT levels. Further analyses with the heart tissues detected reduced myocardial fiber damage, decreased number of apoptotic cells and the protein expressions of Cyt c and cleaved caspase 3, and the elevated level of Endo G and AIF after EAP intervention. At the same time, the protein expressions of antiapoptotic molecules, including Xiap, BclxL, and Bcl2, were obviously increased. *Conclusions.* The present study suggested that EAP protected the myocardium from I/R injury at least partially through the activation of endogenous antiapoptotic signaling.

1. Introduction

Acute myocardial ischemia (AMI) is the most common cause of mortality and morbidity in the developed countries and rapidly becoming a common malady in the developing countries. Early and fast restoration of blood flow is the most ideal approach to prevent further tissue injury [1]. In fact, thrombolytic therapy via drug administration or primary percutaneous coronary intervention (PCI) is the most effective strategy to reduce the size of myocardial infarct and improve clinical outcome. Unfortunately, however, prompt reperfusion can also induce myocardial injury, and the phenomenon is termed myocardial ischemia/reperfusion injury (MIRI) [2].

The damage from reperfusion is triggered by the increased production of oxygen-free radicals at the time of reperfusion and the impaired antioxidant ability of the heart, leading to cell apoptosis and increased infarct size [3, 4]; this accounts for up to 50% of the final size of a myocardial infarct [5]. To reduce MIRI, various methods and drugs have been used in experimental and clinical studies [6], such as remote ischemic preconditioning [7], exenatide

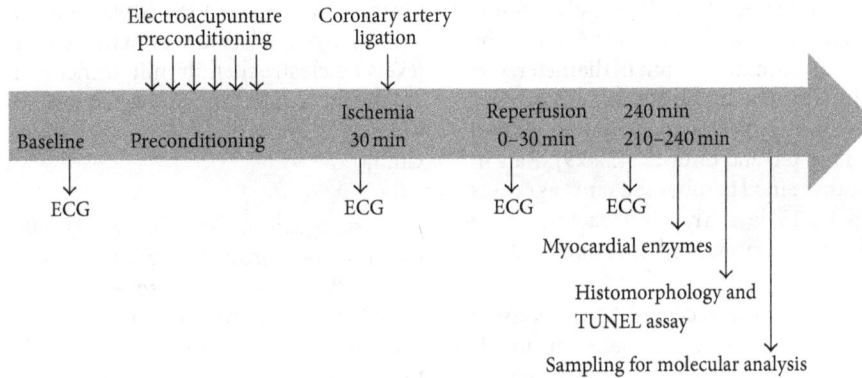

FIGURE 1: The timeline of the experimental process. Six preconditioning groups of rats were used (n = 15/each group). ECG indicates electrocardiogram.

[8], and atorvastatin pretreatment [9]. However, effective therapies to prevent reperfusion injury have proven elusive. Despite an improved understanding of the pathophysiology of this process and encouraging preclinical trials of multiple agents, most of the clinical trials to reduce MIRI have yielded disappointing results [10, 11]. Adjunctive therapies and new treatments to limit reperfusion injury remain an active area of investigation.

Acupuncture has been practiced in China for over two thousand years as an effective approach to improve the symptoms of angina and palpitation by promoting physiologically endogenous protection system [12–15]. According to Chinese medicine theory, Neiguan acupoint (PC6) on the pericardium meridian is considered as the main acupoint for improving heart function and energy metabolism, promoting ischemia tolerance, eliminating free radical, and protecting against cell death [16–24]. Growing evidence, including our previous study, experimentally shows that EAP could alleviate I/R injury of brain and heart tissues [15, 25–27]. Simultaneously, EAP also plays protective roles against cardiac I/R injury in adult patients undergoing heart valve replacement surgery by reducing the level of serum cardiac troponin I, the inotrope score, and by shortening time spent in the intensive care unit [22], and also by reducing PCI-related myocardial injury [28]. However, detailed mechanisms have not been fully elucidated.

The importance of apoptosis in cell death following reperfusion has been demonstrated in in vivo rodent models, which also allows for the evaluation of pharmacological, growth factor-mediated, and genetic interventions [2, 6]. Our previous study has used RNA-seq technology to show that apoptotic molecules were involved in the myocardial protection of EAP at PC6 on the I/R animal model [27], suggesting that cardioprotective effect of EAP may be closely related to antiapoptotic signaling. Therefore, the aims of our present study are to determine, through rat I/R models, whether EAP protects myocardium, along with its antiapoptotic mechanism. The results show that EAP could regulate both pro- and antiapoptotic molecules, suggesting that EAP might be an appropriate alternative treatment for myocardial

ischemia patients who will be undergoing a thrombolytic therapy or primary percutaneous coronary intervention.

2. Methods

2.1. Antibodies and Reagents.
Antibodies for Cyt c, Smac/Diablo, HtrA2/Omi, Endo G, AIF, caspase 3, cleaved caspase 3, Xiap, BclxL, and Bcl2 were obtained from cell signaling. Antibodies for GAPDH were purchased from Abcam (Cambridge, UK). For assessing apoptosis, the in situ cell death detection kit, POD (TUNEL) was obtained from Roche (Lewes, UK).

2.2. Animals and Grouping.
Male adult Sprague-Dawley (SD) rats (280 ± 20 g), supplied by the Vital River Laboratory Animal Technology Co. Ltd. (Beijing, China), were randomly divided into six groups after adaptive feeding for a week: sham operation control group (SO), EAP at PC6 + SO (ES), EAP at nonacupoint + SO (NS), myocardial ischemia/reperfusion model group (I/R), EAP at PC6 + I/R (EA), and EAP at nonacupoint + I/R (NA). A timeline of the study is shown in Figure 1. The study was approved by the Institute for Animal Care and Use Committee at Nanjing University of Chinese Medicine, and all experimental procedures were designed and conducted according to the Guide for the Care and Use of Laboratory Animals published by National Institutes of Health (NIH Publication Number 80-23, revised 1996).

2.3. EAP Intervention.
Prior to the MIRI experiment, rats among ES, NS, EA, and NA groups were pretreated with electroacupuncture for a total of 12 days in the waking state, with one day of rest after six consecutive days of treatment. Both EA and ES groups were pretreated at the PC6, located in the forelimbs [25]. Two acupuncture needles were separately inserted into the PC6 located on each upper limb which were located at a point 1.5 cm proximal to the palm crease just above the median nerve as previously described [16, 25], and an electrical current was provided to the needles for a period of 20 minutes through an electrical stimulator with

a stimulus isolation unit (Han Acuten, WQ1002F, Beijing, China) at 2/15 Hz, with an intensity level of 1 mA [20]. The acupuncture needle, 7 mm long and 0.16 mm in diameter, was inserted 2-3 mm into the subcutis. In the NA and NS groups, the same pretreatments were applied at nonacupoint, located at the junction between the tail and buttock [27, 29]. Rats in SO and I/R groups were restrained in tubes the same as others groups for 20 min daily for 12 days. The electroacupuncture procedure was carried out by a specialized acupuncturist.

2.4. In Vivo MIRI.
Rats that had accepted 12 sessions of EAP were anesthetized with mechanical ventilation using 5% isoflurane and maintained by inhalation of 1-2% isoflurane in 100% oxygen with a mixture of 70% N_2O and 30% O_2 after endotracheal intubation. Tidal volume and respiratory rate were set at 1.0 mL/100 g body weight and 45–60 breaths per minute, respectively. Adequate anesthesia was ensured by monitoring heart rate and the absence of a withdrawal response to a paw pinch. Lead II electrocardiogram (ECG) was monitored and recorded. The left carotid artery was cannulated for blood pressure measurement. Body temperature was maintained with a servo-controlled heating pad at 37°C.

The heart was exposed via a left thoracotomy between the 4th and 5th intercostal space. Following pericardiotomy, the left anterior descending (LAD) coronary artery was ligated with a 6.0 silk suture for 30 min to induce ischemia, followed by 240 min of reperfusion [29]. Successful coronary artery occlusion was confirmed by elevation of the ST segment in the ECG and an immediate 15–30 mmHg fall in arterial blood pressure. The chest was closed 30 min after the LAD was reperfused, and the rats were kept warm and allowed to recover. Buprenorphine HCl (0.05 mg/kg) was employed to minimize pain and distress by intramuscular injection after operation immediately [30].

2.5. Electrocardiogram (ECG) Recording and Scoring of Arrhythmia.
A standard limb lead II ECG was successively monitored and recorded before, during myocardial ischemia, and after reperfusion under anesthesia by the use of a computerized PowerLab system (ADInstruments, Australia), and then monitored again from 210 min to 240 min under anesthesia [27]. The arrhythmias were assessed during the 30 min period of ischemia and the 30 min of reperfusion. The arrhythmia scores were accessed by an electrocardiogram specialist physician and assigned as described previously [27] according to the system described by Curtis and Walker [31] as follows: 0 = no arrhythmia; 1 ≤ 10 s premature ventricular contraction (PVC) and/or ventricular tachycardia (VT); 2 = 11–30 s PVC and/or VT; 3 = 31–90 s PVC and/or VT; 4 = 91–180 s PVC and/or VT or reversible ventricular fibrillation (VF) of <10 s; 5 ≥ 180 s PVC and/or VT, >10 s reversible VF; and 6 = irreversible VF. In addition, the survival rate of animals was also calculated.

2.6. Myocardial Enzyme Analysis.
Following a four-hour reperfusion period, blood was collected from the jugular vein and centrifuged (10,000 g, 10 minutes, and 4°C). Serum lactate dehydrogenase (LDH), creatine kinase (CK) and creatine kinase-MB (CK-MB) levels were analyzed with a biochemistry analyzer. Plasma was extracted and analyzed for cTnT levels by electrochemiluminescence immune-assay method. All the myocardial enzyme detections were performed by the Medical laboratory of Jiangsu Province Hospital (Nanjing, China).

2.7. Histological and Morphological Analyses.
After sacrificing the animals through intravenous injection of high-dose (150 mg/kg) of pentobarbitone at the end of the experiment, cardiac tissues were fixed in 4% paraformaldehyde (Sigma-Aldrich, Inc.) and embedded in paraffin. The embedded tissues were sectioned and stained with TUNEL assay kit as described previously [32, 33], which was employed to observe the positive apoptotic cells in myocardial tissue.

2.8. Apoptotic Molecules Analysis.
After sacrificing the rats, the hearts were quickly removed and placed into liquid nitrogen. Then, total proteins were extracted for the further western blot (WB) assays. Our study has shown that electroacupuncture at PC6 could change gene expression profiles of I/R heart, and that EAP can markedly modify the expression levels of numerous genes involved in apoptotic pathways [27]. Therefore, in this study, we examined the protein expression of caspase 3, cytochrome c (Cyt c), Smac/Diablo, HtrA2/Omi, Endo G, AIF, Bcl2, BclxL, and Xiap to evaluate the status of apoptotic signaling.

2.9. Western Blot Analysis.
WB was performed as described previously [34]. Briefly, after detecting the concentrations by the BCA protein assay (Pierce), equivalent amounts of protein (30 µg/lane) were separated by SDS-polyacrylamide gel electrophoresis and transferred onto PVDF membranes. Each PVDF membranes were incubated with the appropriate primary antibodies anti-Cyt c (1:1000), anti-Smac/Diablo (1:1000), anti-HtrA2/Omi (1:1000), anti-Endo G (1:1000), anti-AIF (1:1000), anti-caspase 3 (1:1000), anti-cleaved caspase 3 (1:1000), anti-Xiap (1:1000), anti-BclxL (1:1000), anti-Bcl2 (1:1000), and anti-GAPDH (1:2000) and followed by incubation with peroxidase-conjugated secondary antibodies. Proteins were quantified using the SuperSignal West Pico Chemiluminescent substrate (Pierce).

2.10. Statistical Analysis.
All values were expressed as a mean ± standard deviation (SD). Statistical analyses were performed using SPSS 17.0. Multiple group comparisons were performed by one-way ANOVA. Tukey's procedure was used for multiple-range tests. Differences were considered significant when $P < 0.05$.

3. Results

3.1. EAP at PC 6 Protected Rat Myocardium from MIRI.
To investigate protective effects of EAP at the PC6 on MIRI, we first observed ECG's ST segments, arrhythmic scores, and serum enzyme levels. The ECG recordings showed that the ST segments were noticeably elevated in I/R, EA, and NA groups during the 30 min after myocardial ischemia (MI) operation,

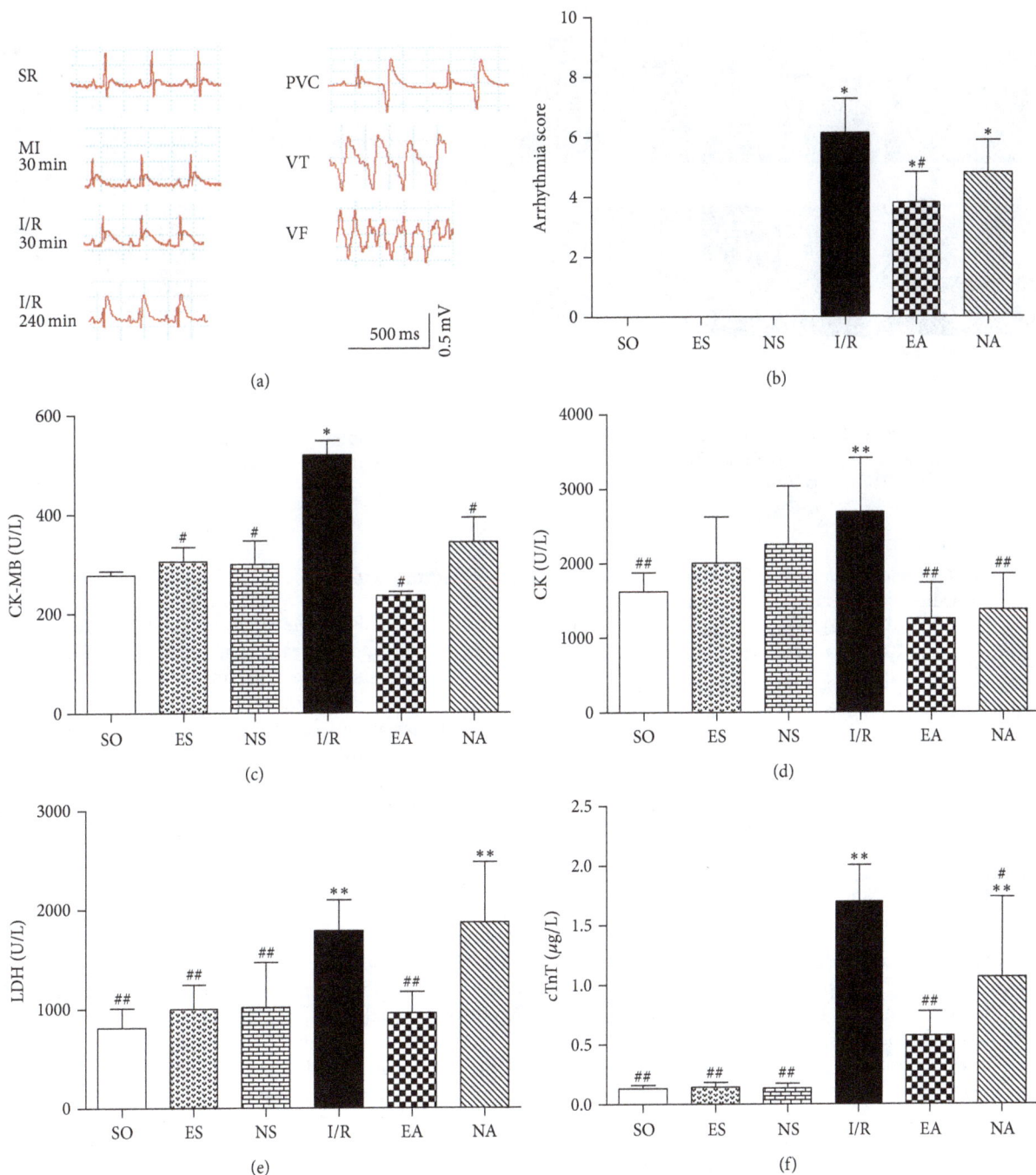

FIGURE 2: Effects of EAP on MIRI. (a) Representative ECG recording in standard limb lead II. PVC, premature ventricular contraction, VT, ventricular tachycardia, and VF, ventricular fibrillation. (b) Quantitative analysis for arrhythmia sores in each group. (c–f) CK, CK-Mb, LDH, and cTnT levels by biochemistry analyzer after myocardial I/R experiment in each group. Data were expressed as mean ± SD, $n = 8$–15/each group. $^{*}P < 0.05$ and $^{**}P < 0.01$ versus SO group; $^{#}P < 0.05$ and $^{##}P < 0.01$ versus I/R group.

and premature ventricular contraction (PVC), ventricular tachycardia (VT), and ventricular fibrillation (VF) were observed during the four-hour reperfusion period (Figure 2(a)), suggesting a successful I/R model. The arrhythmia scores were decreased in both EA and NA groups, especially in EA group compared to that in the I/R group (Figure 2(b)). The (LDH, levels of serum enzymes CK, CK-Mb, and

cTnT), which reflect acute myocardial damage, significantly increased in the I/R group compared to the SO group, but returned to the levels of the SO group after EAP ($P < 0.05$) (Figures 2(c)–2(f)). Meanwhile, the survival rate in the EA group increased significantly to above 70%, compared to 50% in the I/R group (Figure S1 in Supplementary Material available online at http://dx.doi.org/10.1155/2016/4609784).

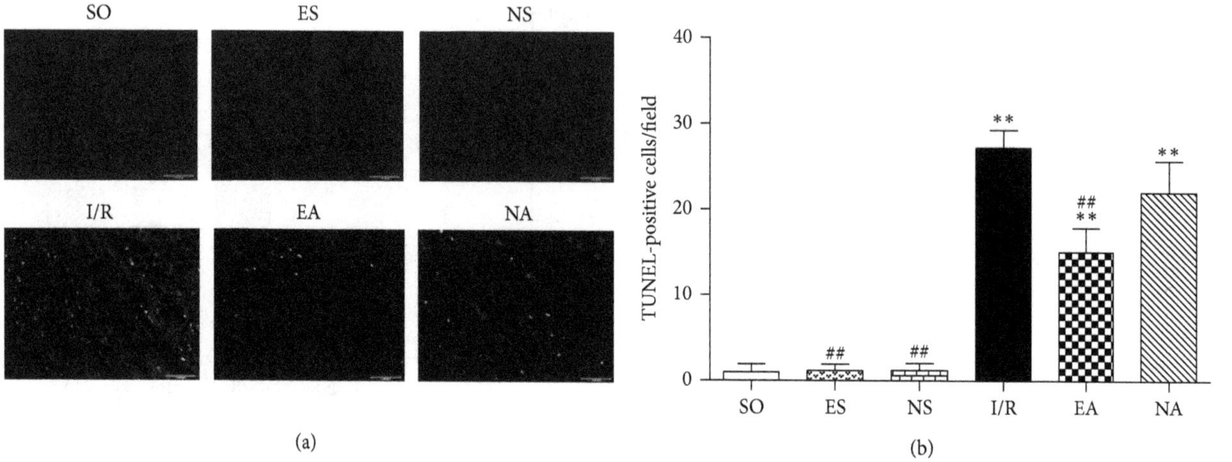

FIGURE 3: EAP promoted cardiomyocyte survival. (a) Representative images of TUNEL staining of each group. Green dots indicate TUNEL-positive cells. (b) Quantification of TUNEL-positive cells in each group. Data were expressed as mean ± SD, $n = 8$–15/each group. $^{**}P < 0.01$ versus SO group; $^{##}P < 0.01$ versus I/R group.

3.2. EAP at PC6 Promoted Survival of Cardiomyocytes against I/R Injury.

Cardiomyocyte survival is a vital factor for cardiac function. In the face of I/R injury, the myocardium has the ability to develop numerous strategies to evade apoptosis. Expectedly, our study detected noticeably increased TUNEL-positive cells in the I/R heart, but the number of these cells was significantly decreased in the EA group (Figures 3(a) and 3(b)). Meanwhile, we also assessed the extent of myocardial fiber damage by ferroalumen hematoxylin staining [35, 36]. Our results showed that injury of myocardial fibers was obvious in I/R group, in which the cells were stained black. Myocardial cells from the EA group, however, did not pick up the stain (Figure S2).

3.3. EAP at PC6 Promotes Antiapoptotic Signaling and Inhibits Proapoptotic Signaling.

Apoptosis plays an important role in lethal reperfusion injury as indicated by numerous studies in various animal models [6, 37]. To further verify what we observed in the previous study by RNA-seq that apoptosis is a possible mechanism relevant to the myocardioprotective effects of EAP, caspase-dependent and caspase-independent apoptotic signaling in the heart tissues was examined by western blotting for caspase 3, Cyt c, Smac/Diablo, HtrA2/Omi, Endo G, and AIF. As shown in Figures 4(a) and 4(b), the expression of proteins of Cyt c, Endo G, and AIF increased in the I/R group but markedly decreased in the EA group ($P < 0.05$), suggesting an antiapoptotic mechanism involved in the cardioprotective effects of EAP against I/R injury. Interestingly, though the expression level of total caspases 3 was decreased in the I/R heart and EAP increased it significantly, the level of cleaved caspase 3, a biologically active caspase 3 enzyme, was elevated in the I/R group, and was evidently decreased in the EA group ($P < 0.05$, Figures 4(c) and 4(d)). Similarly, we detected reduction in antiapoptotic molecules, including Xiap, BclxL, and Bcl2 upon I/R injury, and a significant increase in these proteins after EAP ($P < 0.05$, Figures 4(e) and 4(f)).

4. Discussion

Acupuncture at PC6 is generally prescribed for the treatment of heart and chest disease symptoms, such as palpitation, chest distress, thoracalgia, gastralgia, and nausea and vomiting, based on the theory of Chinese medicine. Previous research has indicated that acupuncture at PC6 acupoint can attenuate cardiac injury, through reducing arrhythmias, apoptosis, and myocardial enzymes [16, 18, 20, 38, 39]. Our previous studies had demonstrated that electroacupuncture could effectively promote angiogenesis and protect myocardial tissue against ischemia injury [33]. EAP, one of acupuncture treatment approaches, has been demonstrated to be protective against I/R injury in brain or heart of the animal models [16, 25, 26, 40, 41]. The cardioprotective effects of EAP in patients undergoing heart valve replacement surgery or PCI operation have also been proved in a randomized controlled trial [22, 28], but the mechanism remains unclear.

As we all know, myocardial injury is often accompanied by changes in ECG and serum enzymes. ST segment elevation and heart rate disorders appear to be the most typical in the ECG detection. And the levels of serum enzymes (LDH, CK, and CK-Mb), especially cTnT [42], reflect acute myocardial damage effectively [43]. Our study, by using rat I/R model, suggested that EAP increased survival rate, reduced the ST segment, the arrhythmia score, and the release of serum enzyme from myocardium, alleviated myocardial fiber damage, and reduced the infarct size of MIRI measurement by TTC staining (the corresponding period results have published) [27], therefore protecting myocardial cells from I/R injury. These findings were consistent with the previous studies [16, 25, 37].

Our previous study and the literature have demonstrated numerous mechanisms that may contribute to MIRI [5, 27, 41–46], such as necrosis, apoptosis, and dysfunction of organelles. Apoptosis has been known to play an important role in the initial stages of reperfusion injury and serve as a mechanism of cellular self-destruction for a variety of

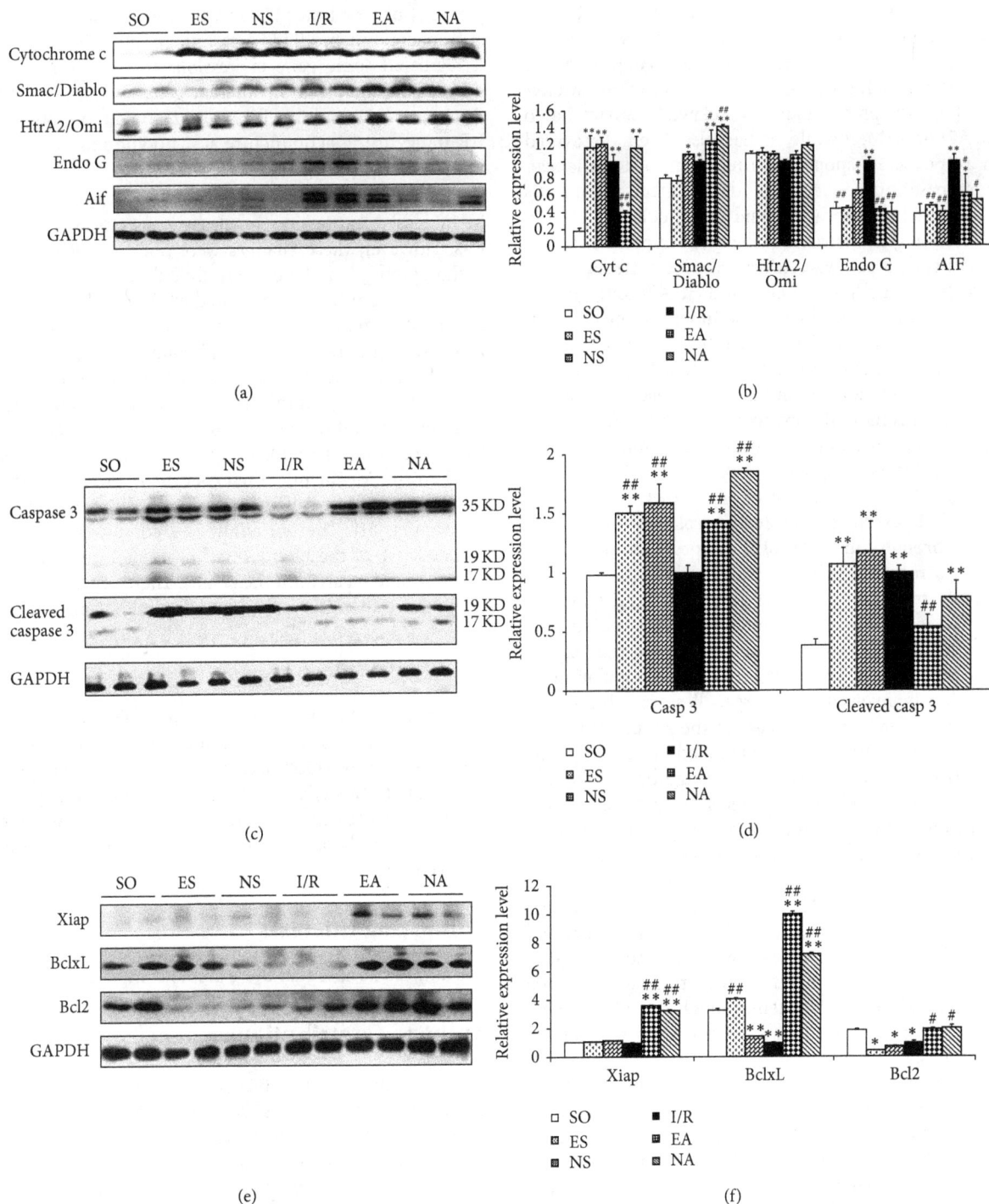

(a)

(b)

(c)

(d)

(e)

(f)

FIGURE 4: EAP regulated apoptotic signaling. Representative western blot results of proapoptotic, antiapoptotic, and histone acetylation proteins in each group ((a), (c), and (e)). Quantitative analysis of proapoptotic, antiapoptotic, and histone acetylation proteins in each group ((b), (d), and (f)). Data were expressed as mean ± SD, n = 8–15/each group. $^*P < 0.05$ and $^{**}P < 0.01$ versus SO group; $^{#}P < 0.05$ and $^{##}P < 0.01$ versus I/R group.

processes [36]. Our data indicated a marked decrease in the number of TUNEL-positive cells as a result of EAP, and the extent of myocardial fiber damage was relieved in the EA group compared with the I/R group (Figure S2). The results suggested that EAP can effectively protect the myocardial

cells from death, consistent with our previous studies on the reduction of myocardial infarction area by EAP [27]. Apoptosis is initiated by unbalancing pro- and antiapoptotic machineries [47–49]. Many studies have demonstrated the importance of caspase-dependent cell death pathways in injuries or diseases [50]. The most widely studied form of intrinsic apoptosis is stress-mediated release of Cyt c from the mitochondria that results in the formation of the apoptosome, which leads to the activation of the executioner caspase 3 [50]. The process may be regulated by Smac/Diablo and HtrA2/Omi. Meanwhile, it has also been discovered that in response to apoptotic stimuli, mitochondria can release caspase-independent cell death effectors such as apoptosis inducing factor (AIF) and Endonuclease G (Endo G) [51], resulting in caspase-independent apoptosis. In the caspase-dependent pathway, cleaved caspase 3-mediated signaling, such as Cyt c, Smac/Diablo, and HtrA2/Omi, directly activates cell death, whereas caspase-independent pathway, mainly including Endo G and AIF, causes cell death through DNA cleavage [52]. Our results showed that EAP decreased the Cyt c level and indirectly inhibited caspase 3 activation. EAP can also promote the expression of Smac/Diablo but not HtrA2/Omi, which indirectly negatively regulates caspase 3 via the inhibitors of apoptosis proteins (IAPs) [50, 53]. Additionally, this is, to the best of our knowledge, the first report of EAP exerting a protective role on myocardial I/R injury through inhibition of the expression of Endo G and AIF. As reported in other studies, the mitochondrial permeability transition pore (MPTP) is a central player of cell fate and is responsible for mitochondrial swelling with the consequent release of proapoptotic factors (i.e., Cyt c, AIF, and Smac/Diablo) [54]. When a large population of mitochondria is involved, these organelles are subjected to swelling, which leads to the release of the apoptotic factors [55]. In the present study, we demonstrated that EAP significantly decreased the opening of MPTP (Figure S3), therefore reducing the release of proapoptotic factors from the I/R heart. Unexpectedly, increased proteins expression levels of some proapoptotic molecules (Cyt c and cleaved caspase 3) and decreased antiapoptotic proteins (Xiap and Bcl2) were observed in the ES and NS groups, at a similar pattern in the I/R group. This observation needs to be addressed mechanistically in our future study, but it suggests that needling at nonacupoint might be also stimulation for the body to respond to certain extent, though the effectiveness of NA was not significant. This result is consistent with our previous finding [27].

The death of a cell was associated with autophagy and MAPK signaling. Early studies have indicated that apoptosis is caused by the activation of an autophagic process, which could be inhibited by chemical inhibitors of autophagy, and it was shown to depend on the autophagic genes APG5 and beclin [56]. We detected decreased beclin1 protein level in the heart treated by EAP (Figure S4). We also observed activated signal transduction of mitogen-activated protein kinases (MAPKs) in myocardial tissue, which had been reported as an important mediator of ischemic-related events [57]. The levels of p-JNK, p-P38, p-P44/42, and Ras were upregulated, and p-P38 level was downregulated in the I/R group, and all of them were reversed by undergoing EAP (Figure S5). Furthermore, to a certain extent, the EAP at nonacupoint also results in similar changes at molecular level as seen in the EA group (Figure 4), but its cardiprotective effect was inferior to the EA group. This is consistent with our

previous observation [27], in which we described that EAP at nonacupoint modified less functional pathways, though it regulated some gene expressions to certain extent. The detailed mechanisms of different gene and protein expression patterns resulting from pretreatment on myocardial I/R injury using acupuncture at acupoint and nonacupoint remain to be investigated.

Interestingly, EAP on the sham operation rats resulted in increased expression of cleaved caspase 3, Cyt c, and Ras. However, these changes were not correlated with any pathological phenotype even though the levels of these proteins were as high as those in the I/R rats. This finding also is consistent with our previous study on ischemia-induced myocardial injury [27]. This phenomenon suggested that EAP might produce a similar stimulation on the heart, as does myocardial injury, mimicking an ischemic preconditioning or remote conditioning [44, 58–60]. A further study might be of significance to confirm this observation and explore its mechanism. Meanwhile, the experimental model is affected by a phenomenon called "nonreflow," which can influence the results [61]. The nonreflow is a condition where there is a collapse of the blood vessel even after coronary artery opening, and it can limit the results. Therefore, it is necessary to pay more attention to the nonreflow in the follow-up study.

5. Conclusions

In summary, the present study demonstrates that EAP effectively protects the myocardium from I/R injury. And suppression of proapoptosis and promotion of antiapoptosis contribute to this effect. Thus, EAP could be an appropriate alternative treatment for patients with MI who will receive thrombolytic therapy or primary percutaneous coronary intervention.

Competing Interests

The authors declare that there are no competing interests.

Authors' Contributions

Bing-mei Zhu, Sheng-feng Lu, and Yan Huang conceived and designed the experiments. Yan Huang, Sheng-feng Lu, Wei-xing Shen, Shu-ping Fu, Qian Li, Xia Chen, and Xin-yue Jing performed the experiments. Bing-mei Zhu, Yan Huang, Sheng-feng Lu, and Ning Wang analyzed the data. Sheng-feng Lu, Bing-mei Zhu, Mei-ling Yu, and Wan-xin Liu wrote the paper. All authors read and approved the final paper. Sheng-feng Lu and Yan Huang contributed equally to this work.

Acknowledgments

This work was supported by grants from the National Basic Research program of China (973 Program, no. 2012CB518501), the National Natural Science Foundation of China (nos. 81574062, 81574063, 81273838, and 81403478), and Natural Science Foundation of Jiangxi province (no. BK20151569).

References

[1] J. L. Anderson, H. W. Marshall, B. E. Bray et al., "A randomized trial of intracoronary streptokinase in the treatment of acute myocardial infarction," *The New England Journal of Medicine*, vol. 308, no. 22, pp. 1312–1318, 1983.

[2] A. Frank, M. Bonney, S. Bonney, L. Weitzel, M. Koeppen, and T. Eckle, "Myocardial ischemia reperfusion injury: from basic science to clinical bedside," *Seminars in Cardiothoracic and Vascular Anesthesia*, vol. 16, no. 3, pp. 123–132, 2012.

[3] G. Ambrosio, J. L. Zweier, C. Duilio et al., "Evidence that mitochondrial respiration is a source of potentially toxic oxygen free radicals in intact rabbit hearts subjected to ischemia and reflow," *The Journal of Biological Chemistry*, vol. 268, no. 25, pp. 18532–18541, 1993.

[4] N. Marczin, N. El-Habashi, G. S. Hoare, R. E. Bundy, and M. Yacoub, "Antioxidants in myocardial ischemia-reperfusion injury: therapeutic potential and basic mechanisms," *Archives of Biochemistry and Biophysics*, vol. 420, no. 2, pp. 222–236, 2003.

[5] D. M. Yellon and D. J. Hausenloy, "Myocardial reperfusion injury," *The New England Journal of Medicine*, vol. 357, no. 11, pp. 1121–1135, 2007.

[6] F. Eefting, B. Rensing, J. Wigman et al., "Role of apoptosis in reperfusion injury," *Cardiovascular Research*, vol. 61, no. 3, pp. 414–426, 2004.

[7] M. Thielmann, E. Kottenberg, P. Kleinbongard et al., "Cardioprotective and prognostic effects of remote ischaemic preconditioning in patients undergoing coronary artery bypass surgery: a single-centre randomised, double-blind, controlled trial," *The Lancet*, vol. 382, no. 9892, pp. 597–604, 2013.

[8] J. S. Woo, W. Kim, S. J. Ha et al., "Cardioprotective effects of exenatide in patients with ST-segment-elevation myocardial infarction undergoing primary percutaneous coronary intervention: results of exenatide myocardial protection in revascularization study," *Arteriosclerosis, Thrombosis, and Vascular Biology*, vol. 33, no. 9, pp. 2252–2260, 2013.

[9] M. Chen, H. Li, and Y. Wang, "Protection by atorvastatin pretreatment in patients undergoing primary percutaneous coronary intervention is associated with the lower levels of oxygen free radicals," *Journal of Cardiovascular Pharmacology*, vol. 62, no. 3, pp. 320–324, 2013.

[10] R. Bolli, L. Becker, G. Gross, R. Mentzer Jr., D. Balshaw, and D. A. Lathrop, "Myocardial protection at a crossroads: the need for translation into clinical therapy," *Circulation Research*, vol. 95, no. 2, pp. 125–134, 2004.

[11] R. O. Cannon III, "Mechanisms, management and future directions for reperfusion injury after acute myocardial infarction," *Nature Clinical Practice Cardiovascular Medicine*, vol. 2, no. 2, pp. 88–94, 2005.

[12] F. H. Xu and J. M. Wang, "Clinical observation on acupuncture combined with medication for intractable angina pectoris," *Zhongguo Zhen Jiu*, vol. 25, no. 2, pp. 89–91, 2005.

[13] J. Hu, "Acupuncture treatment of palpitation," *Journal of Traditional Chinese Medicine*, vol. 28, no. 3, pp. 228–230, 2008.

[14] J. Meng, "The effects of acupuncture in treatment of coronary heart diseases," *Journal of Traditional Chinese Medicine*, vol. 24, no. 1, pp. 16–19, 2004.

[15] J. P. Cao, "The basis for acupuncture treatment of coronary heart disease is humoral factors-mediated favorable regulation," *Zhen Ci Yan Jiu*, vol. 31, no. 3, pp. 185–189, 2006.

[16] J. Gao, L. Zhang, Y. Wang et al., "Antiarrhythmic effect of acupuncture pretreatment in rats subjected to simulative global ischemia and reperfusion—involvement of adenylate cyclase, protein kinase A, and L-type Ca^{2+} channel," *Journal of Physiological Sciences*, vol. 58, no. 6, pp. 389–396, 2008.

[17] J. Li, J. Li, F. Liang et al., "Electroacupuncture at PC6 (Neiguan) improves extracellular signal-regulated kinase signaling pathways through the regulation of neuroendocrine cytokines in myocardial hypertrophic rats," *Evidence-Based Complementary and Alternative Medicine*, vol. 2012, Article ID 792820, 9 pages, 2012.

[18] H. L. Lujan, V. J. Kramer, and S. E. DiCarlo, "Electroacupuncture decreases the susceptibility to ventricular tachycardia in conscious rats by reducing cardiac metabolic demand," *American Journal of Physiology—Heart and Circulatory Physiology*, vol. 292, no. 5, pp. H2550–H2555, 2007.

[19] X. Ni, Y. Xie, Q. Wang et al., "Cardioprotective effect of transcutaneous electric acupoint stimulation in the pediatric cardiac patients: a randomized controlled clinical trial," *Paediatric Anaesthesia*, vol. 22, no. 8, pp. 805–811, 2012.

[20] M.-T. Tsou, C.-H. Huang, and J.-H. Chiu, "Electroacupuncture on PC6 (Neiguan) attenuates ischemia/reperfusion injury in rat hearts," *American Journal of Chinese Medicine*, vol. 32, no. 6, pp. 951–965, 2004.

[21] S.-B. Wang, S.-P. Chen, Y.-H. Gao, M.-F. Luo, and J.-L. Liu, "Effects of electroacupuncture on cardiac and gastric activities in acute myocardial ischemia rats," *World Journal of Gastroenterology*, vol. 14, no. 42, pp. 6496–6502, 2008.

[22] L. Yang, J. Yang, Q. Wang et al., "cardioprotective effects of electroacupuncture pretreatment on patients undergoing heart valve replacement surgery: a randomized controlled trial," *Annals of Thoracic Surgery*, vol. 89, no. 3, pp. 781–786, 2010.

[23] H. Zhang, L. Liu, G. Huang et al., "Protective effect of electroacupuncture at the Neiguan point in a rabbit model of myocardial ischemia-reperfusion injury," *Canadian Journal of Cardiology*, vol. 25, no. 6, pp. 359–363, 2009.

[24] Z. Jin, J. Liang, J. Wang, and P. E. Kolattukudy, "Delayed brain ischemia tolerance induced by electroacupuncture pretreatment is mediated via MCP-induced protein 1," *Journal of Neuroinflammation*, vol. 10, article 63, 2013.

[25] J. Gao, W. Fu, Z. Jin, and X. Yu, "Acupuncture pretreatment protects heart from injury in rats with myocardial ischemia and reperfusion via inhibition of the β1-adrenoceptor signaling pathway," *Life Sciences*, vol. 80, no. 16, pp. 1484–1489, 2007.

[26] X. Li, P. Luo, Q. Wang, and L. Xiong, "Electroacupuncture pretreatment as a novel avenue to protect brain against ischemia and reperfusion injury," *Evidence-Based Complementary and Alternative Medicine*, vol. 2012, Article ID 195397, 12 pages, 2012.

[27] Y. Huang, S.-F. Lu, C.-J. Hu et al., "Electro-acupuncture at Neiguan pretreatment alters genome-wide gene expressions and protects rat myocardium against ischemia-reperfusion," *Molecules*, vol. 19, no. 10, pp. 16158–16178, 2014.

[28] Q. Wang, D. Liang, F. Wang et al., "Efficacy of electroacupuncture pretreatment for myocardial injury in patients undergoing percutaneous coronary intervention: a randomized clinical trial with a 2-year follow-up," *International Journal of Cardiology*, vol. 194, pp. 28–35, 2015.

[29] H. S. Hwang, Y. S. Kim, Y. H. Ryu et al., "Electroacupuncture delays hypertension development through enhancing NO/NOS activity in spontaneously hypertensive rats," *Evidence-Based Complementary and Alternative Medicine*, vol. 2011, Article ID 130529, 7 pages, 2011.

[30] Y. Birnbaum, Y. Ye, S. Rosanio et al., "Prostaglandins mediate the cardioprotective effects of atorvastatin against ischemia-reperfusion injury," *Cardiovascular Research*, vol. 65, no. 2, pp. 345–355, 2005.

[31] M. J. Curtis and M. J. A. Walker, "Quantification of arrhythmias using scoring systems: an examination of seven scores in an in vivo model of regional myocardial ischaemia," *Cardiovascular Research*, vol. 22, no. 9, pp. 656–665, 1988.

[32] F. Labat-Moleur, C. Guillermet, P. Lorimier et al., "TUNEL apoptotic cell detection in tissue sections: critical evaluation and improvement," *Journal of Histochemistry and Cytochemistry*, vol. 46, no. 3, pp. 327–334, 1998.

[33] Y. Tian, W. Zhang, D. Xia, P. Modi, D. Liang, and M. Wei, "Postconditioning inhibits myocardial apoptosis during prolonged reperfusion via a JAK2-STAT3-Bcl-2 pathway," *Journal of Biomedical Science*, vol. 18, no. 1, article 53, 2011.

[34] S.-P. Fu, S.-Y. He, B. Xu et al., "Acupuncture promotes angiogenesis after myocardial ischemia through H3K9 acetylation regulation at VEGF gene," *PLoS ONE*, vol. 9, no. 4, Article ID e94604, 2014.

[35] Y. K. Liu, Z. J. Zhong, X. Ban, and R. S. Bonser, "A compare of three histological stain method for the diagnosis in early myocardial ischemia," *Journal of Harbin Medical University*, vol. 36, no. 3, pp. 238–240, 2002.

[36] M. P. K. Shoobridge, "A new principle in polychrome staining: a system of automated staining, complementary to hematoxylin and eosin, and usable as a research tool," *Stain Technology*, vol. 58, no. 5, pp. 245–258, 1983.

[37] S. Q. Liu, D. Roberts, A. Kharitonenkov et al., "Endocrine protection of ischemic myocardium by FGF21 from the liver and adipose tissue," *Scientific Reports*, vol. 3, article 2767, 2013.

[38] J. Gao, W. Fu, Z. Jin, and X. Yu, "A preliminary study on the cardioprotection of acupuncture pretreatment in rats with ischemia and reperfusion: involvement of cardiac β-adrenoceptors," *Journal of Physiological Sciences*, vol. 56, no. 4, pp. 275–279, 2006.

[39] W. Zhou, Y. Ko, P. Benharash et al., "Cardioprotection of electroacupuncture against myocardial ischemia-reperfusion injury by modulation of cardiac norepinephrine release," *American Journal of Physiology—Heart and Circulatory Physiology*, vol. 302, no. 9, pp. H1818–H1825, 2012.

[40] J. Gao, Y. Zhao, Y. Wang et al., "Anti-arrhythmic effect of acupuncture pretreatment in the rats subjected to simulative global ischemia and reperfusion—involvement of intracellular Ca^{2+} and connexin 43," *BMC Complementary and Alternative Medicine*, vol. 15, no. 1, article 5, 2015.

[41] P.-Y. Liu, Y. Tian, and S.-Y. Xu, "Mediated protective effect of electroacupuncture pretreatment by miR-214 on myocardial ischemia/reperfusion injury," *Journal of Geriatric Cardiology*, vol. 11, no. 4, pp. 303–310, 2014.

[42] V. Novack, M. Pencina, D. J. Cohen et al., "Troponin criteria for myocardial infarction after percutaneous coronary intervention," *Archives of Internal Medicine*, vol. 172, no. 6, pp. 502–508, 2012.

[43] M. Kemp, J. Donovan, H. Higham, and J. Hooper, "Biochemical markers of myocardial injury," *British Journal of Anaesthesia*, vol. 93, no. 1, pp. 63–73, 2004.

[44] J. Vinten-Johansen, R. Jiang, J. G. Reeves, J. Mykytenko, J. Deneve, and L. J. Jobe, "Inflammation, proinflammatory mediators and myocardial ischemia-reperfusion injury," *Hematology/Oncology Clinics of North America*, vol. 21, no. 1, pp. 123–145, 2007.

[45] W. Shi and J. Vinten-Johansen, "Endogenous cardioprotection by ischaemic postconditioning and remote conditioning," *Cardiovascular Research*, vol. 94, no. 2, pp. 206–216, 2012.

[46] D. J. Hausenloy and D. M. Yellon, "Myocardial ischemia-reperfusion injury: a neglected therapeutic target," *The Journal of Clinical Investigation*, vol. 123, no. 1, pp. 92–100, 2013.

[47] A. Busca, M. Saxena, M. Kryworuchko, and A. Kumar, "Anti-apoptotic genes in the survival of monocytic cells during infection," *Current Genomics*, vol. 10, no. 5, pp. 306–317, 2009.

[48] D. S. Ziegler, A. L. Kung, and M. W. Kieran, "Anti-apoptosis mechanisms in malignant gliomas," *Journal of Clinical Oncology*, vol. 26, no. 3, pp. 493–500, 2008.

[49] S. Fulda, "Tumor resistance to apoptosis," *International Journal of Cancer*, vol. 124, no. 3, pp. 511–515, 2009.

[50] L. Portt, G. Norman, C. Clapp, M. Greenwood, and M. T. Greenwood, "Anti-apoptosis and cell survival: a review," *Biochimica et Biophysica Acta—Molecular Cell Research*, vol. 1813, no. 1, pp. 238–259, 2011.

[51] S. P. Cregan, V. L. Dawson, and R. S. Slack, "Role of AIF in caspase-dependent and caspase-independent cell death," *Oncogene*, vol. 23, no. 16, pp. 2785–2796, 2004.

[52] E. Wang, R. Marcotte, and E. Petroulakis, "Signaling pathway for apoptosis: a racetrack for life or death," *Journal of Cellular Biochemistry*, supplement 32-33, pp. 95–102, 1999.

[53] S. Kalimuthu and K. Se-Kwon, "Cell survival and apoptosis signaling as therapeutic target for cancer: marine bioactive compounds," *International Journal of Molecular Sciences*, vol. 14, no. 2, pp. 2334–2354, 2013.

[54] A. Vianello, V. Casolo, E. Petrussa et al., "The mitochondrial permeability transition pore (PTP)—an example of multiple molecular exaptation?" *Biochimica et Biophysica Acta (BBA)—Bioenergetics*, vol. 1817, no. 11, pp. 2072–2086, 2012.

[55] S. Grimm and D. Brdiczka, "The permeability transition pore in cell death," *Apoptosis*, vol. 12, no. 5, pp. 841–855, 2007.

[56] S. Shimizu, T. Kanaseki, N. Mizushima et al., "Role of Bcl-2 family proteins in a non-apoptopic programmed cell death dependent on autophagy genes," *Nature Cell Biology*, vol. 6, no. 12, pp. 1221–1228, 2004.

[57] L. A. King, A. H. Toledo, F. A. Rivera-Chavez, and L. H. Toledo-Pereyra, "Role of p38 and JNK in liver ischemia and reperfusion," *Journal of Hepato-Biliary-Pancreatic Surgery*, vol. 16, no. 6, pp. 763–770, 2009.

[58] L. Zhao, X. Liu, J. Liang et al., "Phosphorylation of p38 MAPK mediates hypoxic preconditioning-induced neuroprotection against cerebral ischemic injury via mitochondria translocation of Bcl-xL in mice," *Brain Research*, vol. 1503, pp. 78–88, 2013.

[59] X.-C. Sun, X.-H. Xian, W.-B. Li et al., "Activation of p38 MAPK participates in brain ischemic tolerance induced by limb ischemic preconditioning by up-regulating HSP 70," *Experimental Neurology*, vol. 224, no. 2, pp. 347–355, 2010.

[60] T. C. Zhao, G. Cheng, L. X. Zhang, Y. T. Tseng, and J. F. Padbury, "Inhibition of histone deacetylases triggers pharmacologic preconditioning effects against myocardial ischemic injury," *Cardiovascular Research*, vol. 76, no. 3, pp. 473–481, 2007.

[61] C. Bouleti, N. Mewton, and S. Germain, "The no-reflow phenomenon: state of the art," *Archives of Cardiovascular Diseases*, vol. 108, no. 12, pp. 661–674, 2015.

11

Protective Effect of *Mangifera indica* Linn., *Cocos nucifera* Linn., and *Averrhoa carambola* Linn. Extracts against Ultraviolet B-Induced Damage in Human Keratinocytes

Chalinee Ronpirin,[1] Nattaporn Pattarachotanant,[2] and Tewin Tencomnao[2]

[1]*Department of Preclinical Science, Faculty of Medicine, Thammasat University, Pathumthani 12120, Thailand*
[2]*Department of Clinical Chemistry, Faculty of Allied Health Sciences, Chulalongkorn University, Bangkok 10330, Thailand*

Correspondence should be addressed to Tewin Tencomnao; tewin.t@chula.ac.th

Academic Editor: Luciana Dini

This study was aimed at investigating the antioxidant activity of *Mangifera indica* Linn., *Cocos nucifera* Linn., and *Averrhoa carambola* Linn. and their biological effect on human keratinocytes affected by the ultraviolet B (UVB), a major cause of cell damage and skin cancer through induction of DNA damage, production of reactive oxygen species (ROS), and apoptosis. The richest antioxidant activity was found in ethanol fraction of *M. indica* (21.32 ± 0.66 mg QE/g dry weight), while the lowest one was found in aqueous fractions of *M. indica* and *C. nucifera* (1.76 ± 2.10 and 1.65 ± 0.38 mg QE/g dry weight, respectively). Ethanol and aqueous fractions of *A. carambola* ($250\,\mu g/mL$) significantly reduced the number of apoptotic cells. The expression of cleaved caspase 3 in UVB-treated group was significantly greater than that in untreated group. Both fractions of *A. carambola* ($50, 100$, and $250\,\mu g/mL$) significantly decreased the expression of cleaved caspase 3. Regarding the induction of DNA repair, ethanol (100 and $250\,\mu g/mL$) and aqueous ($50, 100$ and $250\,\mu g/mL$) fractions of *A. carambola* significantly decreased the percentage of cyclobutane pyrimidine dimers (CPD). Taken together, our results suggest that both fractions of *A. carambola* may be potentially developed for dermal applications.

1. Introduction

Ultraviolet B (UVB) is a well-known risk factor playing a role in photoaging and skin cancer in epidermis through triggering DNA damage or generating reactive oxygen species (ROS). ROS are chemically reactive molecules containing oxygen and play the important roles in cell signaling and homeostasis. In environmental stress such as UV or heat exposure, ROS levels can dramatically increase causing cell structures and DNA damage and apoptosis [1, 2]. Prevention of UVB-induced damage in skin by lowering ROS production is an evidence-based strategy against photoaging and skin cancer.

Thailand is rich in fruits that are not only diversified but also inexpensive and delicious. Unfortunately, there have been a few researches with evidence-based findings that demonstrate the health benefits of these fruits. For example,

resveratrol mostly found in grapes and red wine could exert photoprotective properties on UVB-irradiated cells. To reduce cell death in UVB-damaged skin, resveratrol reduced the production of ROS and attenuated the activation of caspase 3 and caspase 8 that play a major role in apoptosis [3]. Moreover, the extracts of *Elaeocarpus hygrophilus* (makoknum) and *Phyllanthus emblica* (makampom) had high antimicrobial and strong antioxidant activities [4].

Caspase 3 is an effector caspase protein frequently activated in mammalian cell apoptosis [5–7]. It is associated with the initiation of the death cascade. Pathways to caspase 3 activation are either extrinsic or intrinsic apoptotic pathways by interacting with caspase 8 and caspase 9, respectively. Besides apoptotic pathway, caspase 3 is essential for cell survival that converges on many events such as cell shrinkage, blebbing, chromatin condensation, and DNA fragmentation [7–10].

The other pathway through which UVB damages cells is DNA damage. UV induction of DNA damage is a factor that influences the normal life process of all organisms. Minor DNA damage is to allow effective repair, while more severe damage can induce apoptosis and cell cycle arrest. There are two types of UVB-induced DNA damage such as cyclobutane pyrimidine dimers (CPD) and pyrimidine (6-4) pyrimidone photoproducts (6-4PP). Two results (CPDs and 6-4PPs) are the transition of C to T and CC to TT. CPD contains a four-membered ring which is from the coupling of the double bonds (C=C) of pyrimidines. CPD is the major source of UV-induced mutations because these dimers interfere with base pairing during DNA replication. CPD is usually at a 5 to 10 folding higher frequency than 6-4PPs. In minor DNA damage, CPD is repaired by exogenous CPD photolyase [1, 2, 11].

Previous study provided the evidence to support the protective effect of Thailand native herb extracts on UVB-induced toxicity in human keratinocyte. It found that the extracts of turmeric and ginger could protect human keratinocyte from UVB-induced DNA damage and apoptosis through the attenuation of caspase 3 activity and CPD formation [12].

This objective of this study was to evaluate the protective effect of three Thai fruit species, *Mangifera indica* Linn., *Cocos nucifera* Linn., and *Averrhoa carambola* Linn., on UVB-induced damage in human keratinocytes. All fruits selected in this investigation were evaluated for their antioxidant activities as potential mechanisms for antiapoptotic activity and induction of DNA repair in human keratinocyte cell line (HaCaT). Development of natural products for dermal applications is our future goal based on the findings of this work.

In traditional medicine, *M. indica* was used to clear digestion and acidity. It is antidiuretic, antidiarrheal, antiemetic, and cardiac herb. Its fruits are known as a potential source of natural antioxidants containing phenolic compounds, ascorbate, and β-carotene [13].

The aqueous extract of *C. nucifera* was found to contain a free amino acid, L-arginine, which reduced the free radical generation. Moreover, vitamin C significantly reduced lipid peroxidation and increased antioxidant enzymes. *C. nucifera* could reduce lipid peroxidation content due to the high content of L-arginine. Besides, the high content of polyphenol could maintain the normal levels of lipid in tissue and serum. The aqueous extract of *C. nucifera* may be a new source of antineoplastic and antimultidrug resistance activities [14].

A. carambola or star fruits contain high polyphenol contents which were contributed significantly in ferric reducing capacity and radical scavenging capacity. Their antioxidant capacities were significantly increased with ripening and associated with flavonol, flavones, and hydrolysable tannins [15].

2. Materials and Methods

2.1. Chemicals and Reagents. All reagents used in this study were of analytical grade. Dimethyl sulfoxide (DMSO) and ethanol were purchased from Merck (Darmstadt, Germany). 1,4-Dithiothreitol (DTT) was purchased from Bio Basic Inc. (Ontario, Canada). Phenylmethyl sulphonyl fluoride (PMSF)

was purchased from United States Biochemicals (Cleveland, OH, USA). Kodak processing chemicals for autoradiography films, Amersham ECL Select Western blotting detection reagent, and Hyperfilm ECL were purchased from GE Healthcare (Piscataway, NJ, USA). Dulbecco's modified Eagle medium (DMEM)/high glucose were purchased from Sigma Aldrich Co. (St. Louis, MO, USA). Fetal bovine serum (FBS) and penicillin-streptomycin solution (10,000 units/mL of penicillin and 10,000 μg/mL of streptomycin) were purchased from HyClone (Logan, UT, USA).

A solution of 30% acrylamide/bis-acrylamide (37.5:1) was purchased from Biorad (Hercules, CA, USA). Ammonium persulfate (APS) was purchased from EMD Millipore (Billerica, MA, USA). The monoclonal rabbit anticaspase 3 (8G10, cat#9665) and polyclonal rabbit anti-GAPDH (14C10, cat#2118) were purchased from Cell Signaling Technology (Beverly, MA, USA). FITC Annexin V Apoptosis Detection kit with PI was purchased from Biolegend (CA, USA). OxiSelect™ Cellular UV-Induced DNA Damage ELISA Kit (CPD) was purchased from Cell Biolabs (CA, USA).

Folin Ciocalteu's phenol reagent, gallic acid, Aluminium Chloride ($AlCl_3$), Sodium Acetate (NaOAc), and Sodium Carbonate (Na_2CO_3) were purchased from Sigma Aldrich (USA).

2.2. Cell Line. HaCaT cells, an immortalized human epidermal keratinocyte cell line, were purchased from cell line service (Heidelberg, Germany). They were cultured in DMEM/high glucose containing 10% FBS and antibiotics (100 U/mL penicillin and 100 μg/mL streptomycin) at 37°C in a humidified atmosphere at 5% CO_2.

2.3. Plant Materials. Thai fruits were collected from Pathumthani and Nakornpathom provinces. They were authenticated based on their characteristics by Professor Dr. Thaweesakdi Boonkerd (Department of Botany, Faculty of Science, Chulalongkorn University). The voucher specimens deposited at Professor Kasin Suvatabhandhu Herbarium (Department of Botany, Faculty of Science, Chulalongkorn University) were A015246 (BCU), A015247 (BCU), and A015251 (BCU) for *A. carambola*, *M. indica*, and *C. nucifera*, respectively.

2.4. Thai Fruit Extraction. The dried fruits were extracted by maceration method using absolute ethanol (ratio 1:2) at 4°C for 48 h and filtered. For extraction using water, the mixture (ratio 1:2) was incubated at 100°C for 30 min and filtered. The residues were extracted twice. The two filtrates were combined and concentrated by evaporation at 45°C. The crude extracts were dissolved in DMSO or kept at -80°C until further investigation.

2.5. Antioxidant Determination by Folin Ciocalteu Phenol Assay and Total Flavonoid of Determination

2.5.1. Folin Ciocalteu Phenol Assay (FCP). Thai fruit extracts (50 μL) and 10% Folin Ciocalteu phenol reagent (50 μL) were mixed and incubated in the dark at room temperature for 30 min. Na_2CO_3 solution (35 μL) was added, mixed, and incubated in the dark at room temperature for 20 min. The absorbance of reaction was measured with a spectrophotometer at 750 nm. Gallic acid was used as a standard. The amount of phenolic compound is in gallic acid equivalent (GE) mg/g of dry weight.

2.5.2. Detection of Total Flavonoid.
Thai fruit extracts (50 μL) were mixed with the solution (150 μL of 100% ethanol, 10 μL of 1 M NaOAc, and 10 μL of AlCl$_3$). The mixture was incubated in the dark at room temperature for 40 min and the absorbance was measured with a spectrophotometer at 415 nm. Quercetin was used as a standard. The content of flavonoid is in Quercetin equivalent (QE) mg/g of dry weight.

2.6. The Effect of Thai Fruits Extracts on Cell Viability by MTT Assay.
Cells were seeded at 10,000 cells/well in 96-well plates and incubated at 37°C for 24 hours. Cells were treated with Thai fruit extracts at different concentrations ranging from 0 to 500 μg/mL for 48 hours. MTT working solution was added at 20 μL/well and incubated at 37°C for 4 hours. In this step, formazan product was formed. The cytotoxicity was detected by removing media carefully and dissolving formazan product with 150 μL of 100% DMSO. Supernatant was collected by centrifuge and transferred to a new 96-well plate and the absorbance was measured at 550 nm. The percentage of cell viability was calculated by using the formula

$$\% \text{ cell viability} = \frac{(\text{Abs}_{\text{treated cells}} - \text{Abs}_{\text{blank}})}{(\text{Abs}_{\text{untreated cells}} - \text{Abs}_{\text{blank}})} \times 100. \quad (1)$$

2.7. The Effect of UVB on Cell Viability by Trypan Blue Exclusion.
Cells were seeded in 6-well plates at 200,000 cells/well and cultured for 24 hours. Media were removed and cells were treated with UVB at different doses (0, 200, 400, 800, and 1600 mJ/cm^2). After UVB treatment, media were added and cells were cultured for 24 hours. To determine cell viability Trypan blue dye (ratio 1:10) was used.

2.8. The effect of Thai Fruit Extracts on Cell Apoptosis by Flow Cytometer.
Cells were seeded at 200,000 cells/well in 6-well plates and incubated at 37°C for 24 hours. Having been incubated, media were removed and cells were treated with UVB 200 mJ/cm^2. After treatment, cells were treated with Thai fruit extracts at the concentrations of 50, 100, and 250 μg/mL for 24 hours. Having been treated, media were removed and cold PBS was added to wash cells twice. Cells were harvested and recentrifuged at 400 g for 5 min. The supernatant was discarded and cells were resuspended in 100 μL of 1x annexin-binding buffer. Cell suspension was added with 2.5 μL of Alexa Fluor 488 annexin V and 5 μL of PI and incubated at room temperature for 15 min. Having been incubated, 400 μL of 1x annexin-binding buffer was added and cells were kept on ice. Cell apoptosis was analyzed by flow cytometry.

2.9. The Effect of Thai Fruit Extracts on Caspase 3 Protein Expression by Western Blotting.
Cells were seeded at 200,000 cells/well in 6-well plates and incubated at 37°C for 24 hours. Having been incubated, media were removed and cells were treated with UVB 200 mJ/cm^2. After treatment, Thai fruit extracts at the concentrations of 50, 100, and 250 μg/mL were treated for 24 hours. In the following day, protein extraction was carried out using 1 mM of DTT and 1 mM of PMSF in NP-40 lysis buffer. Total protein (20 μg) was mixed with Laemmli buffer (ratio 1:1) and boiled for 5 min. Protein was separated by 10% sodium dodecyl sulfate-polyacrylamide gel electrophoresis (SDS-PAGE) and transferred onto polyvinylidene difluoride (PVDF) membranes. Membranes were blocked with 5% nonfat milk either for 1 hour at room temperature or overnight at 4°C. Membranes were incubated with caspase 3 and GAPDH primary antibodies for 1 hour at room temperature or overnight at 4°C. After incubation, membranes were washed by 1x TBS-Tween 20 (TBST) for 15 min 3 times, incubated with secondary antibodies (anti-rabbit IgG, HRP-linked antibody) for 45 min at room temperature, and washed by TBST for 15 min 3 times. Protein bands were visualized by adding the enhanced chemiluminescence detection reagent and visualized by using Amersham Hyperfilm ECL and Kodak processing chemicals for autoradiography films. Each band was normalized against GAPDH as an internal control.

2.10. The Effect of Thai Fruit Extracts on UV-Induced DNA Damage.
Cells were seeded at 200,000 cells/well in 6-well plates and incubated at 37°C for 24 hours. Having been incubated, media were removed and cells were treated with UVB 200 mJ/cm^2. After treatment, cells were treated with Thai fruit extracts at the concentrations of 50, 100, and 250 μg/mL for 24 hours.

2.10.1. Fixation and Denaturation.
Media were removed and 100 μL of 75% methanol/25% acetic acid was added. Cells were incubated at room temperature for 30 min. Wells were aspirated and 100 μL of 70% ethanol was added and then they were incubated at room temperature for 30 min. Wells were aspirated and 100 μL of Denaturation Solution A was added and then they were incubated at room temperature for 5 min. Cells were gently washed with 200 μL of Dulbecco's Phosphate-Buffered Saline (DPBS) containing magnesium and calcium. After aspirating wells, 100 μL of Denaturation Solution B was added and then they were incubated at room temperature for 10 min. Wells were aspirated and 200 μL of Assay Diluent was added and they were incubated at room temperature for 30 min.

2.10.2. CPD Detection.
100 μL of diluted anti-CPD antibody was added to wells and they were incubated at room temperature for 1 hour on the orbital shaker. Wells were washed with 1x wash buffer.

2.11. Statistical Analysis.
Data were presented as the mean ± standard error (SD). Means were from three or more independent experiments. Data were analyzed by one-way analysis of variance (one-way ANOVA), followed by post hoc Dunnett's test (P value < 0.05).

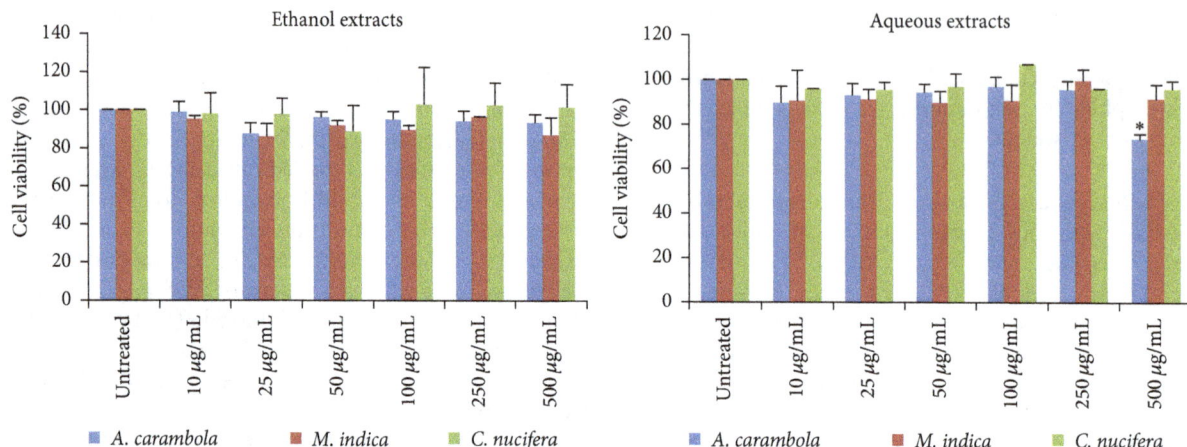

FIGURE 1: The effect of *M. indica*, *C. nucifera*, and *A. carambola* extracts on viability of HaCaT cells. Detection of cell viability was performed using MTT assay. HaCaT cells were treated with Thai fruit extracts at the concentration of 0–500 µg/mL for 48 h. The aqueous extract of *A. carambola* could significantly decrease cell viability. ∗ The aqueous extract of *A. carambola* at the concentration of 500 µg/mL could significantly decrease cell viability in comparison with the cell viability of untreated group.

3. Results

3.1. Total Phenol and Flavonoid Contents of M. indica, C. nucifera, and A. carambola Extracts.
Results of phenol and flavonoid of *M. indica*, *C. nucifera*, and *A. carambola* extracts were shown in Table 1. In all assays, the richest antioxidant activity was found in ethanol fraction of *M. indica* (21.32 ± 0.66 mg QE/g dry weight by total flavonoid determination). The lowest antioxidant activities were found in aqueous fractions of both *M. indica* and *C. nucifera* (1.76 ± 2.10 and 1.65 ± 0.38 mg QE/g dry weight, resp.).

3.2. The Effect of of M. indica, C. nucifera, and A. carambola Extracts on Cell Viability.
To evaluate the effect of Thai fruit extracts on HaCaT cell viability, MTT assay was employed. Cell was treated with the different concentrations of extracts (0–500 µg/mL). Results of cytotoxicity of all extracts were shown in Figure 1. The aqueous extract of *A. carambola* at the concentration of 500 µg/mL could significantly decrease cell viability (73.42% ± 3.66, $P < 0.05$). Therefore, three concentrations of all extracts used in this study were 50, 100, and 250 µg/mL.

3.3. The Effect of UVB Intensity on Cell Viability.
Evaluating the effect of UVB intensity on cell viability was employed by Trypan blue assay. Cells were treated with different intensities of UVB (0–1,600 mJ/cm^2). The lowest intensity that could significantly decrease cell viability was 200 mJ/cm^2. Results of the effect of all intensity of UVB on cell viability were shown in Figure 2.

3.4. The Protective Effect of All Fractions of M. indica, C. nucifera, and A. carambola Extracts on UVB-Induced Apoptosis by Flow Cytometry.
Results of the protective effect of all fractions on UVB-induced apoptosis were shown in Figures 3(a) and 3(b). Ethanol and aqueous fractions of *A. carambola* (250 µg/mL) could significantly decrease the

TABLE 1: Total phenol and flavonoid contents of *M. indica*, *C. nucifera*, and *A. carambola* extracts derived from ethanol and aqueous solvents.

Extracts	Phenol content (mg GE/g dry weight)		Flavonoid content (mg QE/g dry weight)	
	Ethanol	Aqueous	Ethanol	Aqueous
M. indica	3.04 ± 2.52	3.22 ± 0.11	21.32 ± 0.66	1.76 ± 2.10
A. carambola	4.13 ± 1.51	5.27 ± 2.96	6.34 ± 0.13	5.94 ± 0.60
C. nucifera	2.21 ± 0.11	4.36 ± 0.12	2.89 ± 1.89	1.65 ± 0.38

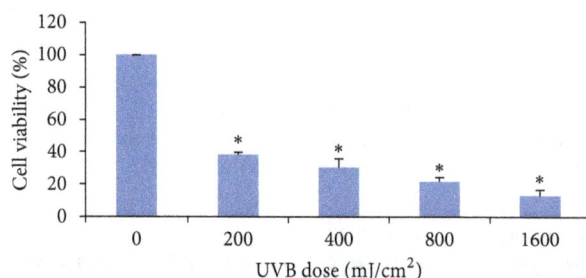

FIGURE 2: The effect of all UVB intensities on cell viability by Trypan blue assay. Cell viability values shown as mean ± SD were derived from 3 independent experiments. ∗ The cell viability in UVB-treated groups (200-1,600 mJ/cm^2) significantly decreased when comparing to that in UVB-untreated group (0 mJ/cm^2).

number of apoptotic cells in comparison with the number of apoptotic cells in the UVB-treated group ($P < 0.05$).

3.5. The Effect of M. indica, C. nucifera, and A. carambola Extracts on Caspase 3 Expression by Western Blot.
Since caspase 3 plays a major role in caspase-dependent apoptosis, the effect of Thai fruit extracts on the reduction of cleaved caspase 3 expression was investigated in this investigation. Using Western blot analysis, the aqueous extract (Figure 4(a))

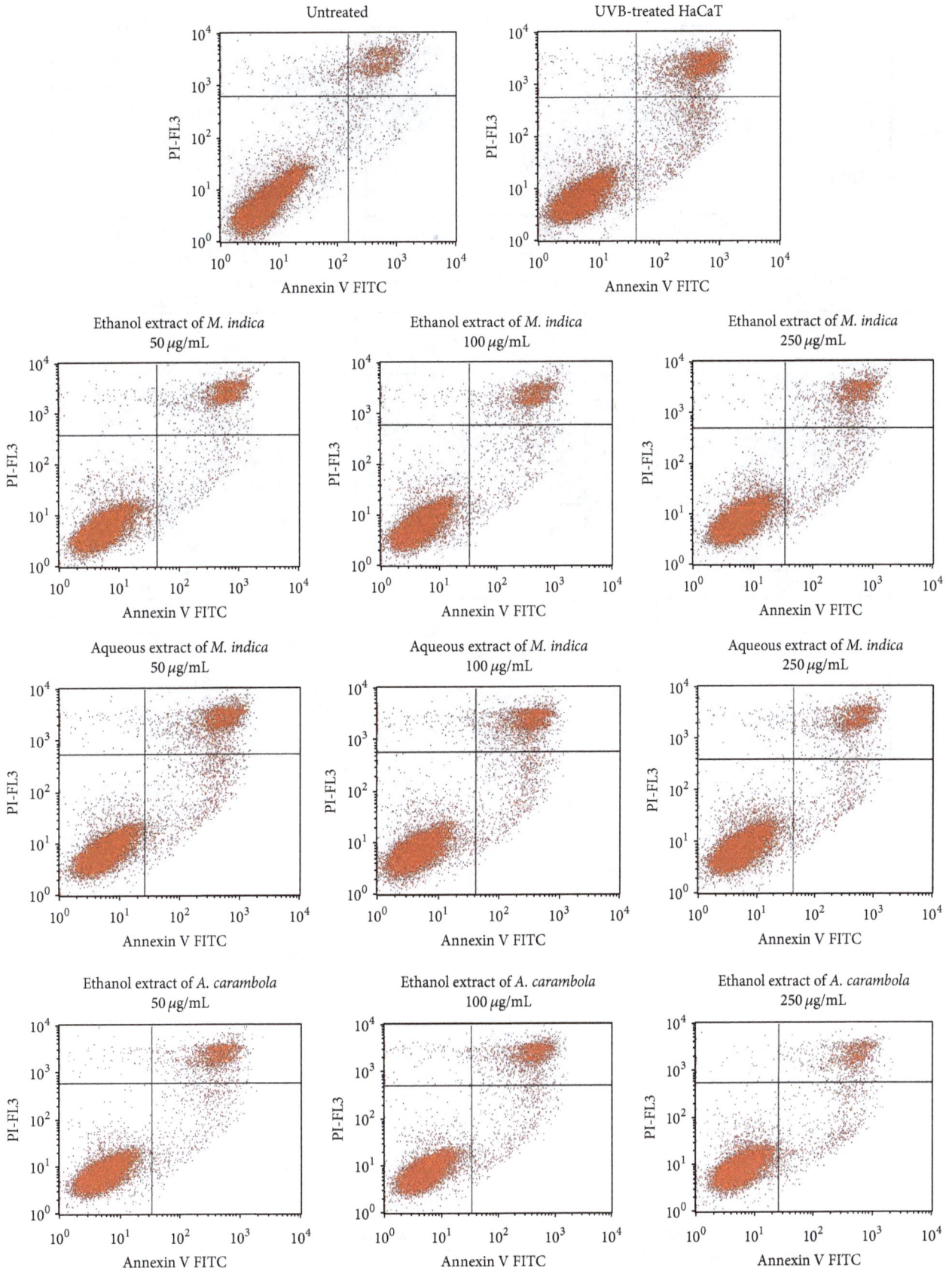

FIGURE 3: Continued.

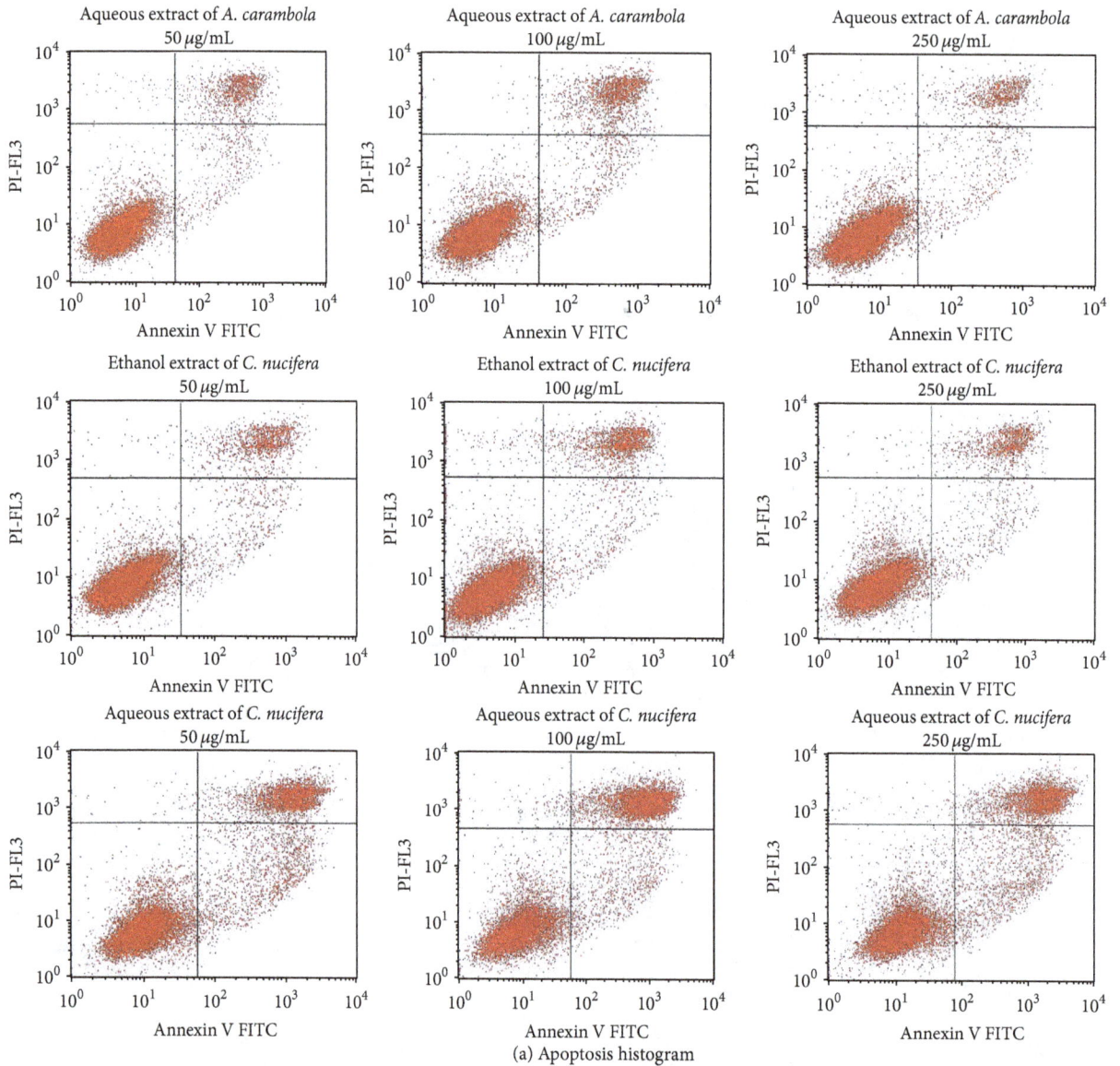

(a) Apoptosis histogram

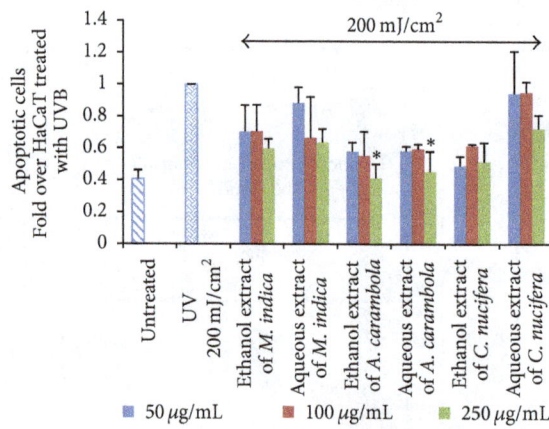

(b) The number of apoptotic cells

FIGURE 3: The effect of *M. indica*, *C. nucifera*, and *A. carambola* extracts on apoptosis of UVB-treated HaCaT cells. HaCaT cells were treated with UVB intensity at $200 \, \text{mJ/cm}^2$ and Thai fruit extracts at the concentration of 50, 100, and $250 \, \mu\text{g/mL}$ for 24 h. Apoptotic cell images were shown as histogram (a) and apoptotic values were shown as mean ± SD derived from 3 independent experiments (b). ∗ The extracts of both fractions of *A. carambola* ($250 \, \mu\text{g/mL}$) could significantly decrease the number of apoptotic cells in comparison with the number of apoptotic cells in the UVB-treated group.

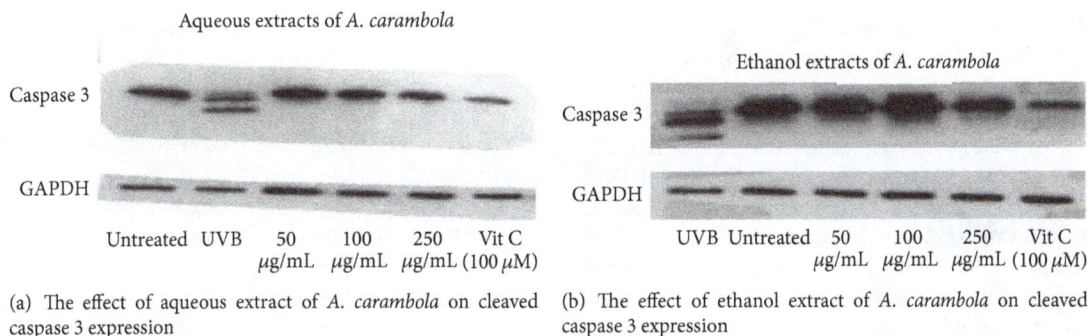

Aqueous extracts of *A. carambola*

Ethanol extracts of *A. carambola*

(a) The effect of aqueous extract of *A. carambola* on cleaved caspase 3 expression

(b) The effect of ethanol extract of *A. carambola* on cleaved caspase 3 expression

FIGURE 4: The effect of both aqueous (a) and ethanol (b) extracts of *A. carambola* on cleaved caspase 3 expression. Cleaved caspase 3 expression was increased when cells were treated with UVB ($200 \, mJ/cm^2$). After UVB stimulation, cells were treated with extracts for 24 h. Both extracts of *A. carambola* could significantly decrease cleaved caspase 3 expression.

and the ethanol extract (Figure 4(b)) of *A. carambola* could decrease the cleavage of caspase 3 expression after 24 hours of extract treatment. Vitamin C was used as a standard.

3.6. The Effect of M. indica, C. nucifera, and A. carambola Extracts on the Induction of DNA Repair by Cyclobutane Pyrimidine Dimers (CPD) Detection.

CPD is the product of UVB-induced DNA lesions. In this study, UVB ($200 \, mJ/cm^2$) treatment could significantly increase CPD expression. After the treatment of Thai fruit extracts, the result showed that ethanol (100 and 250 μg/mL) and aqueous (50, 100, and 250 μg/mL) fractions of *A. carambola* could significantly decrease the percentage of CPD ($P < 0.05$). The results were shown in Figure 5.

4. Discussion

UVB is a major cause of cell damage and skin cancer through inducing DNA damage and apoptosis. There are two pathways that decrease UVB-induced cell damage such as antiapoptosis and DNA damage repair. The effect of these extracts on apoptosis was detected by flow cytometry and Western blot analysis.

According to the flow cytometric data, the percentage of apoptotic cells in the untreated group was significantly different from that in the UVB-treated group, suggesting that UVB at $200 \, mJ/cm^2$ could lead to the increase in apoptotic cells. In addition, both ethanol and aqueous extracts of *A. carambola* at the concentration of 250 μg/mL could significantly decrease the percentage of the number of apoptotic cells ($P < 0.05$).

To confirm the effect of both extracts on protecting UV-induced apoptosis, the expression of caspase 3 was detected by Western blot. Many studies indicated that caspase 3 (35 kDa) in UVB-treated cells was cleaved. Cleaved caspase 3 (17 and 19 kDa) is an important factor which plays a role in the induction of cell apoptosis through apoptotic pathway [7, 16–21].

It was recently reported that vitamin C exerted antiapoptotic activity by attenuating caspase 3 expression [22, 23]. Therefore, vitamin C was used as a control in this study.

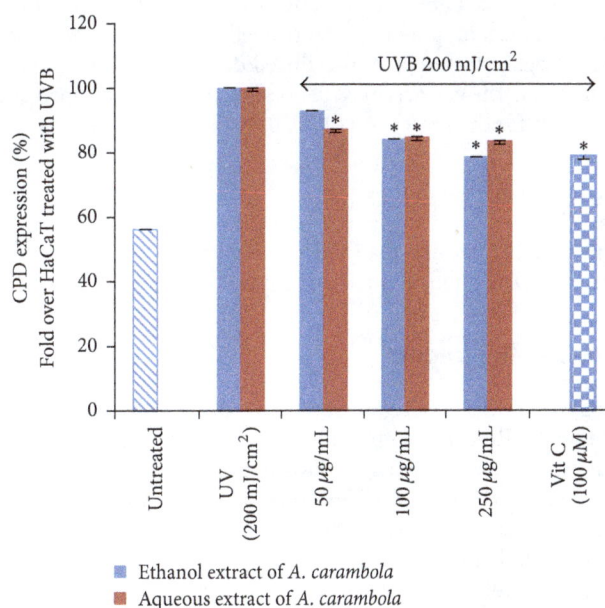

FIGURE 5: CPD expression in cells treated with UVB $200 \, mJ/cm^2$; both extracts of *A. carambola* and 100 μM of vitamin C. The level of CPD expression was low in untreated group. UVB could induce DNA damage causing CPD expression to increase. After extract treatment for 24 h, CPD expression was significantly decreased. Values of CPD expression were shown as mean ± SD derived from 3 independent experiments. ∗ The ethanol (100 and 250 μg/mL) and aqueous (50, 100, and 250 μg/mL) fractions of *A. carambola* could significantly decrease the percentage of CPD in comparison with the percentage of CPD in the UVB-treated group.

Results of the expression of cleaved caspase 3 decreasing in both ethanol and aqueous fractions of *A. carambola*-treated and vitamin C-treated cells implied that the attenuation of cleaved caspase 3 was involved in cell survival after UVB irradiation [20, 24, 25].

The results showed that the level of CPD expression was increased when treated with UVB. After UVB radiation, CPD level in *A. carambola*-treated group was significantly decreased ($P < 0.05$).

The extract of *A. carambola* has been used in the traditional medicine for treating many diseases such as diabetes and diabetic nephropathy. Many studies indicated that it could inhibit apoptotic pathway by attenuating the activation of caspase 3, caspase 8, and caspase 9 [26, 27]. Level of active caspase 3 can affect the formation of DNA fragmentation, since caspase 3 is a primary activator which induces the cleavage of DNA fragmentation factor (DFF) complex. Cleaved DFF causes DNA damage and cell death [9, 28]. To date, there are not many studies to investigate the effect of *A. carambola* extract on DNA damage and cytotoxicity.

Collectively, our results showed that both ethanol and aqueous fractions of *A. carambola* could attenuate UVB-induced damage in human keratinocytes by inhibiting the cleavage of caspase 3 and CPD formation in the HaCaT keratinocyte cell line. The present study is the first to provide the evidence of potent protective effect of *A. carambola* extract against ultraviolet B-induced damage in human keratinocytes. The extracts of *A. carambola* may be developed as the agent for the protection of UVB-induced damage in skin.

Conflict of Interests

The authors declare that there is no conflict of interests regarding the publication of this paper.

Acknowledgments

This work was finally supported by the Royal Thai Government's Research Fund (to Chalinee Ronpirin) and the Ratchadapisek Sompoch Endowment Fund (2015) of Chulalongkorn University, CU-58-003-HR (to Tewin Tencomnao). The authors would like to acknowledge Professor Dr. Thaweesakdi Boonkerd, Department of Botany, Faculty of Science, Chulalongkorn University, for herbal authentication and Department of Immunology, Faculty of Dentistry, Chulalongkorn University, for allowing the authors to access the flow cytometry facility.

References

[1] R. P. Rastogi, Richa, A. Kumar, M. B. Tyagi, and R. P. Sinha, "Molecular mechanisms of ultraviolet radiation-induced DNA damage and repair," *Journal of Nucleic Acids*, vol. 2010, Article ID 592980, 32 pages, 2010.

[2] H.-L. Lo, S. Nakajima, L. Ma et al., "Differential biologic effects of CPD and 6-4PP UV-induced DNA damage on the induction of apoptosis and cell-cycle arrest," *BMC Cancer*, vol. 5, article 135, 2005.

[3] D. L. Narayanan, R. N. Saladi, and J. L. Fox, "Review: ultraviolet radiation and skin cancer," *International Journal of Dermatology*, vol. 49, no. 9, pp. 978–986, 2010.

[4] S. Nanasombat, K. Khanha, J. Phan-im et al., "Antimicrobial and antioxidant activities of Thai local fruit extracts: application of a selected fruit extract. *Phyllanthus emblica* Linn. as a natural preservative in raw ground pork during refrigerated storage," *The Online Journal of Science and Technology*, vol. 2, no. 1, pp. 1–7, 2012.

[5] D. W. Nicholson and N. A. Thornberry, "Caspases: killer proteases," *Trends in Biochemical Sciences*, vol. 22, no. 8, pp. 299–306, 1997.

[6] M. D. Jacobson, M. Weil, and M. C. Raff, "Review: programmed cell death in animal development," *Cell*, vol. 88, no. 3, pp. 347–354, 1997.

[7] A. G. Porter and R. U. Jänicke, "Review: emerging roles of caspase-3 in apoptosis," *Cell Death & Differentiation*, vol. 6, no. 2, pp. 99–104, 1999.

[8] R. U. Jänicke, M. L. Sprengart, M. R. Wati, and A. G. Porter, "Caspase-3 is required for DNA fragmentation and morphological changes associated with apoptosis," *The Journal of Biological Chemistry*, vol. 273, no. 16, pp. 9357–9360, 1998.

[9] B. B. Wolf, M. Schuler, F. Echeverri, and D. R. Green, "Caspase-3 is the primary activator of apoptotic DNA fragmentation via DNA fragmentation factor-45/inhibitor of caspase-activated DNase inactivation," *The Journal of Biological Chemistry*, vol. 274, no. 43, pp. 30651–30656, 1999.

[10] S. Sahara, M. Aoto, Y. Eguchi, N. Imamoto, Y. Yoneda, and Y. Tsujimoto, "Acinus is a caspase-3-activated protein required for apoptotic chromatin condensation," *Nature*, vol. 401, no. 6749, pp. 168–173, 1999.

[11] R. Drouin and J.-P. Therrien, "UVB-induced cyclobutane pyrimidine dimer frequency correlates with skin cancer mutational hotspots in p53," *Photochemistry and Photobiology*, vol. 66, no. 5, pp. 719–726, 1997.

[12] V. Thongrakard, N. Ruangrungsi, M. Ekkapongpisit, C. Isidoro, and T. Tencomnao, "Protection from UVB toxicity in human keratinocytes by thailand native herbs extracts," *Photochemistry and Photobiology*, vol. 90, no. 1, pp. 214–224, 2014.

[13] S. M. Rocha Ribeiro, J. H. De Queiroz, M. E. Lopes Ribeiro de Queiroz, F. M. Campos, and H. M. Pinheiro Sant'Ana, "Antioxidant in mango (*Mangifera indica* L.) pulp," *Plant Foods for Human Nutrition*, vol. 62, no. 1, pp. 13–17, 2007.

[14] M. DebMandal and S. Mandal, "Coconut (*Cocos nucifera* L.: Arecaceae): in health promotion and disease prevention," *Asian Pacific Journal of Tropical Medicine*, vol. 4, no. 3, pp. 241–247, 2011.

[15] Y. S. Lim and S. T. Lee, "In vitro antioxidant capacities of star fruit (*Averrhoa carambola*), an underutilised tropical fruit," *Journal of Biology*, vol. 1, no. 1, pp. 21–24, 2013.

[16] C.-H. Lee, S.-B. Wu, C.-H. Hong, H.-S. Yu, and Y.-H. Wei, "Molecular mechanisms of UV-induced apoptosis and its effects on skin residential cells: the implication in UV-based phototherapy," *International Journal of Molecular Sciences*, vol. 14, no. 3, pp. 6414–6435, 2013.

[17] K. Park and J.-H. Lee, "Photosensitizer effect of curcumin on UVB-irradiated HaCaT cells through activation of caspase pathways," *Oncology Reports*, vol. 17, no. 3, pp. 537–540, 2007.

[18] S. Namura, J. Zhu, K. Fink et al., "Activation and cleavage of caspase-3 in apoptosis induced by experimental cerebral ischemia," *Journal of Neuroscience*, vol. 18, no. 10, pp. 3659–3668, 1998.

[19] A. M. Roy, M. S. Baliga, C. A. Elmets, and S. K. Katiyar, "Grape seed proanthocyanidins induce apoptosis through p53, bax, and caspase 3 pathways," *Neoplasia*, vol. 7, no. 1, pp. 24–36, 2005.

[20] N. Mendelev, S. Witherspoon, and P. A. Li, "Overexpression of human selenoprotein H in neuronal cells ameliorates ultraviolet irradiation-induced damage by modulating cell signaling pathways," *Experimental Neurology*, vol. 220, no. 2, pp. 328–334, 2009.

Protective Effect of Mangifera indica Linn., Cocos nucifera Linn., and Averrhoa carambola Linn. Extracts...

99

[21] Y.-K. Park and B.-C. Jang, "UVB-induced anti-survival and pro-apoptotic effects on HaCaT human keratinocytes via caspase- and PKC-dependent downregulation of PKB, HIAP-1, Mcl-1, XIAP and ER stress," *International Journal of Molecular Medicine*, vol. 33, no. 3, pp. 695–702, 2014.

[22] B. Cheng, Y. Zhang, A. Wang, Y. Dong, and Z. Xie, "Vitamin C attenuates isoflurane-induced caspase-3 activation and cognitive impairment," *Molecular Neurobiology*, vol. 52, no. 3, pp. 1580–1589, 2014.

[23] O. Ozmen and F. Mor, "Effects of vitamin C on pathology and caspase-3 activity of kidneys with subacute endosulfan toxicity," *Biotechnic & Histochemistry*, vol. 90, no. 1, pp. 25–30, 2014.

[24] K. Park and J.-H. Lee, "Protective effects of resveratrol on UVB-irradiated HaCaT cells through attenuation of the caspase pathway," *Oncology Reports*, vol. 19, no. 2, pp. 413–417, 2008.

[25] L. Jing, S. Kumari, N. Mendelev, and P. A. Li, "Coenzyme Q10 ameliorates ultraviolet B irradiation induced cell death through inhibition of mitochondrial intrinsic cell death pathway," *International Journal of Molecular Sciences*, vol. 12, no. 11, pp. 8302–8315, 2011.

[26] Q. Wen, T. Liang, F. Qin et al., "Lyoniresinol 3α-O-β-D-glucopyranoside-mediated hypoglycaemia and its influence on apoptosis-regulatory protein expression in the injured kidneys of streptozotocin-induced mice," *PLoS ONE*, vol. 8, no. 12, Article ID e81772, 2013.

[27] X. Xu, T. Liang, Q. Wen et al., "Protective effects of total extracts of *Averrhoa carambola* l. (oxalidaceae) roots on streptozotocin-induced diabetic mice," *Cellular Physiology and Biochemistry*, vol. 33, no. 5, pp. 1272–1282, 2014.

[28] E. Sharif-Askari, A. Alam, E. Rhéaume et al., "Direct cleavage of the human DNA fragmentation factor-45 by granzyme B induces caspase-activated DNase release and DNA fragmentation," *The EMBO Journal*, vol. 20, no. 12, pp. 3101–3113, 2001.

12

Chinese Herbal Medicine for Functional Abdominal Pain Syndrome: From Clinical Findings to Basic Understandings

Tao Liu,[1] Ning Wang,[2] Li Zhang,[1] and Linda Zhong[3]

[1]*Institute of Digestive Diseases, Longhua Hospital, Shanghai University of Traditional Chinese Medicine, Shanghai 200032, China*
[2]*School of Chinese Medicine, Li Ka Shing Faculty of Medicine, University of Hong Kong, Pok Fu Lam, Hong Kong*
[3]*School of Chinese Medicine, Hong Kong Chinese Medicine Study Centre, Hong Kong Baptist University, Kowloon Tong, Hong Kong*

Correspondence should be addressed to Li Zhang; zhangli.hl@163.com and Linda Zhong; ldzhong@hkbu.edu.hk

Academic Editor: Raffaele Capasso

Functional abdominal pain syndrome (FAPS) is one of the less common functional gastrointestinal disorders. Conventional therapy has unsatisfactory response to it so people turn to Chinese medicine for help. Currently, we reviewed the whole picture of Chinese herbal medicine (CHM) clinical and basic application in the treatment of FAPS, especially the traditional Chinese medicine (TCM) syndrome, the single herb, and Chinese medicine formulae, thus to provide a solid base to further develop evidence-based study for this common gastrointestinal complaint in the future. We developed the search strategy and set the inclusion and exclusion criteria for article search. From the included articles, we totally retrieved 586 records according to our searching criteria, of which 16 were duplicate records and 291 were excluded for reasons of irrelevance. The full text of 279 articles was retrieved for detailed assessment, of which 123 were excluded for various reasons. The number one used single herb is Radix Ginseng. The most common syndrome was *liver qi depression*. The most frequently used classic formula was Si-Mo-Tang. This reflected the true situation of clinical practice of Chinese medicine practitioners and could be further systematically synthesized as key points of the therapeutic research for FAPS.

1. Introduction

Functional abdominal pain syndrome (FAPS) is one of the less common functional gastrointestinal disorders [1]. It also has less investigation compared to other functional digestive disorders, namely, irritable bowel disorder (IBS) and functional constipation (FC). The disorder is characterized by continuous, almost continuous, or at least frequently recurrent abdominal pain that is poorly related to bowel habits and often not well localized [2]. Until currently, the definition and diagnosis of FAPS have only been recognized. The Rome III classification has symptom-based criteria to diagnose FAPS [3]. Diagnostic criteria (criteria fulfilled for the last 3 months with symptom onset at least 6 months before diagnosis) for functional abdominal pain syndrome must include all of the following:

(1) Continuous or nearly continuous abdominal pain.

(2) No or only occasional relationship of pain with physiological events (e.g., eating, defecation, or menses).

(3) Some loss of daily functioning.

(4) The pain is not feigned (e.g., malingering).

(5) Insufficient symptoms to meet criteria for another functional gastrointestinal disorder that would explain the pain.

Another feature about it is that FAPS appears highly related to alterations in endogenous pain modulation systems, which is consistent with dysfunction of descending pain modulation and cortical pain modulation circuits.

The epidemiology of FAPS is very limited because of the lack of available data and the difficulties in establishing a diagnosis that can be differentiated from other more common functional gastrointestinal disorders [4]. Some research indicated that the prevalence of FAPS ranges from 0.5% to 2% in North America and a female predominance was noted (F : M = 1 : 1.5). A substantial proportion of patients are referred to gastroenterology practices and medical centers; they have a disproportionate number of health care visits and often undergo numerous diagnostic procedures and treatments.

The clinical manifestation is characterized by the presence of continuous or frequently recurrent abdominal pain associated with loss of daily functioning [3]. FAPS is better understood as an abnormal perception of normal (regulatory) gut function, instead of a true motility disorder. Therefore, patients with FAPS will not typically experience relief of pain after defecation (a pattern that is characteristic for irritable bowel syndrome [IBS]), supporting the contention that disturbances in bowel motility do not fully explain the pain [1, 2, 4, 5]. In contrast to other functional gastrointestinal disorders, treatments for patients with conventional medicine are empirical and not based on results from well-designed clinical trials. It focuses on establishing an effective patient-physician relationship, following a general treatment approach, and offering more specific management that often encompasses a combination of treatment options [1–7]. So far, there is no satisfactory therapy for FAPS and many people seek Chinese medicine (CM) for help.

According to CM, FAPS usually belongs to the CM syndrome of "abdominal pain," which related to exogenous evils, intemperate diet, yang deficiency, and liver qi stagnation. In summary, FAPS in CM could be classified into two main types. One is excessive syndrome, including exogenous evils, intemperate diet, dampness-heat, and qi stagnation; the other is deficient syndrome, including yang deficiency and qi deficiency. When exogenous cold and wind attack the abdomen or excessive raw and cold foods injure the stomach or abdomen, all these will impair and block qi movement. Such blockage will lead to abdominal pain. Dampness and heat will also invade and lodge qi movement [8].

The treatment of CM for FAPS is based on the criteria of syndrome differentiation [9]. In general, herbal treatment and acupuncture are the main two approaches. In this paper, we will focus on Chinese herbal medicine (CHM), especially the single herb, Chinese medicine formulae, CM syndromes, and their related Chinese medicine syndrome. The key clinical syndromes of FAPS include five main types, which are *blockage by cold, qi stagnation, dampness-heat, yang deficiency,* and *qi deficiency*. The first three types belong to excessive syndromes and the latter two types belong to deficient syndrome. When treating abdominal pain, be careful to identify the affected meridian, ascertain whether it is due to qi or to cold or heat, and differentiate between excessive and deficient syndrome. For abdominal pain of excessive syndrome emphasize expulsion of disease evil and relief of blockage [10–12]. For abdominal pain of deficient syndrome emphasize warm-augmentation of yang and qi [13–15]. Based on these principles, syndrome-based CHM treatments given to FAPS patients generally include (i) warming the interior organ and dispelling cold; (ii) unblocking the liver, reliving stagnation, and regulating qi movement; (iii) cooling heat, dry dampness, relieving stagnation; (iv) warming the stomach and intestine, augmenting qi, and strengthening the spleen to stop pain; (v) nourishing the vital energy of spleen qi [16–20].

In this review article, we mainly presented a Chinese medical view about the etiology and therapy of FAPS, investigate the clinical study on CM for FAPS to reveal the single herbs, Chinese medicine formula, internal application of CM, and so forth, and tried to discuss the scientific basis of CM so as to provide a better understanding of CM for FAPS.

2. Material and Methods

Many CHM interventions have been applied for the treatment of FAPS. However, these reports of the clinical study lacked the benefits of individual interventions or individual types of interventions. Another problem is that since the field of FAPS is still not emphasized by both scientists and clinicians, the research in FAPS has very low quality. There is limited evidence-based information from studies specifically designed for the treatment of FAPS. In order to investigate the whole picture of CHM applications in the treatment of FAPS based on syndrome-based differentiation, especially the single herbs, Chinese medicine formula, and CM syndrome, we systematically reviewed all the available data from current databases including clinical trials, clinical observational studies, case studies, and case reports. Based on the large data sets of conventional medicine literature (PubMed, Ovid, etc.) and traditional Chinese medicine literature (SinoMed, CNKI, etc.), we also applied data slicing algorithm in text mining [20]. Through all the comprehensive data searching and synthesis, we aim to investigate the current clinical practice situation of CHM for FAPS and also the basic research of CHM for FAPS.

2.1. Literatures Search. Primary electronic database search is listed as below: all EBM reviews, including Cochrane DSR, ACP Journal Club, DARE, CCTR, CMR, HTA, and NHSEED (from inception to Dec. 2015); Embase 1980–Dec. 2015; Embase Classic 1947 to Dec. 2015; PubMed (from inception to Dec. 2015); Ovid MEDLINE(R) 1950–Dec. 2015; Ovid OLDMEDLINE(R) 1948–1965; SinoMed (1978–Dec. 2015); China Journals Full-Text Database (1994–Dec. 2015); CBM Disc (1979–Dec. 2015). Secondary hand search included bibliographic references of identified literatures, textbooks, review articles, and meta-analyses. The search strategy in the study included (abdominal pain* OR chronic abdominal pain* OR functional abdominal pain*) AND (herb* OR herbal medicine* OR traditional Chinese medicine OR Chinese medicine OR herbal medicine OR complementary medicine OR naturopathy).

All Chinese-to-English translations were deduced primarily from *the World Health Organization (WHO) Evidence-Based Complementary and Alternative Medicine International Standard Terminologies on Traditional Medicine in the Western Pacific Region* [21].

2.2. Interventions to Be Included. Studies of CHM interventions including but not limited to all forms of herbal treatment (single herb, classical formulae, new formulae, herb-derived products, and combination products) should be included.

2.3. Trials to Be Included. The trials to be included were as follows: (1) quasi or randomized controlled trials;

(2) observational clinical studies; (3) case series or case reports; (4) other types of appropriate research methods.

2.4. Data to Be Considered. The data to be considered was as follows: (1) study subjects of any age and gender with FAPS; (2) objective measures by laboratory or imaging techniques; (3) measurement from other informants or nursing staff or patients.

2.5. Data Extraction. Two authors searched the databases and selected the relevant publications independently. If there were any disagreements about the eligibility of a study, the two authors would check the study against the selection criteria, discuss its eligibility, and come to a further decision. One author extracted the data and the other checked the extracted data. For each study, the following variables were extracted: study design, sample size, mode of recruitment, sampling and diagnostic procedure, inclusion and exclusion criteria, and participants' characteristics including age, gender, and duration. TCM patterns, TCM treatment principles, treatment regimen, and outcome of TCM treatments were obtained.

2.6. Quality Assessment. For RCTs of CHM, methodological quality will be assessed using the Jadad scale. The Jadad scale evaluates a study in terms of the description of randomization, blinding, and dropouts. Points are awarded if the study is described as randomized, 1 point; has an appropriate randomization method, 1 point; is described as double-blind, 1 point; uses appropriate blinding method, 1 point; and has description of withdrawals and dropouts, 1 point. The Jadad scale ranges from 1 to 5, and RCTs with a score from 3 to 5 are regarded as better quality trials.

2.7. Text Data Mining. Besides the systematic literature searching, we also conducted text data mining. The text data mining was conducted by filtering the biomedical literature on FAPS in SinoMed (http://www.sinomed.ac.cn/) on Feb. 25, 2016, and we downloaded associated literature data set containing items. We also applied dictionary-based data slicing algorithm which is constructed on the principle of cooccurrence; we filtered the downloaded literature data with traditional Chinese medicine associated keywords, for example, Chinese herbal medicine, Chinese patent medicine, and TCM syndrome which are collected from textbooks and the Internet [20]. This data mining is a good supplement for literature searching since it will provide some insights into the quantitative relationship between the individual herbs and formula in the treatment of FAPS.

3. Results and Discussion

3.1. Clinical Study and Chinese Medicine Interventions for FAPS. Totally, we accessed 586 records according to our searching criteria, of which 16 were duplicate records and 291 were excluded for reasons of irrelevance. The full text of 279 articles was retrieved for detailed assessment, of which 123 were excluded for various reasons (Figure 1). Of the included 156 studies which fulfilled the inclusion and

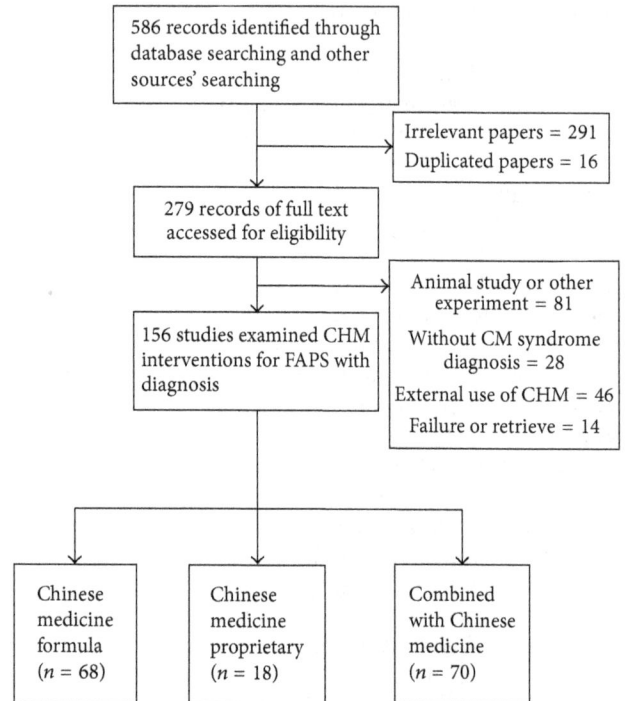

FIGURE 1: Flowchart of literature selection logistics.

exclusion criteria, 68 were on Chinese medicine formula, 18 were on Chinese medicine proprietary, and 70 were on a combination of Chinese herbal medicine with conventional treatment. Sample size of the 156 studies ranged from 30 to 210.

3.2. TCM Syndrome Category and Treatment Criteria. From the included articles, we totally retrieved 53 different TCM syndrome diagnoses from 156 individual studies. The most common pattern was *liver qi depression*, which was diagnosed in 407 subjects (frequency among all the studies = 37, percentage among the top five diagnoses = 32.5%); it was followed by *liver qi invading the stomach* (subjects = 217, frequency = 24, 21.1%), *liver depression and spleen deficiency* (subjects = 189, frequency = 21, 18.4%), *qi stagnation due to cold* (subjects = 167, frequency = 16, 14.0%), and *spleen-stomach deficiency cold* (subjects = 148, frequency = 14.0%). The results were listed in Table 1.

In all the commonly applied TCM syndromes, we could analyze that, among the top five syndromes, three belonged to excessive syndrome and the other could be categorized as combination of deficiency and sufficiency or deficient syndrome. The result was consistent with other studies by other researchers of syndrome distribution among FAPS patients, especially the elderly and children [17–19].

3.3. TCM Single Herbs and TCM Syndrome-Based Chinese Herbal Formulae. The top ten most frequently used herbs and their action were listed in Table 2. The top ten single herbs are Radix Ginseng, Rhizoma Atractylodis Macrocephalae, Pericarpium Citri Reticulatae, Semen Arecae, Lignum

TABLE 1: Top five most commonly used TCM syndromes for FAPS.

TCM syndrome	Therapeutic principle	Number of subjects diagnosed with the diagnosis	Number of frequency among all the studies	Percentage among the total syndrome (53)/top 5 syndrome diagnoses
Liver qi depression 肝气郁结	Soothe the liver and regulate qi	407	37	69.5%/32.5%
Liver qi invading the stomach 肝胃不和	Harmonize the liver and stomach	217	24	45.3%/21.1%
Liver depression and spleen deficiency 肝郁脾虚	Soothe the liver and fortify the spleen	189	21	39.6%/18.4%
Qi stagnation due to cold congealing 寒凝气滞	Dissipate cold and move qi	167	16	30.2%/14.0%
Spleen-stomach deficiency cold 脾胃虚寒	Warm the middle and dissipate cold	148	16	30.2%/14.0%

Aquilariae Resinatum, Radix Linderae, Rhizoma Corydalis, Radix Aucklandiae, Rhizoma Zingiberis Recens, and Radix Glycyrrhizae. Among 68 studies on Chinese herbal formulae, the most frequently used Chinese herbal formulae based on syndrome diagnosis were Si-Mo-Tang and its modification (number of frequency among all the studies, $N = 28$, percentage among the top five formulae, $p = 24.6\%$). It was the same as Tong-Xie-Yao-Fang ($N = 28$, $p = 24.6\%$) and followed by Wen-Dan-Tang ($N = 21$, $p = 18.4\%$), Xiang-Sha-Liu-Jun-Zi-Tang ($N = 19$, $p = 16.7\%$), and Xiao-Yao-San ($N = 18$, $p = 15.8\%$). The most five commonly used TCM syndrome-based Chinese herbal formulae and their indications were summarized in Table 3. From this summary, we could clearly notice that the frequency of single herbs is consistent with the combination of the mostly used Chinese herbal formulae. The data mining of Chinese herbal formulae and single herbs was very helpful for us to further discover the mechanisms of TCM in the treatment of FAPS and its potential new combination.

Attention should also be paid to the fact that many studies regarding Chinese herbal formula or Chinese herbal medicine proprietary did not provide the standard criteria or even the complete diagnosis criteria of the syndrome. The results from these studies could not be compared or repeated if the diagnostic criteria varied or were penurious.

3.4. Pharmacological Study of Chinese Herbal Medicine on FAPS. Although abundant clinical studies, which has been elaborated as above, have investigated the efficacy of Chinese herbal medicine in treating FAPS, studies on its scientific evidence are not yet available. This may be due to the insufficient understanding of the pathophysiology of FAPS, as well as a scientifically convincing preclinical model being available. Few pathophysiological studies were conducted particularly on clinical FAPS patients, as it is not easy, in a biomedical aspect, to completely discriminate the pathological features of FAPS from those of severe IBS. Indeed, patients with FAPS have a great similarity in symptoms to those with severe IBS. Both FAPS and IBS patients are commonly suffering

chronic abdominal pain, which is a multidimensional sensation of sensory, emotional, and cognitive experience. The chronic pain could be explained by the neurophysiological malfunction at the afferent, spinal, and central nerve systems (CNS) [22]. Illustration of the neurophysiological basis of chronic pain in FAPS is scarce; however, data derived from studies on patients with severe IBS revealed that perception of chronic pain comes from a central hypersensitivity and hypervigilance of central turnup of abnormal peripheral input of the gut. The perception of pain can be peripheral or central in alternative scenarios, which reflect either evaluated transmission by gut afferents in response to various stimuli or evoked interpretation of normal transmit accurate information by the CNS [4]. Compared with IBS, with which patients have a certain degree of disorder in peripheral input, FAPS is rendered by predominantly central pathophysiology. A recent study conducted with adults with IBS and FAPS observed that an IBS patient has lowered rectal thresholds in response to rectal balloon distention, while a FAPS patient renders normal perceptual thresholds, indicating the great role of CNS upregulation of incoming afferent signals in perception of chronic pain in FAPS patients [23]. Grover and Drossman summarized the following mechanisms that dominate pathophysiology of chronic pain: (1) ascending visceral pain transmission; (2) peripheral amplification of afferent signals; (3) descending pain modulation; and (4) central amplification and psychiatric factors [2].

Scanty information is available about establishment of an animal model of FAPS, which imposes restriction on the pharmacological study of potential therapy for the disorder. An animal model has been established by slow-release emulsion of morphine (10 mg/kg) for 8 days to develop narcotic bowel-like syndrome [24]. Although it was claimed to be a successful animal model recently [4], this established model does not specifically imitate the pathophysiological condition of FAPS as far as possible [24]. The insufficient development of a preclinical FAPS model largely limits the scientific study of Chinese herbal medicine. Although clinical experiences of ancient and modern Chinese medicine physicians have

Table 2: Action and indication of the ten most frequently used herbs for FAPS.

Chinese name in pinyin	Latin name	Frequency of usage	Action	Indication
Ren Shen	Radix Ginseng	78	Replenish the primordial qi; tonify the spleen and lung; promote fluid production and induce tranquilization	(1) Prostration syndrome of primordial qi (2) Lung qi deficiency syndrome (3) Spleen qi deficiency syndrome (4) Thirst due to qi deficiency and consumption of fluid in febrile disease (5) Palpations, fearful throbbing, insomnia, and dream–disturbed sleep
Bai Zhu	Rhizoma Atractylodis Macrocephalae	53	Invigorate spleen and replenish qi; dry dampness and induce diuresis; stop sweating; prevent abortion	(1) Spleen qi deficiency syndrome (2) Edema, phlegm-fluid retention (3) Spontaneous sweating due to qi deficiency (4) Threatened abortion due to spleen deficiency
Chen Pi	Pericarpium Citri Reticulatae	43	Regulate qi and invigorate spleen; dry dampness and resolve phlegm	(1) Qi stagnation of spleen and stomach (2) Retention of dampness and cough with profuse sputum
Bing Lang	Semen Arecae	41	Expel worms and remove food stagnation; move qi; induce diuresis	(1) Intestinal parasitic disease (2) Dyspepsia and qi stagnation manifested as dysentery with tenesmus (3) Edema and beriberi with the manifestations of swelling and pain
Chen Xiang	Lignum Aquilariae Resinatum	29	Promote qi flow to relieve pain; warm the middle energizer to stop vomiting; warm kidney to improve inspiration	(1) Distending pain in the chest and abdomen (2) Stomach cold causing vomiting (3) Dyspnea of deficiency type
Wu Yao	Radix Linderae	26	Promote qi flow to relieve pain; warm kidney to disperse cold	(1) Chest and abdomen pain syndromes (2) Frequent urination and enuresis
Yan Hu Suo	Rhizoma Corydalis	26	Activate blood; move qi; relieve pain	Stagnation of qi and blood stasis causing pain
Mu Xiang	Radix Aucklandiae	23	Promote qi flow to stop pain; regulate the middle energizer	(1) Spleen and stomach qi stagnation syndromes (2) Large intestine qi stagnation syndrome (3) Liver and gallbladder qi stagnation
Sheng Jiang	Rhizoma Zingiberis Recens	19	Dispel cold, release superficies; warm the middle; arrest vomiting; resolve phlegm and stop cough	(1) Exterior contraction of wind-cold (2) Stomach cold and vomiting (3) Lung cold and cough
Gan Cao	Radix Glycyrrhizae	19	Tonify spleen and replenish qi; dispel phlegm and arrest cough; relieve spasm and pain; clear heat and relieve toxicity; harmonize all medicinals	(1) Spleen qi deficiency syndrome (2) Heart qi insufficient syndrome (3) Cough and dyspnea (4) Spasm in the abdomen and extremities (5) Heat-toxin with ulcers and sore throat; medical or food poisoning (6) Moderating the properties of medicinals

TABLE 3: Summary of the top five most frequently used Chinese herbal formulae for FAPS based on syndrome diagnosis.

English name in pinyin	Composition in pinyin	TCM syndrome	Number of frequency among all the studies	Actions in Chinese medicine
Si-Mo-Tang	Ren Shen Bin Lang Chen Xiang Wu Yao	Liver qi depression	28	Activate qi; lower adverse qi; ease the chest and disperse stagnation
Tong-Xie-Yao-Fang	Bai Zhu Bai Shao Chen Pi Fang Feng	Liver depression and spleen deficiency	28	Reinforce the spleen; reduce the liver; relieve pain and stop diarrhea
Wen-Dan-Tang	Ban Xia Ju Hong Fu Ling Gan Cao Sheng Jiang Zhu Ru Zhi Shi Da Zao		21	Regulate qi; remove phlegm; clear gallbladder heat and harmonize the stomach
Xiang-Sha-Liu-Jun-Zi-Tang	Ren Shen Bai Zhu Fu Lin Ban Xia Chen Pi Mu Xiang Sha Ren Gan Cao		19	Replenish qi to invigorate the spleen; activate qi and eliminate phlegm
Xiao-Yao-San	Chai Hu Dang Gui Bai Shao Bai Zhu Fu Ling Gan Cao Bo He Sheng Jiang	Liver depression and spleen deficiency	18	Soothe the liver to relieve depression; invigorate the spleen and nourish blood

addressed the effective use of medicinal herbs in treating FAPS, most of preclinical study cannot well discriminate the pharmacological effect of Chinese herbal medicine in pathophysiological context. In this case, we include laboratory tests that were studied on the relief of FAPS-associated symptoms by Chinese herbal medicine. Both pure compounds naturally occurring in medicinal herbs, extracts of single herb and composite herbal formula, were included.

3.4.1. Chinese Herbal Medicine as Antinociceptive with Central Regulation. In a study with classical Chinese medicine formula Tong-Xie-Yao-Fang (TXYF), Hu and colleagues revealed that the formula can significantly relieve experimental visceral hypersensitivity. TXYF significantly decreased serotonin (5-HT) levels in serum and corticotrophin releasing factor (CRF) concentrations in the brain. The pharmacological effect of TXYF is largely dependent on the substance P (SP) expression in the colon mucosa, indicating that the activity of TXYF is associated with central mechanism of brain-gut axis regulation through decreasing the expression of 5-HT and SP in the periphery and that of CRF in the center [25]. Methanol extract of *Kaempferia galangal*

(200 mg/kg, p.o.) markedly demonstrated the antinociceptive action to relieve abdominal pain. Both central and peripheral mechanism are involved. The extracts may act as agonist of opioid receptors [26]. Extract of *Hedyotis corymbosa* (Linn.) Lam. (50–200 mg/kg, p.o.) exhibits antinociceptive effect and can relieve abdominal pain in an opioid receptor-dependent manner, which indicates an involvement of central and peripheral mechanism of action [27]. The fractions (ethanol, ethyl acetate, chloroform, and n-hexane) and crude ethyl acetate extract of *Carpolobia lutea* (Polygalaceae) (770 mg/kg, i.p.) can potently relieve abdominal pain in an animal model. Its mechanism of action can be both central and peripheral. The neurogenic (0–5 min) algesia was significantly blocked by the extract, indicating that it can act through opioid receptors which were more centrally than peripherally located. However, reduction on proinflammatory factors by *Carpolobia lutea* treatment reveals its peripheral antinociceptive effect [28]. *Senecio rufinervis* essential oil has central and peripheral analgesic effect to relieve abdominal pain. However, the central effect of this essential oil is not as potent as the peripheral one because it does not exhibit any sedative or muscle relaxant property [29]. Carvacrol (5-isopropyl-2-methylphenol), a monoterpenic phenol present

in the essential oil of oregano and thyme, exhibited suppression of abdominal pain in an animal model (50–100 mg/kg, p.o.). Mechanistic study revealed that though the pharmacological effect of carvacrol is not mediated by opioid receptor or NO, it can definitely reduce centrally associated intestine neurogenic pain, indicating its antinociceptive effect might involve central regulation [30]. Wang et al. studied the antinociceptive effect of tanshinone IIA on visceral pain induced by chronic pancreatitis (CP). Tanshinone IIA attenuates CP-induced pain via downregulation of spinal high mobility group box 1 (HMGB1) protein and Toll-like receptor 4 (TLR4) expression in the spinal cord, indicating a central regulation underlying its antinociceptive effect [31].

3.4.2. Chinese Herbal Medicine Alleviates Abdominal Pain Majorly by Peripheral Mechanism. Tjong and colleague found that extract of Coptidis Rhizoma can reduce irritable bowel syndrome- (IBS-) associated pain. Coptidis Rhizoma increased pain threshold response and attenuated Electromyogram (EMG) activity via lowering 5-HT release and cholecystokinin (CCK) expression in the colon, which in turn peripherally reduced visceral perception [32]. *Lepidium sativum* crude extract (100–300 mg/kg, p.o.) exhibits antispasmodic activities. Study on an isolated rat ileum indicated that this effect could be regional and blockade of muscarinic receptors and calcium channels may be involved [33]. Oral administration of *Cyperus rotundus* extracts (400 mg/kg, p.o.) reduces abdominal pain in mice, which may be associated with a peripheral inhibition of the effect or the release of endogenous substances (arachidonic acid metabolites) that excite pain nerve endings [34]. Friedelin (40 mg/kg, p.o.) isolated from *Azima tetracantha* Lam. can suppress abdominal pain in an animal model. This effect could not be blocked by naloxone, indicating that opioid receptor is not involved and the antinociceptive effect of friedelin may be peripheral [35]. Marrubiin (30.0 μmol/kg, i.p.) isolated from *Marrubium vulgare* has potent antinociceptive effect in relieving abdominal pain. This effect of marrubiin cannot be related to the inhibition of cyclooxygenase products derived from the arachidonic acid pathway or the participation of the opioid system. Analysis using different models revealed that the pharmacological effect of marrubiin may involve peripheral mechanism [36].

3.4.3. Chinese Herbal Medicine That Directly Treats Visceral Pain. A Chinese medicine compound formula, Sunqingwan watered pill (SWP), can reduce abdominal pain caused by ulcerative colitis. The anticolitis effect of SWP may be largely dependent on its protection on the colon through anti-inflammatory mechanisms [37]. Another Chinese medicine formula SWT5 and its component herbs *Angelica* root, chamomile flower, and liquorice root produce antispasmodic activities to relieve upper abdominal pain. The mechanism underlying its effect is independent of the nerve system as fast sodium channel blocker tetrodotoxin, the synaptic transmission blocker ω-conotoxin GVIA, or muscarinergic antagonist atropine has minimal block on its pharmacological action. It may involve a direct regulation of smooth muscle cells

of the stomach to exert multiple, region-specific effects on gastric motility [38]. *Ganoderma lucidum* polysaccharides have potent activity in relieving chronic pancreatitis-induced abdominal pain, which could be associated with reduced production of inflammatory cytokines such as interleukin-1 beta (IL-1β) and interferon-gamma (INF-γ) [39]. Glycycoumarin, a known component of Radix Glycyrrhizae, exhibits potent antispasmodic activities on the smooth muscle of the mouse jejunum. This pharmacological effect may be associated with intracellular accumulation of cAMP through the inhibition of PDEs, especially isozyme 3 [40]. Isoliquiritigenin, one of the antispasmodic principles of *Glycyrrhiza uralensis* roots, has similar antispasmodic effect on the mouse jejunum, the mechanism of which is yet independent of accumulation of cAMP/cGMP or inhibition of PDEs [41].

3.4.4. Anti-Inflammation-Mediated Relief of Abdominal Pain by Chinese Herbal Medicine. Ethanolic extract from *Pluchea sagittalis* (Lam.) Cabrera (500–700 mg/kg) exhibits antinociceptive effect at inflammatory phase but not neurogenic phase, as demonstrated by the differential pharmacological activities of the extract in acetic acid-induced abdominal pain model and formalin- or glutamate-induced nociception model. The effect of this extract may be associated with its blockade of expression of proinflammatory factors and activation of its downstream pathways [42]. Extract of *Patrinia villosa* (50–100 mg/kg, p.o.) showed inhibition of acetic acid-induced abdominal pain in mice, which could be associated with reduced liberation of inflammatory cytokines including interleukin-6 (IL-6), interleukin-8 (IL-8), and tumour necrosis factor-alpha (TNF-α) [43]. Hydroalcoholic extract (1000 mg/kg) of *Neurolaena lobata* (L.) R. Br. and its chloroform- and hexane-partitioned fractions (100 mg kg/kg) can relieve abdominal pain. This effect is not similar to the action of morphine, indicating a mechanism independent of central or peripheral regulation may be involved. It has been postulated that inhibition of inflammatory factors, such as 5-HT, PEG, and histamine, may mediate its pharmacological effect [44]. Crude extract, fractions, and compounds isolated from *Piper tuberculatum* (3–300 mg/kg p.o.) have antinociceptive effect in reducing acetic acid-induced abdominal constriction. This pharmacological action could be due to inhibition of the release of TNF-α, IL-1β, and IL-8 by resident peritoneal cells [45]. Triglycerides (TFC) of the fermented mushroom of *Coprinus comatus* (10–30 mg/kg, p.o.) have potent analgesic activity on abdominal pain. This is not related to noninflammatory, central perception of pain but may be dependent on the peripheral reduction of proinflammatory cytokines such as TNF-α, IL-1β, VEGF-α, and IL-17 [46].

4. Conclusion

The investigation of CHM treatment for FAPS patients was very limited due to the lack of the clinical studies and also the situation is the same as the basic research so far. In order to describe the enough information in this disorder, we retrieved the data from different designs of clinical studies, ranging from case reports and cohort studies to quasi or randomized controlled trials; the quality of these studies was various and we could not make quantitative comparison. Despite the limitations, our study for the first time summarized the important and practicable data concerning the whole picture of CHM applications in the treatment of FAPS. More high quality studies both clinical and basic research concerning the integration of CM syndrome differentiation and disease with standard and repeatable treatment procedure should be further conducted.

Competing Interests

The authors declare that they have no competing interests.

Acknowledgments

This work was supported by the National Natural Science Foundation of China (no. 81202626).

References

[1] D. A. Drossman, "Functional abdominal pain syndrome," *Clinical Gastroenterology and Hepatology*, vol. 2, no. 5, pp. 353–365, 2004.

[2] M. Grover and D. A. Drossman, "Functional abdominal pain ," *Current Gastroenterology Reports*, vol. 12, no. 5, pp. 391–398, 2010.

[3] D. Drossman, E. Corazziari, M. Delvaux et al., *Rome III: The Functional Gastrointestinal Disorders*, Degnon Associates, Inc., McLean, Va, USA, 2006.

[4] A. D. Sperber and D. A. Drossman, "Review article: the functional abdominal pain syndrome ," *Alimentary Pharmacology & Therapeutics*, vol. 33, no. 5, pp. 514–524, 2011.

[5] R. E. Clouse, E. A. Mayer, Q. Aziz et al., "Functional abdominal pain syndrome," *Gastroenterology*, vol. 130, no. 5, pp. 1492–1497, 2006.

[6] H. Törnblom and D. A. Drossman, "Centrally targeted pharmacotherapy for chronic abdominal pain," *Neurogastroenterology and Motility*, vol. 27, no. 4, pp. 455–467, 2015.

[7] A. Kaminski, A. Kamper, K. Thaler, A. Chapman, and G. Gartlehner, "Antidepressants for the treatment of abdominal pain-related functional gastrointestinal disorders in children and adolescents," *Cochrane Database of Systematic Reviews*, vol. 6, no. 7, Article ID CD008013, 2011.

[8] B. Zhang, J. Dong, and Z. Zhou, *Traditional Chinese Internal Medicine*, Shang Hai Science and Technology Press, Shanghai, China, 1985.

[9] Q. Wang, T. Liu, X. Fei et al., "Record of clinical teaching round for functional abdominal pain syndrome," *Shanghai Journal of Traditional Chinese Medicine*, vol. 49, no. 12, pp. 15–17, 2015.

[10] L. He, "Clinical observation on 215 children with functional abdominal pain treated with huaji granules," *World Chinese Medicine*, vol. 10, no. 11, pp. 1295–1297, 2013.

[11] X. Huo and C. Song, "Treatment experience of functional abdominal pain syndrome with modified kaiyu daoqi decoction," *Guangming Journal of Chinese Medicine*, vol. 26, no. 11, pp. 2243–2244, 2007.

[12] H. Zhang, "Modified huixiang juhe pill for functional abdominal pain: 27 cases," *Hebei Journal of Traditional Chinese Medicine*, vol. 29, no. 4, p. 312, 2007.

[13] H. Xu and H. Shao, "Clinical research on treating functional abdominal pain in children with the Liqi Jianzhong decoction," *Clinical Journal of Chinese Medicine*, vol. 4, no. 8, p. 78, 2012.

[14] Y. Chen, *Chai Hujian Decoction in the Treatment of Functional Abdominal Pain in 36 Cases*, vol. 28 of *Medical Information*, 2013.

[15] D. Liu, J. Wang, and M. Li, "Clinical observation of self-designed Wenwei powder with moxibustion for children functional abdominal pain: 56 cases," *Youjiang Medical Journal*, vol. 40, no. 1, pp. 34–35, 2012.

[16] M. Fu, H. Liu, and S. Yang, "Prof. Chen Baiyi's six treament principle for children abdominal pain," *Shaanxi Journal of Traditional Chinese Medicine*, vol. 34, no. 9, pp. 1202–1203, 2013.

[17] Y. Tu and X. Liu, "Treatment experience of Ni Zhuying for children functional abdominal pain," *Journal of Traditional Chinese Medicine*, vol. 52, no. 21, pp. 1820–1821, 2011.

[18] Y. Yuan and Y. Zhang, "Jialiujin's experiences on functional abdominal pain," *Journal of Shanxi College of Traditional Chinese Medicine*, vol. 15, no. 5, p. 18, 2015.

[19] Q. Wang, "Diagnosis and treatment experience of children recurrent abdominal pain with Traditional Chinese Medicine," *Journal of Emergency in Traditional Chinese Medicine*, vol. 20, no. 10, pp. 1706–1707, 2011.

[20] J. Wang, "Treatment experience of children functional abdominal pain with Traditional Chinese Medicine," *Shaanxi Journal of Traditional Chinese Medicine*, vol. 29, no. 8, p. 1102, 2008.

[21] WHO Regional Office for the Western Pacific, *WHO International Standard Terminologies on Traditional Medicine in the Western Pacific Region*, WHO Regional Office for the Western Pacific, Manila, Philippines, 2007.

[22] K. L. Casey, "Match and mismatch: identifying the neuronal determinants of pain," *Annals of Internal Medicine*, vol. 124, no. 11, pp. 995–998, 1996.

[23] C. Ballard-Croft, D. Wang, C. Jones et al., "Physiologic response to a simplified venovenous perfusion-induced systemic hyperthermia system," *ASAIO Journal*, vol. 58, no. 6, pp. 601–606, 2012.

[24] S. Agostini, H. Eutamene, C. Cartier et al., "Evidence of central and peripheral sensitization in a rat model of narcotic bowel-like syndrome," *Gastroenterology*, vol. 139, no. 2, pp. 553–563, 2010.

[25] X.-G. Hu, D. Xu, Y. Zhao et al., "The alleviating pain effect of aqueous extract from Tong-Xie-Yao-Fang, on experimental visceral hypersensitivity and its mechanism," *Biological and Pharmaceutical Bulletin*, vol. 32, no. 6, pp. 1075–1079, 2009.

[26] W. Ridtitid, C. Sae-wong, W. Reanmongkol, and M. Wongnawa, "Antinociceptive activity of the methanolic extract of Kaempferia galanga Linn. in experimental animals," *Journal of Ethnopharmacology*, vol. 118, no. 2, pp. 225–230, 2008.

[27] M. Moniruzzaman, A. Ferdous, and S. Irin, "Evaluation of antinociceptive effect of ethanol extract of Hedyotis corymbosa Linn. whole plant in mice," *Journal of Ethnopharmacology*, vol. 161, pp. 82–85, 2015.

[28] L. L. Nwidu, P. A. Nwafor, V. C. Da Silva et al., "Anti-nociceptive effects of Carpolobia lutea G. Don (Polygalaceae) leaf fractions in animal models," *Inflammopharmacology*, vol. 19, no. 4, pp. 215–225, 2011.

[29] D. Mishra, G. Bisht, P. M. Mazumdar, and S. P. Sah, "Chemical composition and analgesic activity of *Senecio rufinervis* essential oil," *Pharmaceutical Biology*, vol. 48, no. 11, pp. 1297–1301, 2010.

[30] F. H. Cavalcante Melo, E. R. V. Rios, N. F. M. Rocha et al., "Antinociceptive activity of carvacrol (5-isopropyl-2-methylphenol) in mice," *Journal of Pharmacy and Pharmacology*, vol. 64, no. 12, pp. 1722–1729, 2012.

[31] Y.-S. Wang, Y.-Y. Li, L.-H. Wang et al., "Tanshinone IIA attenuates chronic pancreatitis-induced pain in rats via downregulation of HMGB1 and TRL4 expression in the spinal cord," *Pain Physician*, vol. 18, no. 4, pp. E615–E628, 2015.

[32] Y. Tjong, S. Ip, L. Lao et al., "Analgesic effect of Coptis chinensis rhizomes (Coptidis Rhizoma) extract on rat model of irritable bowel syndrome," *Journal of Ethnopharmacology*, vol. 135, no. 3, pp. 754–761, 2011.

[33] N.-U. Rehman, M. H. Mehmood, K. M. Alkharfy, and A.-H. Gilani, "Studies on antidiarrheal and antispasmodic activities of lepidium sativum crude extract in rats," *Phytotherapy Research*, vol. 26, no. 1, pp. 136–141, 2012.

[34] K.-J. Soumaya, M. Dhekra, C. Fadwa et al., "Pharmacological, antioxidant, genotoxic studies and modulation of rat splenocyte functions by *Cyperus rotundus* extracts," *BMC Complementary and Alternative Medicine*, vol. 13, article 28, 2013.

[35] P. Antonisamy, V. Duraipandiyan, and S. Ignacimuthu, "Anti-inflammatory, analgesic and antipyretic effects of friedelin isolated from *Azima tetracantha* Lam. in mouse and rat models," *Journal of Pharmacy and Pharmacology*, vol. 63, no. 8, pp. 1070–1077, 2011.

[36] R. A. P. De Jesus, V. Cechinel-Filho, A. E. Oliveira, and V. Schlemper, "Analysis of the antinociceptive properties of marrubiin isolated from Marrubium vulgare," *Phytomedicine*, vol. 7, no. 2, pp. 111–115, 2000.

[37] N. Han, G. Li, R. Kang et al., "Treatment of Suqingwan watered pill reduces colon injury induced by experimental colitis," *Journal of Ethnopharmacology*, vol. 136, no. 1, pp. 144–148, 2011.

[38] M. Schemann, K. Michel, F. Zeller, B. Hohenester, and A. Rühl, "Region-specific effects of STW 5 (Iberogast®) and its components in gastric fundus, corpus and antrum," *Phytomedicine*, vol. 13, supplement 1, pp. 90–99, 2006.

[39] K. Li, M. Yu, Y. Hu et al., "Three kinds of Ganoderma lucidum polysaccharides attenuate DDC-induced chronic pancreatitis in mice," *Chemico-Biological Interactions*, vol. 247, pp. 30–38, 2016.

[40] Y. Sato, T. Akao, J.-X. He et al., "Glycycoumarin from Glycyrrhizae Radix acts as a potent antispasmodic through inhibition of phosphodiesterase 3," *Journal of Ethnopharmacology*, vol. 105, no. 3, pp. 409–414, 2006.

[41] Y. Sato, J.-X. He, H. Nagai, T. Tani, and T. Akao, "Isoliquiritigenin, one of the antispasmodic principles of *Glycyrrhiza ularensis* roots, acts in the lower part of intestine," *Biological and Pharmaceutical Bulletin*, vol. 30, no. 1, pp. 145–149, 2007.

[42] S. M. Figueredo, F. P. Do Nascimento, C. S. Freitas et al., "Antinociceptive and gastroprotective actions of ethanolic extract from Pluchea sagittalis (Lam.) Cabrera," *Journal of Ethnopharmacology*, vol. 135, no. 3, pp. 603–609, 2011.

[43] Y. Zheng, Y. Jin, H.-B. Zhu, S.-T. Xu, Y.-X. Xia, and Y. Huang, "The anti-inflammatory and anti-nociceptive activities of *Patrinia villosa* and its mechanism on the proinflammatory cytokines of rats with pelvic inflammation," *African Journal of Traditional, Complementary and Alternative Medicines*, vol. 9, no. 3, pp. 295–302, 2012.

[44] J. S. Gracioso, M. Q. Paulo, C. A. Hiruma Lima, and A. R. M. Souza Brito, "Antinociceptive effect in mice of a hydroalcoholic extract of *Neurolaena lobata* (L.) R. Br. and its organic fractions," *Journal of Pharmacy and Pharmacology*, vol. 50, no. 12, pp. 1425–1429, 1998.

[45] R. V. Rodrigues, D. Lanznaster, D. T. Longhi Balbinot, V. D. M. Gadotti, V. A. Facundo, and A. R. S. Santos, "Antinociceptive effect of crude extract, fractions and three alkaloids obtained from fruits of *Piper tuberculatum*," *Biological and Pharmaceutical Bulletin*, vol. 32, no. 10, pp. 1809–1812, 2009.

[46] J. Ren, J.-L. Shi, C.-C. Han, Z.-Q. Liu, and J.-Y. Guo, "Isolation and biological activity of triglycerides of the fermented mushroom of Coprinus Comatus," *BMC Complementary and Alternative Medicine*, vol. 12, article 52, 2012.

13

Shengmai San Ameliorates Myocardial Dysfunction and Fibrosis in Diabetic *db/db* Mice

Juan Zhao, Tong-Tong Cao, Jing Tian, Hui-hua Chen, Chen Zhang, Hong-Chang Wei, Wei Guo, and Rong Lu

Department of Pathology, Shanghai University of Traditional Chinese Medicine, 1200 Cailun Road, Shanghai 201203, China

Correspondence should be addressed to Wei Guo; guowei311@aliyun.com and Rong Lu; lurong@shutcm.edu.cn

Academic Editor: Yuewen Gong

In this study, we mainly investigated the effects of Shengmai San (SMS) on diabetic cardiomyopathy (DCM) in *db/db* mice. The *db/db* mice were randomly divided into model group and SMS group, while C57BLKS/J inbred mice were used as controls. After 24-week treatment, blood glucose, body weight, and heart weight were determined. Hemodynamic changes in the left ventricle were measured using catheterization. The myocardial structure and subcellular structural changes were observed by HE staining and electron microscopy; the myocardium collagen content was quantified by Masson staining. To further explore the protective mechanism of SMS, we analyzed the expression profiles of fibrotic related proteins. Compared to nondiabetic mice, *db/db* mice exhibited enhanced diastolic myocardial dysfunction and adverse structural remodeling. Higher expression of profibrotic proteins and lower levels of extracellular matrix degradation were also observed. After SMS oral administration for 24 weeks, cardiac dysfunction, hypertrophy, and fibrosis in diabetic mice were greatly improved. Moreover, increased profibrotic protein expression was strongly reversed by SMS treatment in *db/db* mice. The results demonstrate that SMS exerts a cardioprotective effect against DCM by attenuating myocardial hypertrophy and fibrosis via a TGF-β dependent pathway.

1. Introduction

Diabetic patients have a 2- to 5-fold increased risk of developing heart failure [1], which is partly driven by diabetic cardiomyopathy (DCM). DCM is characterized by diastolic dysfunction, myocardial fibrosis, and hypertrophy without ischemic heart disease, hypertension, or other comorbidities. The pathogenesis of DCM is complicated, but myocardial fibrosis, which increases ventricle stiffness, is thought to be one of the major causes of myocardial dysfunction [2]. Numerous studies demonstrated that one of the key determinants of myocardial fibrosis is the accumulation of increased extracellular matrix (ECM), which causes irreversible tissue damage and consequent cardiac dysfunction, ultimately resulting in heart failure [3]. Among the cytokines in the regulation of ECM metabolism, transforming growth factor-$\beta 1$ (TGF-$\beta 1$) is the critical factor and has been recognized as a therapeutic target for organ fibrosis [4].

Shengmai San (SMS), a traditional Chinese medical recipe, consists of Radix Ginseng (*Panax ginseng*, Araliaceae), Radix Ophiopogonis (*Ophiopogon japonicas*, Liliaceae), and Fructus Schisandrae (*Schisandra chinensis*, Schisandraceae). SMS is deemed a typical replenishing Qi and nourishing Yin formula in clinic and has been traditionally used in ischemic disease and diabetic patients. In experimental studies, SMS has been reported to have multiple pharmacological activities, such as antioxidant and anti-inflammation activities and being a regulator of lipid metabolism [5, 6]. Recently, one study indicated that SMS exhibited an antimyocardial fibrosis effect in a rat model induced by high-fat diet and STZ injection [7]; however, the exact mechanism remains to be determined. Thus, in the present study, we investigated the effects of SMS on cardiac function and fibrosis in a type 2 diabetic *db/db* mouse model, to further observe the associated signaling mechanism.

2. Materials and Methods

2.1. Shengmai San Preparation. Shengmai San (SMS) was purchased from Tauto Biotech Company (Shanghai, China), which contains ginseng 10 g, ophiopogon root 15 g, and Schisandra chinensis 6 g, and the solution was concentrated to 0.8 g/mL.

2.2. Animals and Treatment. Experimental protocols complied with the National Institutes of Health Guidelines on the Use of Laboratory Animals and were approved by the Animal Care and Use Committee of Shanghai University of Traditional Chinese Medicine. Thirty male BKS·Cg-m+/+LeprdbNJU mice (*db/db* mice), 4–6 weeks age, were randomly divided into two groups: model group and SMS group. Fifteen male C57BL/6J mice were used as age-matched controls. All animals were purchased from the Model Animal Research Center of Nanjing University (Nanjing, China) and raised in the animal research institute of Shanghai University of TCM (Shanghai, China). The mice were kept on a 12 h light/dark cycle and had access to food and water ad libitum. Since 8 weeks age, the mice were treated with SMS at a dose of 4.5 g/kg daily or with same volume of vehicle by oral gavage for 24 weeks.

2.3. Hemodynamic Measurement. At the end of the experiment, mice were fasted for 12 hours and blood samples were collected from the tail vein. Blood glucose levels were tested using a digital blood glucose meter (Optium Xceed, Abbott Laboratories, USA). Body weight and heart weight of mice were measured before or after hemodynamic measurements, respectively. Cardiac function was determined by invasive hemodynamic measurements. Mice were anesthetized with pentobarbital sodium (60 mg/kg, i.p.). With the help of stereoscopic microscope (Stemi DV4, Carl Zeiss, Germany), a SciSence FT-1.2 catheter (Scisence, Canada) was inserted into the right carotid artery and advanced into the left ventricle. The ventricular pressure was recorded and analyzed with Labscribe 2 software (iWorx, Dover, NH, USA). The hemodynamic parameters included maximal ascending and descending rates of left ventricular pressure ($+dp/dt_{max}$ and $-dp/dt_{max}$), left ventricular systolic pressure (LVSP), and left ventricular end-diastolic pressure (LVEDP).

2.4. Hematoxylin and Eosin (H&E) Staining. After hemodynamic measurements, mouse hearts were excised from the chest, trimmed of atria and large vessels, weighed, and transversely cut between the atrioventricular groove and the apex. The specimens were fixed in 4% paraformaldehyde. The tissues were paraffin-embedded and sliced perpendicular to interventricular septum continuously. The sections underwent hematoxylin and eosin staining and then were investigated by optical microscope (Stemi DV4 or Axio Scope A1, Carl Zeiss, Germany).

2.5. Myocardial Ultrastructure Observation. Parts of cardiac tissues were rapidly cut into 1 mm cubes, immersed in 2.5% glutaraldelyde in 0.1 M phosphate buffer (pH 7.4) overnight at 4°C. After fixation, the selections were immersed in 1% buffered osmium tetroxide for 2 h. The specimens were then dehydrated through a graded ethanol series and embedded in epoxy resin. After that, the selections were incised into ultrathin sections (60–70 nm) with an ultramicrotome and

poststained with uranyl acetate and lead citrate. Then sections were examined under a Tecnai-12 Biotwin transmission electron microscope (Philips, Germany).

2.6. Masson's Trichrome Staining and Collagen Volume Fraction (CVF) Analysis. After conventional deparaffin of the paraffin sections, Masson's trichrome staining was performed to evaluate myocardial fibrosis. Myocardial cells were stained red and collagenous fibers stained blue. The collagen deposition was quantitatively analyzed for collagen volume fraction (CVF) via Metamorph image process (Universal Imaging Corp, USA). The calculation formula of CVF in each view of the slice is CVF = collagen area/total area × 100%.

2.7. Western Blotting. Total extracted protein lysates from similar portions of LV tissue were prepared by standard procedures, and protein lysate concentrations were determined via BCA protein assay kit (Beyotime, Shanghai, China). Equivalent amounts of tissue protein (50 μg) were subjected to 10–12% SDS-PAGE, electrotransferred onto polyvinylidene difluoride (PVDF) membranes, and then incubated overnight at 4°C with the primary antibodies, including transforming growth factor-β1 (TGF-β1), transforming growth factor-β receptor II (TGFβRII), p-Smad2, p-Smad3, Smad2, Smad3, Smad4 (Cell Signaling Technology, USA), matrix metallopeptidase-2 (MMP-2), matrix metallopeptidase-9 (MMP-9), tissue inhibitor of metalloproteinases-2 (TIMP-2), and GAPDH (Santa Cruz biotechnology, USA). Next day, membranes were washed and incubated with the corresponding secondary antibodies for 2 h; anti-mouse and anti-rabbit antibodies were from Cell Signaling Technology; protein bands were detected by Fluor Chem E (Protein Simple, USA). Quantitation was performed via Image J software (Bethesda, MD, USA). GAPDH was used as loading controls for total protein expression.

2.8. Statistical Analysis. All values were analyzed with SPSS21.0 and expressed as means ± SEM. Multiple comparisons between groups were examined using one-way analysis of variance (ANOVA) followed by Tukey's post hoc analysis, and $P < 0.05$ were considered statistically significant.

3. Results

3.1. Effects of SMS on Blood Glucose Level, Body Weight, and Heart Weight. Compared to nondiabetic controlmice, *db/db* mice exhibit typical characteristics of type 2 diabetes indicated by hyperglycemia as well as increasing heart and body weight. Blood glucose levels and body weight did not significantly differ between *db/db* mice with or without SMS treatment; however, SMS markedly alleviated the increase of heart weight seen in *db/db* mice (Figure 1).

3.2. SMS Attenuated Diabetes-Induced Myocardial Diastolic Dysfunction. To determine the role of SMS in type 2 diabetic mice, cardiac catheterization was performed to evaluate ventricular function. The results demonstrated that LVSP and $+dp/dt_{max}$ values did not significantly differ between nondiabetic and *db/db* mice, suggesting unaltered systolic function

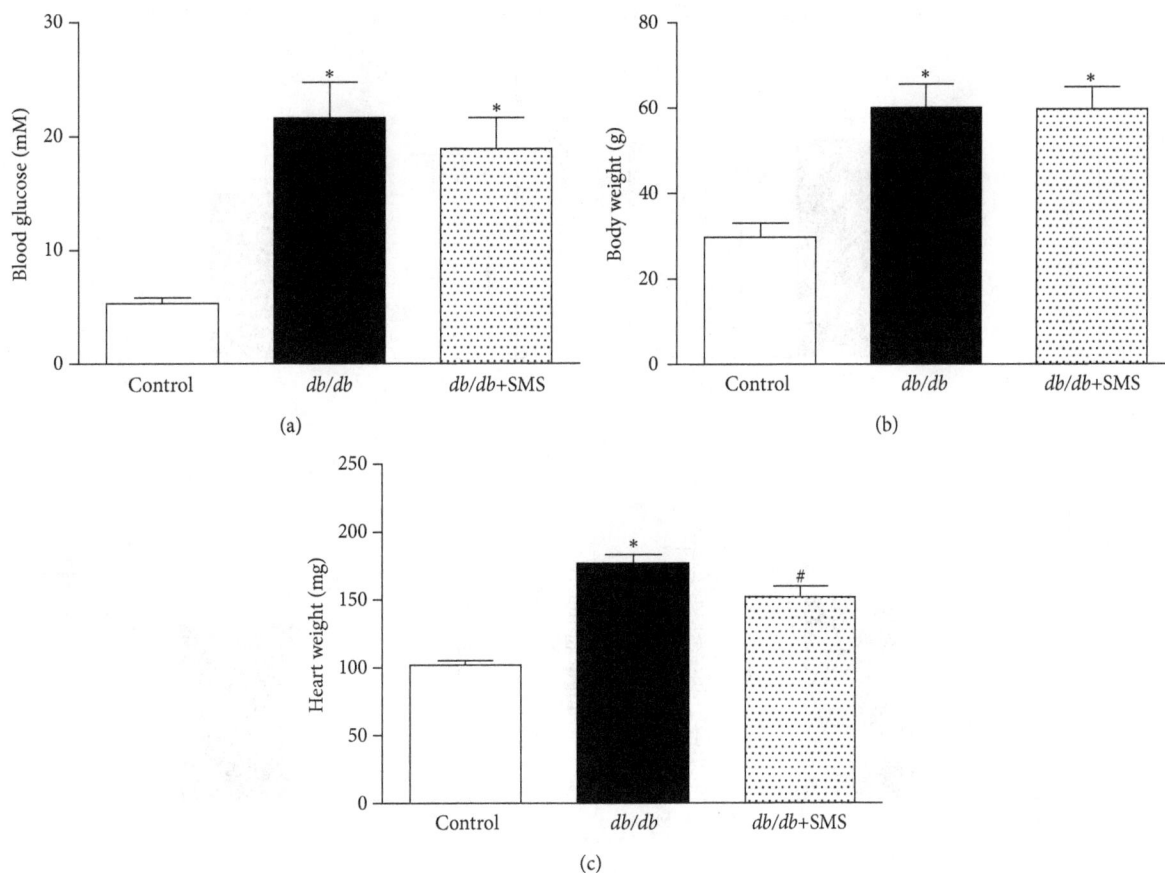

FIGURE 1: Effects of SMS on blood glucose, body weight, and heart weight. After a 24-week treatment, general biochemical parameters were measured (n = 8–10). In the bar figures, values are the mean ± SEM. $^*P < 0.05$ versus Control group; $^{\#}P < 0.05$ versus db/db group. (a) Fast blood glucose level, (b) body weight, and (c) heart weight.

in type 2 DM (Figures 2(a) and 2(c)). In contrast, compared with the control, $-dp/dt_{max}$ value was significantly reduced in db/db mice, accompanied with increased LVEDP level, indicating a marked diastolic dysfunction in db/db mice, although increased LVEDP in db/db mice did not show statistical significance. Moreover, SMS treatment for 24 weeks significantly reversed the diastolic dysfunction in db/db mice (Figures 2(b) and 2(d)).

3.3. Effects of SMS on Histological and Morphological Changes.
To identify the morphological changes in the db/db mice and the protective effects of SMS, heart sections were processed for HE staining and TEM. HE images of the model group displayed remarkably thickened ventricular wall, hypertrophied cardiomyocyte, and disordered cell arrangement. These responses were partly prevented by SMS (Figures 3(a) and 3(b)). TEM images of db/db hearts displayed small finger-like projections on the surface of endothelial cell (Figure 3(c), black arrows) and swollen mitochondria (Figure 3(d), white arrows), which were partly attenuated by SMS treatment.

3.4. Effects of SMS on Myocardial Fibrosis and TGF-β1 Expression.
Using Masson staining and CVF quantifiable analysis,

we found that db/db mice exhibited more severe myocardial fibrosis compared to nondiabetic mice, indicated by increased blue collagenous fibers and higher CVF values. SMS administration for 24 weeks partly ameliorated cardiac hypertrophy and markedly reversed myocardial fibrosis in db/db mice (Figures 4(a) and 4(b)). To observe the underlying mechanism involved in antifibrosis of SMS, the level of TGF-β1 protein expression in heart tissue was determined by Western blotting. The data indicated that TGF-β1 was significantly higher in cardiac tissues of db/db mice compared tonondiabetic mice, suggesting activation of fibrosis associated pathway in diabetic mice. SMS administration significantly decreased the expression level of TGF-β1 protein in db/db mice (Figures 4(c) and 4(d)).

3.5. Effects of SMS on TGF-β Associated Downstream Signaling.
As a critical factor for development of organ fibrosis, the expression of TGF-β1 dramatically increased in db/db mice. Based on the above result, we further analyzed the changes of TGF-β associated downstream signaling. The data shows that the levels of TGF-β receptor II, phospho-Smad2, phospho-Smad3, and Smad4 were significantly higher in cardiac tissues of db/db mice compared to nondiabeticmice, which was inhibited by SMS treatment for 24 weeks (Figure 5). No

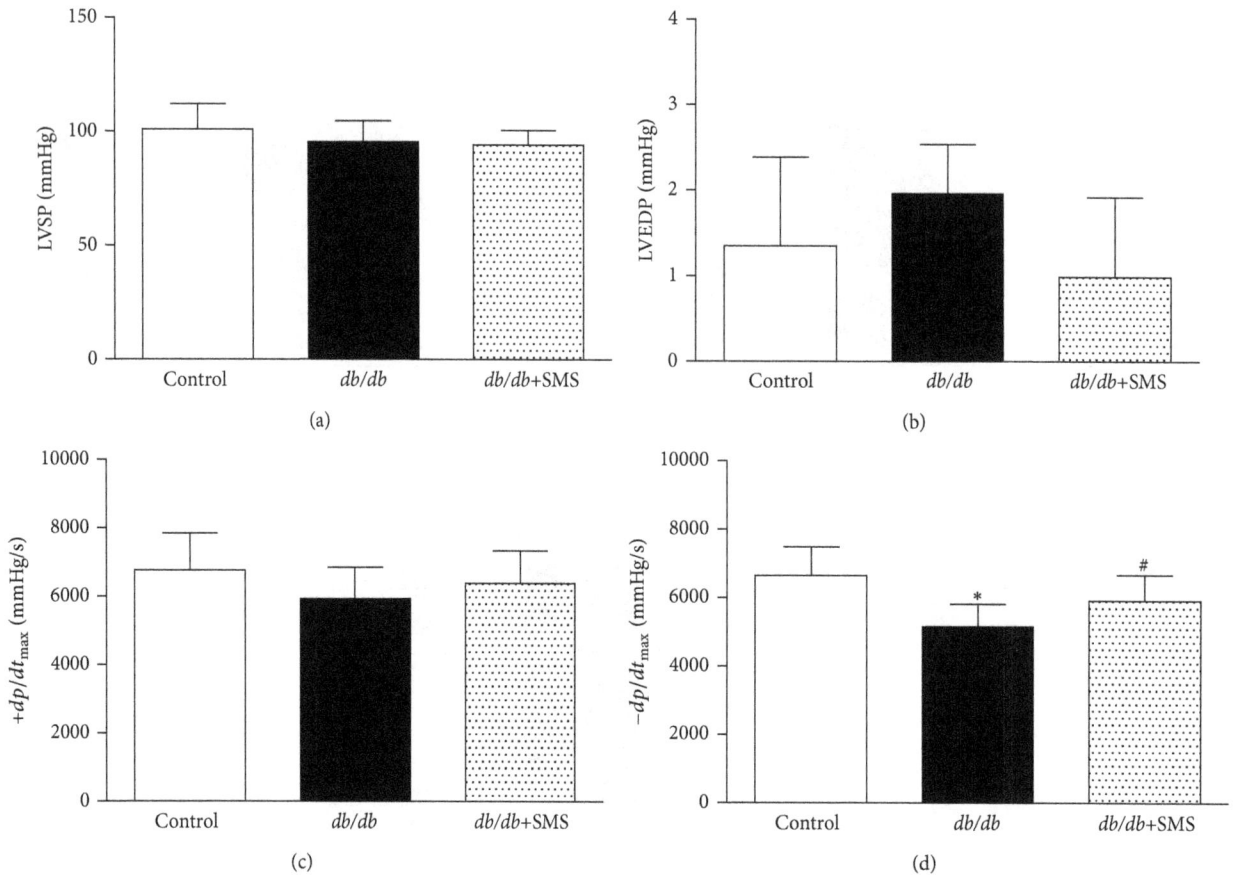

FIGURE 2: Effects of SMS on diabetes-induced myocardial dysfunction. Left ventricular function was assessed by cardiac catheterization in anesthetized mice ($n = 8$–10). In the bar figures, values are the mean ± SEM. $^*P < 0.05$ versus Control group; $^\#P < 0.05$ versus db/db group. (a) Left ventricular systolic pressure (LVSP), (b) left ventricular end-diastolic pressure (LVEDP), (c) maximal ascending rates of left ventricular pressure ($+dp/dt_{max}$), and (d) maximal descending rates of left ventricular pressure ($-dp/dt_{max}$).

significant changes in total Smad2 or Smad3 protein levels were observed.

3.6. Effects of SMS on MMP-2, MMP-9, and TIMP-2 Levels. Myocardial ECM is primarily mediated by MMPs and their role in fibrosis is now well established; thus, we further assessed the expression of MMP-2, MMP-9, and TIMP-2. The data shows that MMP-2 and MMP-9 protein levels in db/db mice were significantly downregulated, whereas TIMP-2 levels were significantly upregulated compared to nondiabetic mice, leading to a lower MMP-2/TIMP-2 ratio in db/db mice. The changes of protein levels presented in diabetic mice were markedly reversed by SMS treatment (Figure 6).

4. Discussion

In spite of the clinical importance of diabetic cardiomyopathy (DCM) as a distinct disease, the cellular and molecular mechanisms triggering the adverse changes in diabetic myocardium have not been fully understood. In our study, compared with nondiabetic control mice, the 32-week db/db mice exhibited obvious obesity, hyperglycemia, myocardial hypertrophy, and fibrosis. Using hemodynamic analysis, we

also found distinct diastolic dysfunction in db/db mice, indicated by a significant decreased $-dp/dt_{max}$ and an elevated LVEDP, although increased LVEDP did not reach statistical significance. In contrast, myocardial systolic function in db/db mice was similar tonondiabetic mice, characterized by unaltered LVSP and $+dp/dt_{max}$. In type 2 DM experimental models, cardiac performance has been extensively studied. As a leptin receptor defective animal, most studies support that db/db mice mainly display diastolic dysfunction, while systolic function was preserved well for a long time [8, 9], which was also confirmed by our results. Since myocardial hypertrophy and fibrosis cause increased passive myocardial stiffness, we assumed that the two features, at least in part, result in diastolic dysfunction in db/db mice.

SMS treatment has been proved effective for type 2 diabetes in both clinical and experimental studies. Some clinical researches indicated that SMS promotes the beneficial effects of oral hypoglycemic drugs and improves diabetic complications [10]. In experimental studies, multiple pharmacological activities of SMS have also been reported, such as antioxidant, anti-inflammation, and regulating lipid metabolism activities. In our study, SMS treatment for 24 weeks significantly reversed the myocardial diastolic dysfunction shown

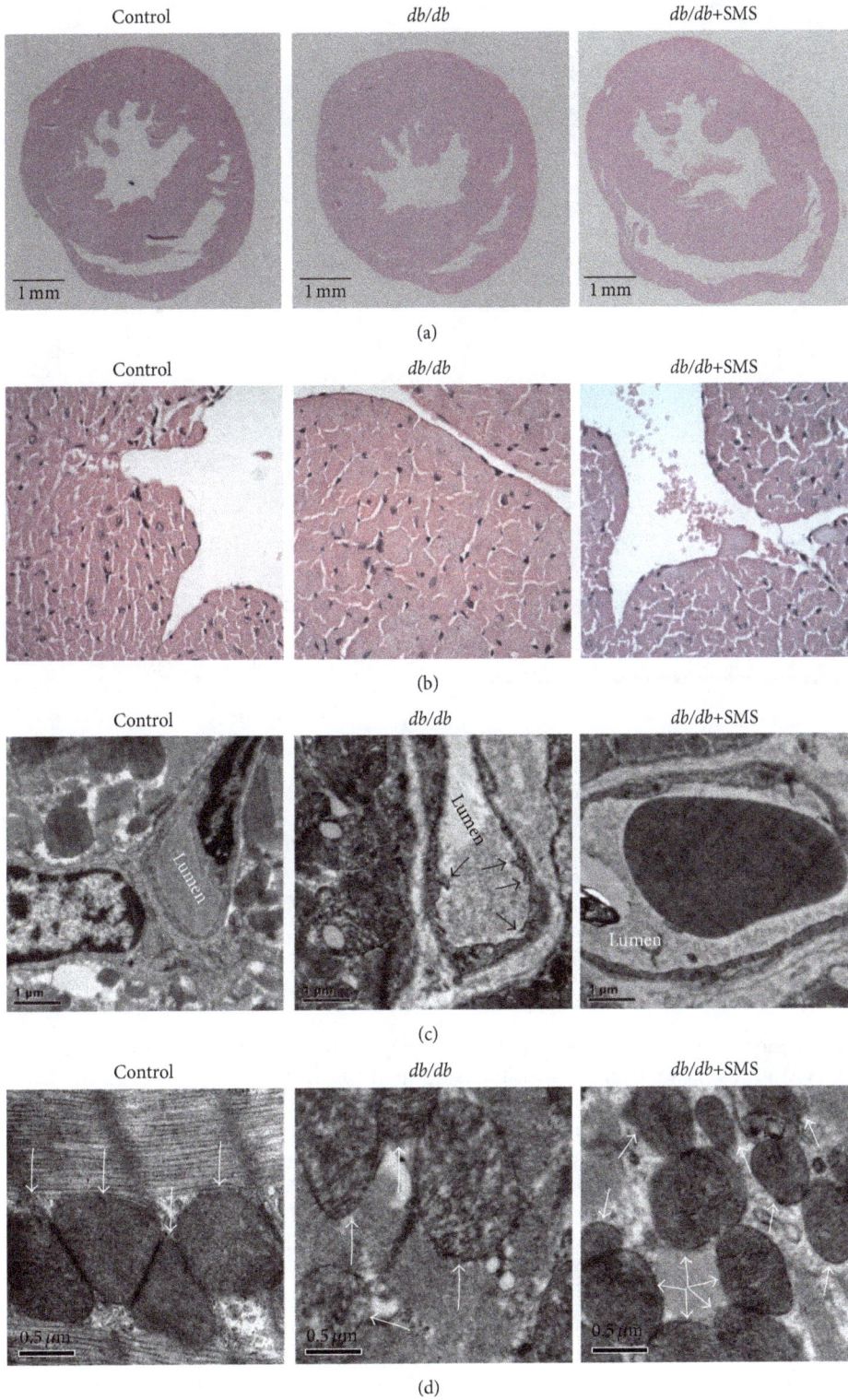

FIGURE 3: Effects of SMS on histological and ultrastructure changes. To assess histological and morphological features in each group, H&E staining and transmission electron microscopy (TEM) observation were performed. (a) Low-power (8-fold) and (b) high-power (200-fold) via light microscope; (c) and (d) myocardial ultrastructure images from TEM. (Black arrows indicate finger-like projections, while white arrows indicate mitochondria.)

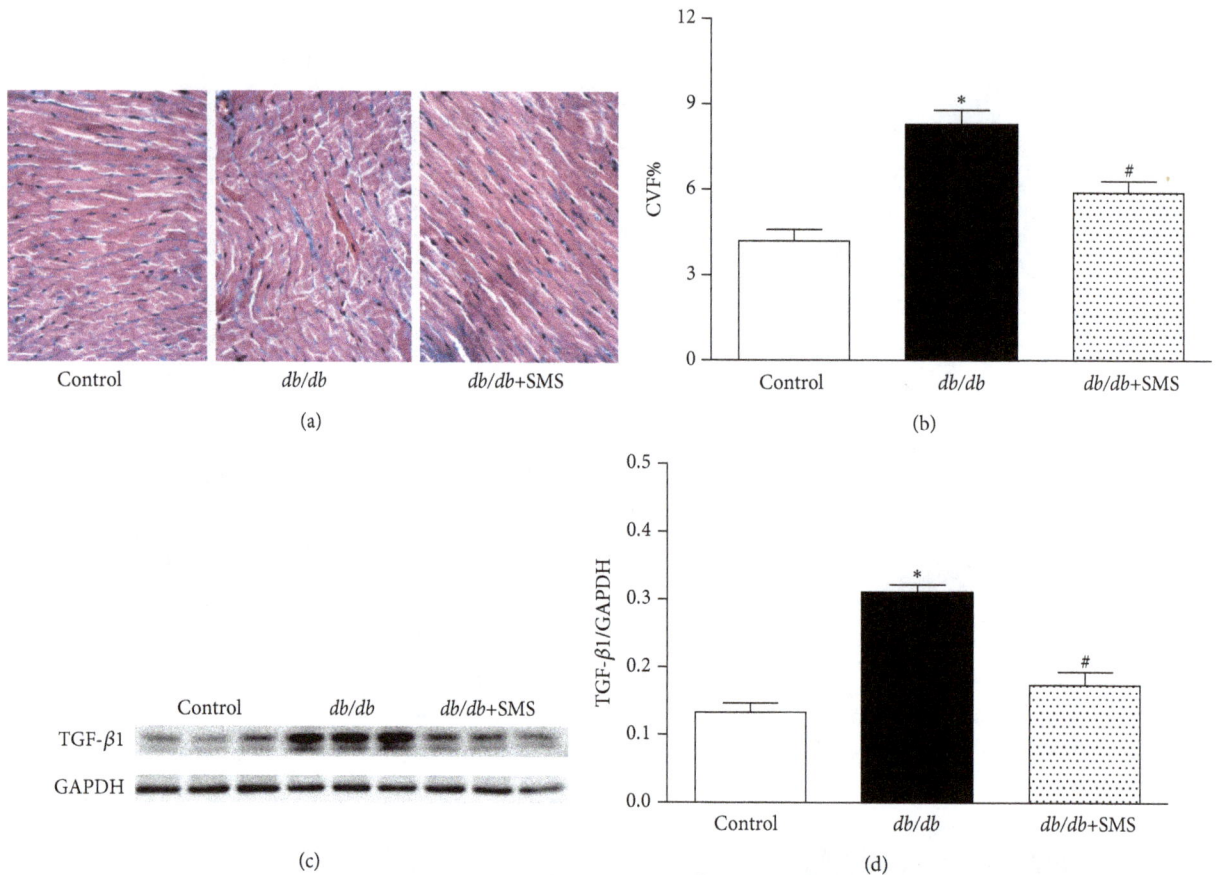

FIGURE 4: Effects of SMS on myocardial fibrosis and TGF-β1 expression. To detect the role of SMS in myocardial remodeling, Masson's trichrome staining was performed to evaluate fibrosis, the myocardial cells were stained for red, and collagenous fibers were blue. The collagen deposition was quantitatively analyzed via CVF, which equals collagen area/total area × 100% (a and b). To observe the underlying mechanism involved in antifibrosis of SMS, the level of transforming growth factor-β1 (TGF-β1) protein expression in heart tissue was determined using Western blotting (3 heart tissues from each group) (c and d). Data are presented as mean ± SEM. $^{*}P < 0.05$ versus Control group; $^{\#}P < 0.05$ versus db/db group.

in db/db mice. Furthermore, SMS apparently prevented cardiac hypertrophy and ultrastructural injury, which was confirmed by histological and morphological assessment. We found that heart weight was significantly increased in db/db mice, with markedly enlarged cardiomyocyte cross-sectional area, accompanied by swollen mitochondria, all of which were alleviated by SMS administration. Masson staining and CVF analysis revealed that SMS also reversed the increased myocardial fibrosis shown in db/db hearts. It is noteworthy that blood glucose and body weight did not significantly differ between db/db and db/db treated with SMS, suggesting that hypoglycemic effect may not be involved. In conclusion, our data indicated that SMS attenuate diastolic dysfunction, cardiac hypertrophy, and fibrosis in type 2 diabetic db/db mice model.

Fibrotic remodeling of the myocardium has been reported to play a critical role in pathophysiologic progress in DCM [11, 12]. The potential causes of myocardial fibrotic remodeling include the imbalance between extracellular matrix synthesis and degradation and interstitial collagen

deposition and disorder of collagen proportions, which gradually lead to myocardial stiffness and eventually cardiac dysfunction [13–16]. Our data shows that SMS remarkably abrogated the accumulation of collagen. Consistent with our results, recent evidence implicates that SMS contribute to antimyocardial fibrosis in a rat model induced by high-fat diet and STZ injection [7]. However, the exact mechanism of antifibrosis of SMS is still unclear.

Among numerous fibrotic signals, TGF-β1 is reported to be a key fibrogenic mediator. Excessive activation of TGF-β1 leads to dysfunction of extracellular matrix synthesis and degradation, which results in fibrotic remodeling [17, 18]. It is now clear that the binding of TGF-β1 to its receptors promotes Smad2 and Smad3 phosphorylation, after forming heterotrimers with co-Smad (Smad4), then translocating into the nucleus to regulate gene transcription. Smad2 and Smad3 are well-documented downstream mediators of TGF-β1 induced fibrosis, and activation of Smad2 and Smad3 is found to stimulate matrix-component synthesis, such as fibronectin (Fn), collagens, and proteoglycan [19–22]. Moreover, TGF-β1

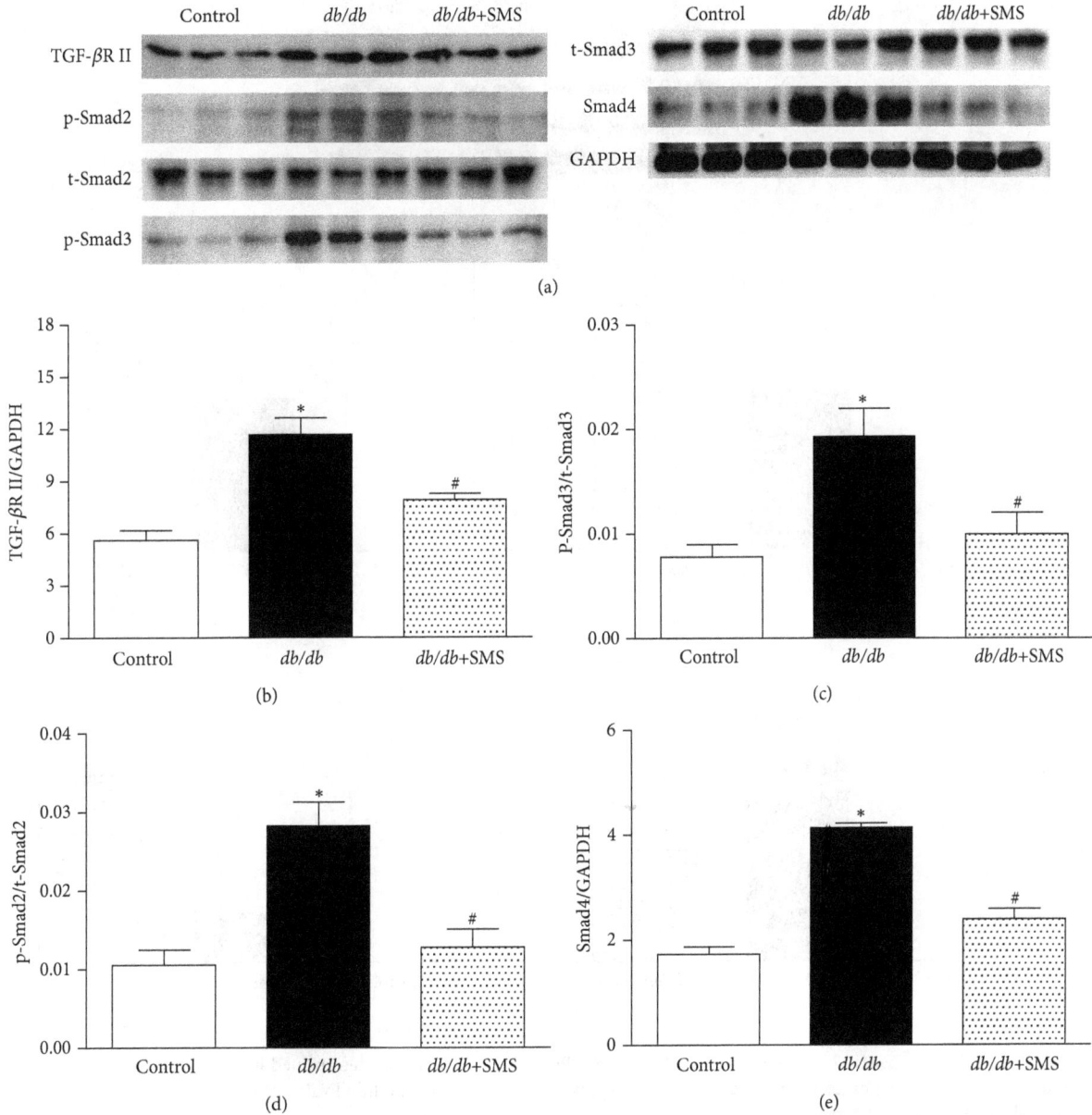

FIGURE 5: Effects of SMS on TGF-β associated downstream signaling. Protein expression was determined in the whole cell lysate via Western blotting and quantified by densitometric analysis. (a) Protein expression band. (b–e) Quantified value of protein expression. Data presented are means ± SEM (3 heart tissues from each group). $^*P < 0.05$ versus Control group; $^\#P < 0.05$ versus db/db group. TGF-β1, transforming growth factor-β1; TGFβRII, transforming growth factor-β receptor II; p-Smad2, phosphorylated Smad2; p-Smad3, phosphorylated Smad3; t-Smad2, total Smad2; t-Smad3, total Smad3; MMP-2, matrix metallopeptidase 2; MMP-9, matrix metallopeptidase 9; TIMP-2, tissue inhibitor of metalloproteinases-2.

can also inhibit the expressions of MMPs, which are the main degrading enzymes of the ECM, by increasing plasminogen activator inhibitors (PAI) and decreasing plasminogen activator (PA), and mediate the synthesis of protein hydrolytic enzyme inhibitors [23–26]. In the present study, we found that as a critical factor for development of organ fibrosis, the expression of TGF-β1 and TGF-β receptor II dramatically increased in db/db mice. We further detected changes in TGF-β associated downstream signaling; the data showed

that the levels of p-Smad2, p-Smad3, and Smad4 were significantly higher in cardiac tissues of db/db mice compared to nondiabeticmice, without significant changes in total Smad2 and Smad3 protein; all changes in protein levels were reversed by SMS treatment. Furthermore, MMP-2 and MMP-9 in db/db mice were markedly downregulated, accompanied by higher level of TIMP-2 than nondiabetic mice, which led to a much lower ratio of MMP-2/TIMP-2 in db/db mice. After SMS administration, the ratio of MMP-2/TIMP-2 nearly

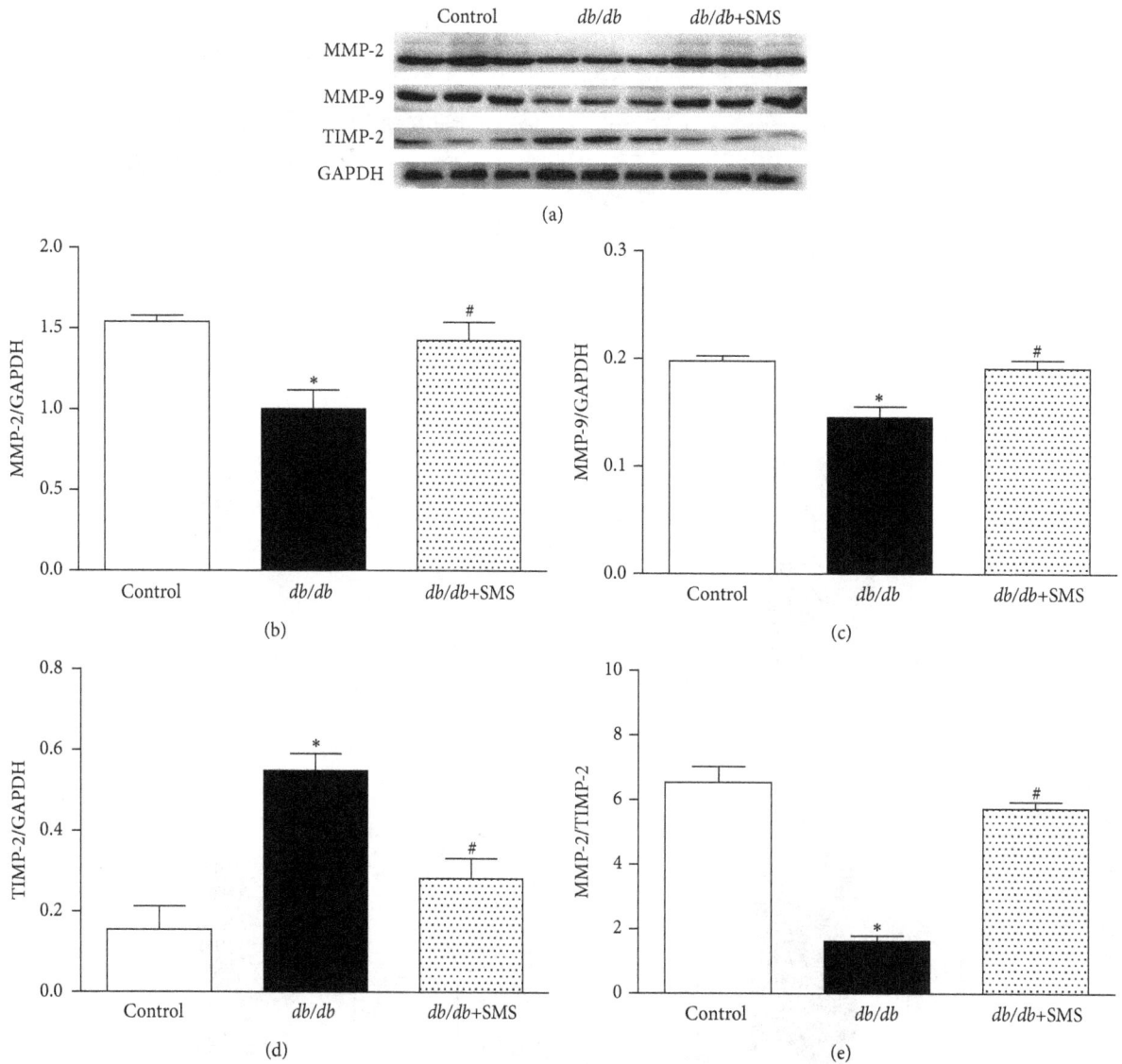

FIGURE 6: Effects of SMS on MMP-2, MMP-9, and TIMP-2 Levels. Protein expression was determined in the whole cell lysate via Western blotting and quantified by densitometric analysis. (a) Protein expression band. (b–e) Quantified value of protein expression. Data presented are means ± SEM (3 heart tissues from each group). $^*P < 0.05$ versus Control group; $^#P < 0.05$ versus db/db group. MMP-2, matrix metallopeptidase 2; MMP-9, matrix metallopeptidase 9; TIMP-2, tissue inhibitor of metalloproteinases-2.

shifted to normal condition. The above data implies that an imbalance of extracellular matrix synthesis and degradation may aggravate fibrotic remodeling in db/db mice, which consequently causes cardiac dysfunction.

Taken together, our results demonstrate that as a traditional Chinese medical recipe, SMS exerts a protective effect against type 2 diabetes-induced myocardial dysfunction and fibrosis through the regulation of TGF-β1/Smads axis. Therefore, SMS should be a potential drug for the treatment of diabetic cardiomyopathy.

Competing Interests

The authors declare that there is no conflict of interests regarding the publication of this paper.

Authors' Contributions

Juan Zhao and Tong-Tong Cao are equal contributors to this work.

Acknowledgments

This work was supported by grants from the National Natural Science Foundation of China (nos. 81373858 and 81473476).

References

[1] D. S. H. Bell, "Heart failure: the frequent, forgotten, and often fatal complication of diabetes," *Diabetes Care*, vol. 26, no. 8, pp. 2433–2441, 2003.

[2] D. N. Brindley, B. P. Kok, P. C. Kienesberger, R. Lehner, and J. R. Dyck, "Shedding light on the enigma of myocardial lipotoxicity: the involvement of known and putative regulators of fatty acid storage and mobilization," *American Journal of Physiology-Endocrinology and Metabolism*, vol. 298, no. 5, pp. E897–E908, 2010.

[3] I. Falcão-Pires and A. F. Leite-Moreira, "Diabetic cardiomyopathy: understanding the molecular and cellular basis to progress in diagnosis and treatment," *Heart Failure Reviews*, vol. 17, no. 3, pp. 325–344, 2012.

[4] C.-J. Li, L. Lv, H. Li, and D.-M. Yu, "Cardiac fibrosis and dysfunction in experimental diabetic cardiomyopathy are ameliorated by alpha-lipoic acid," *Cardiovascular Diabetology*, vol. 11, article 73, 2012.

[5] L.-H. Li, J.-S. Wang, and L.-Y. Kong, "Protective effects of Shengmai San and its three fractions on cerebral ischemia-reperfusion injury," *Chinese Journal of Natural Medicines*, vol. 11, no. 3, pp. 222–230, 2013.

[6] V. V. Giridharan, R. A. Thandavarayan, and T. Konishi, "Antioxidant formulae, Shengmai San, and LingGuiZhuGanTang, prevent MPTP induced brain dysfunction and oxidative damage in mice," *Evidence-Based Complementary and Alternative Medicine*, vol. 2015, Article ID 584018, 10 pages, 2015.

[7] Q. Ni, J. Wang, E.-Q. Li et al., "Study on the protective effect of Shengmai San on the myocardium in the type 2 diabetic cardiomyopathy model rat," *Journal of Traditional Chinese Medicine*, vol. 31, no. 3, pp. 209–219, 2011.

[8] C. Christoffersen, E. Bollano, M. L. S. Lindegaard et al., "Cardiac lipid accumulation associated with diastolic dysfunction in obese mice," *Endocrinology*, vol. 144, no. 8, pp. 3483–3490, 2003.

[9] L. M. Semeniuk, A. J. Kryski, and D. L. Severson, "Echocardiographic assessment of cardiac function in diabetic db/db and transgenic db/db-hGLUT4 mice," *American Journal of Physiology—Heart and Circulatory Physiology*, vol. 283, no. 3, pp. H976–H982, 2002.

[10] W. Ping and W. Yang, "Application of Sheng Mai San in the treatment of diabetes mellitus," *Journal of Tianjin University of Traditional Chinese Medicine*, vol. 30, no. 2, pp. 127–128, 2011.

[11] C. A. Souders, S. L. K. Bowers, and T. A. Baudino, "Cardiac fibroblast: the renaissance cell," *Circulation Research*, vol. 105, no. 12, pp. 1164–1176, 2009.

[12] V. P. Singh, K. M. Baker, and R. Kumar, "Activation of the intracellular renin-angiotensin system in cardiac fibroblasts by high glucose: role in extracellular matrix production," *American Journal of Physiology—Heart and Circulatory Physiology*, vol. 294, no. 4, pp. H1675–H1684, 2008.

[13] M. Tang, M. Zhong, Y. Shang et al., "Differential regulation of collagen types I and III expression in cardiac fibroblasts by AGEs through TRB3/MAPK signaling pathway," *Cellular and Molecular Life Sciences*, vol. 65, no. 18, pp. 2924–2932, 2008.

[14] S. Zibadi, F. Cordova, E. H. Slack, R. R. Watson, and D. F. Larson, "Leptin's regulation of obesity-induced cardiac extracellular matrix remodeling," *Cardiovascular Toxicology*, vol. 11, no. 4, pp. 325–333, 2011.

[15] S. Ares-Carrasco, B. Picatoste, A. Benito-Martín et al., "Myocardial fibrosis and apoptosis, but not inflammation, are present in long-term experimental diabetes," *The American Journal of Physiology—Heart and Circulatory Physiology*, vol. 297, no. 6, pp. H2109–H2119, 2009.

[16] P. Yue, T. Arai, M. Terashima et al., "Magnetic resonance imaging of progressive cardiomyopathic changes in the db/db mouse," *American Journal of Physiology-Heart and Circulatory Physiology*, vol. 292, no. 5, pp. H2106–H2118, 2007.

[17] Y. Wang, Y. Ding, and M. Liu, "The molecular mechanism of myocardial fibrosis induced by different factors," *Medical Review*, vol. 18, no. 17, pp. 2736–2740, 2012.

[18] M. Bonetti, A. Fontana, F. Martinelli et al., "Oxygen ozone therapy for degenerative spine disease in the elderly: a prospective study," *Acta Neurochirurgica Supplement*, vol. 108, pp. 137–142, 2011.

[19] A. Biernacka, M. Dobaczewski, and N. G. Frangogiannis, "TGF-β signaling in fibrosis," *Growth Factors*, vol. 29, no. 5, pp. 196–202, 2011.

[20] M. Bujak, G. Ren, H. J. Kweon et al., "Essential role of Smad3 in infarct healing and in the pathogenesis of cardiac remodeling," *Circulation*, vol. 116, no. 19, pp. 2127–2138, 2007.

[21] K. C. Flanders, "Smad3 as a mediator of the fibrotic response," *International Journal of Experimental Pathology*, vol. 85, no. 2, pp. 47–64, 2004.

[22] M. Dobaczewski, M. Bujak, N. Li et al., "Smad3 signaling critically regulates fibroblast phenotype and function in healing myocardial infarction," *Circulation Research*, vol. 107, no. 3, pp. 418–428, 2010.

[23] R. Derynck and Y. E. Zhang, "Smad-dependent and Smad-independent pathways in TGF-β family signalling," *Nature*, vol. 425, no. 6958, pp. 577–584, 2003.

[24] X. M. Meng, X. R. Huang, A. C. K. Chung et al., "Smad2 protects against TGF-β/Smad3-mediated renal fibrosis," *Journal of the American Society of Nephrology*, vol. 21, no. 9, pp. 1477–1487, 2010.

[25] W. H. Baricos, S. L. Cortez, M. Deboisblanc, and X. Shi, "Transforming growth factor-β is a potent inhibitor of extracellular matrix degradation by cultured human mesangial cells," *Journal of the American Society of Nephrology*, vol. 10, no. 4, pp. 790–795, 1999.

[26] S. Tomooka, W. A. Border, B. C. Marshall, and N. A. Noble, "Glomerular matrix accumulation is linked to inhibition of the plasmin protease system," *Kidney International*, vol. 42, no. 6, pp. 1462–1469, 1992.

14

Osteoporosis Recovery by *Antrodia camphorata* Alcohol Extracts through Bone Regeneration in SAMP8 Mice

Hen-Yu Liu,[1,2] **Chiung-Fang Huang,**[3] **Chun-Hao Li,**[1,4] **Ching-Yu Tsai,**[1,4]
Wei-Hong Chen,[1,4] **Hong-Jian Wei,**[1,4] **Ming-Fu Wang,**[5] **Yueh-Hsiung Kuo,**[6,7]
Mei-Leng Cheong,[8,9] **and Win-Ping Deng**[1,4,10]

[1] *Stem Cell Research Center, Taipei Medical University, Taipei 110, Taiwan*

[2] *School of Dentistry, College of Oral Medicine, Taipei Medical University, Taipei 110, Taiwan*

[3] *Department of Dentistry, Taipei Medical University Hospital, Taipei 110, Taiwan*

[4] *Graduate Institute of Biomedical Materials and Tissue Engineering, Taipei Medical University, Taipei 110, Taiwan*

[5] *Department of Food and Nutrition, Providence University, Taichung 433, Taiwan*

[6] *Department of Chinese Pharmaceutical Sciences and Chinese Medicine Resources, China Medical University, Taichung 404, Taiwan*

[7] *Department of Biotechnology, Asia University, Taichung 413, Taiwan*

[8] *Department of Obstetrics and Gynecology, Cathay General Hospital, Taipei 106, Taiwan*

[9] *College of Medicine, Taipei Medical University, Taipei 110, Taiwan*

[10]*Institute of Medicine, Fu Jen Catholic University, Taipei 242, Taiwan*

Correspondence should be addressed to Mei-Leng Cheong; joymlcheong@gmail.com and
Win-Ping Deng; wpdeng@ms41.hinet.net

Academic Editor: Ki-Wan Oh

Antrodia camphorata has previously demonstrated the efficacy in treating cancer and anti-inflammation. In this study, we are the first to evaluate *Antrodia camphorata* alcohol extract (ACAE) for osteoporosis recovery *in vitro* with preosteoblast cells (MC3T3-E1) and *in vivo* with an osteoporosis mouse model established in our previous studies, ovariectomized senescence accelerated mice (OVX-SAMP8). Our results demonstrated that ACAE treatment was slightly cytotoxic to preosteoblast at 25 μg/mL, by which the osteogenic gene expression (RUNX2, OPN, and OCN) was significantly upregulated with an increased ratio of OPG to RANKL, indicating maintenance of the bone matrix through inhibition of osteoclastic pathway. Additionally, evaluation by Alizarin Red S staining showed increased mineralization in ACAE-treated preosteoblasts. For *in vivo* study, our results indicated that ACAE inhibits bone loss and significantly increases percentage bone volume, trabecular bone number, and bone mineral density in OVX-SAMP8 mice treated with ACAE. Collectively, *in vitro* and *in vivo* results showed that ACAE could promote osteogenesis and prevent bone loss and should be considered an evidence-based complementary and alternative medicine for osteoporosis therapy through the maintenance of bone health.

1. Introduction

Osteoporosis is the most common bone disease and is characterized by low bone mass, microarchitectural deterioration of bone tissue, and subsequent bone fragility with susceptibility to fracture [1]. Bone fracture risk typically increases in the hip, vertebral, and distal forearm bones. These fractures are not only painful but also disabling, leading to the need for nursing home care and increased mortality when compared to age matched populations [2, 3]. Because of the high morbidity and mortality associated with osteoporotic fractures, treatment of osteoporosis prioritizes fracture prevention [4].

Multiple treatment options are currently available to osteoporosis patients including bisphosphonates, cell therapy, and supplementation of calcium and/or vitamin D; however, significant shortcomings and the continued widespread impact of the disease warrants further investigation into alternative treatments [5, 6]. Bisphosphonates effectively prevent bone loss through inhibition of osteoclastic bone resorption, but this tactic is one sided in that it does not affect bone renewal and has several adverse reactions ranging from mild to severe [7–9]. Cell therapy is a promising possibility but has many intrinsic hurdles to overcome such as the lack of bone homing ability in mesenchymal stem cells and the uncertainty of cell fate after implantation [10–12]. Vitamin D and calcium are components of bone renewal, but supplementation has limited and inconsistent effectiveness and is often used in combination with other treatments [13].

Antrodia camphorata (AC) is a traditional herbal medicine that is safe and contains osteogenic precursors that make it a likely candidate for effective osteoporosis therapy. AC is a *Ganoderma*-like fungus of the Polyporaceae Basidiomycota family composed of pharmacologically active components including steroids, triterpenoids, polysaccharides, lignans, phenyl derivatives, fatty acids, and trace elements [14, 15]. Much characterization and evaluation of AC components such as crude extracts, bioactivities, and pure compounds have already been completed [16]. Traditional medicines currently made from the fungus are used to treat digestion, hypertension, and pain along with exhibiting anti-inflammatory, antioxidative, and anticancer effects [17]. Recent studies on AC have also shown promising ability to protect the liver from oxidative stress and tissue injuries [18–21]. Previously, we showed that AC alcohol extracts (ACAE) inhibited non-small-cell lung cancer cell growth by promoting cell cycle arrest and inducing caspase 3-mediated apoptosis [18]. There are currently no studies on how AC affects osteoblasts, but many of the above mentioned components are known individually as factors in bone metabolism [22, 23]. AC was obtained from an artificial culture community for this study and concentrated into an alcohol extract (ACAE) to evaluate its potential as a preventative treatment for osteoporosis. *In vivo*, our study utilizes senescence accelerated mouse prone 8 (SAMP8), which was established through phenotypic inbreeding from a common genetic pool of the AKR/J mouse strain that exhibits osteoporosis and can be enhanced by ovariectomy, as established in our previous study. Therefore, ovariectomized-SAMP8 mice (OVX-SAMP8) were an appropriate animal model for *in vivo* study of ACAE on bone [10]. We hypothesized that ACAE treatment is slightly cytotoxic and could induce osteogenesis in preosteoblast *in vitro* and in osteoporotic mice *in vivo*. Subsequently, ACAE treatment may be an effective and safe alternative osteoporosis therapy.

2. Materials and Methods

2.1. Experimental Animals and ACAE Treatment. The female SAMP8 mice experiment protocol was approved by the Institutional Animal Care and Use Committee of Taipei Medical University. All applicable institutional and/or national guidelines for the care and use of animals were followed. The mice were maintained in the animal room under maintained conditions of 25°C and 50% relative humidity. The ovariectomized-SAMP8 female mouse was established by our previous study as an osteoporotic mouse model [10]. Female SAMP8 mice were ovariectomized at 4 months after birth to induce osteoporosis for experiments with 6 animals

per group. The operation was performed on a SHAM-operated group of SAMP8 female mice at 4 months of age excluding removal of the ovaries. For 4 months following the ovariectomy operation 450 mg/kg/day by oral gavage was administered to the ACAE group, while the control group received phosphate buffered solution (PBS).

2.2. Cell Culture. MC3T3-E1 preosteoblastic (ATCC CRL-2593) cells were cultured in alpha minimum essential media (α-MEM) (Gibco) supplemented with 10% fetal bovine serum (FBS) (Gibco) and 1% Penicillin-Streptomycin-Amphotericin B (PSA) in a 10 cm culture dish.

2.3. Preparation of ACAE. AC fruiting bodies were cultured artificially and provided by Well Shine Biotechnology Development Co. (Taipei, Taiwan.) Finely powdered AC was combined with 95% ethanol in a 1 : 20 (w/v) ratio and shaken for 24 h at room temperature. The supernatant was extracted and filtered at a pore size of 0.2 mm (Millex GP Carrigtwohill, Cork, Ireland) and then centrifuged at 3000 rpm for 30 min to remove the precipitate. The extracts were lyophilized and stored at −20°C before use.

2.4. MTT Assay. MTT 3-(4,5-dimethylthiazol-2-yl)-2,5-diphenyltetrazolium bromide assay with tetrazolium salt reagent (Roche) was performed to determine the cytotoxicity of ACAE and EtOH on MC3T3-E1 preosteoblasts (EtOH data not shown). MC3T3-E1 cells were seeded into a 96-well plate at a density of 2×10^3 cells/well and, after 24 hours, the media were changed to different concentrations of ACAE in media along with a control group that was cultured in α-MEM complete culture media only. MTT reagent was added into each well 24 hours after the treatment media. Four hours after the addition of MTT, the reagent was replaced with DMSO, and the optical density values were analyzed using Multiskan PC (Thermo Lab), and cell survival curves were plotted.

2.5. Alizarin Red S Staining for Osteogenesis. Osteogenesis was verified using Alizarin Red S staining. Cells were fixed with 10% formaldehyde (Merk) followed by 2% Alizarin Red S (pH 4.2) (Sigma) staining for 15 min at room temperature. For quantification, the bound staining was eluted with 10% cetylpyridinium chloride, and the absorbance of supernatants was measured at 540 nm [24].

2.6. RT-PCR Analysis. Total RNA was isolated from the test groups of MC3T3-E1 cells cultured in different concentrations of ACAE media using Trizol reagent (Invitrogen). Gene expression levels were measured by RT-PCR. Primer sequences were indicated as follows: Osteocalcin (OCN) forward primer 5′-CAGCTTGGTGCACACCTA-AGC-3′; reverse primer 5′-AGGGTTAAGCTCACACTG-CTCC-3′; temperature 55°C; Osteopontin- (OPN-) forward primer 5′-ATGA-GATTGGCAGTGATT-3′; reverse primer 5′-GTTGACCTCAGAAGATGA-3′; temperature 48.8°C; Runt-related transcription factor 2 (RUNX2) forward primer 5′-ACTTTCTCCAGGAAGACTGC-3′; reverse primer 5′-GCTGTTGTTGCTGTTGCTGT-3′; temperature 55°C; Receptor Activator of Nuclear Factor Kappa B

(RANK) forward primer 5′-TCCAGGTCACTCCTCCAT-GC-3′; reverse primer 5′-GTTCCAGTGGTAGCCAGCCG-3′; temperature 66°C; glyceraldehyde 3-phosphate dehydrogenase (GAPDH) which was used as an internal control (CTRL) forward primer 5′-GCTCTCCAGAACATCATC-CCTGCC-3′; reverse primer 5′-CGTTGTCATACCAGG-AAATGAGCTT-3′; temperature 55°C. PCR products were separated by electrophoresis on 1% agarose gels (Agarose I; AMRESCO) and visualized with DNA View (Biotools, Taipei, Taiwan) staining.

2.7. Bone Imaging.
Dual-energy X-ray absorptiometry (DEXA) (XR-36; Norland Corp.; host software revision 2.5.3, scanner software revision 2.0.0) analysis was used to establish measurements of bone mineral density in the spine and femur after 4 months of treatment. Bone samples from all groups were collected and imaged using a SkyScan-1076 MicroCT System (Skyscan, Belgium). The following three-dimensional (3D) parameters were measured: bone volume, total volume, and trabecular bone numbers. For trabecular bone analysis and 3D image construction, a MicroCT scanner (Skyscan-1076, Skyscan, Belgium) was operated at 50 kV, 200 μA, 0.4 μ of rotation step, 0.5 mm Al filter, and 9 μm/pixel of scan resolution. The data collected was quantitatively represented as the percentage of bone volume/total volume and the trabecular bone number (1/mm) [25].

2.8. Statistical Analysis.
All results were represented as mean ± standard deviation (SD). Significant differences between two groups were determined by Student's t-test, P value <0.05. Figures were graphed using Sigma Plot 10.0.

3. Results

3.1. Dose Dependent Cytotoxicity of ACAE on Preosteoblasts.
To determine the cytotoxicity of ACAE, the preosteoblasts MC3T3-E1 were exposed to ACAE at concentrations of 0, 25, 50, and 100 μg/mL. The results indicated slight cytotoxic effect of ACAE on preosteoblast viability at 25 μg/mL of ACAE: a 10% decrease in survival rate at 50 μg/mL and a 13% decrease in survival rate at 100 μg/mL (Figure 1). Therefore, ACAE at 25 μg/mL was used as the experimental dosage for the subsequent study.

3.2. Osteogenesis of Preosteoblasts Treated with ACAE.
To further examine the degree of osteogenic differentiation in preosteoblasts in the presence of ACAE, Alizarin Red S staining and RT-PCR were performed. PCR was used to detect the degree of gene expression for the osteogenic markers: RUNX2, OCN, and OPN from a culture of preosteoblasts in α-MEM with 25 μg/mL ACAE to compare to a control culture without ACAE. Stronger expression of all 3 osteogenic markers when cultured with ACAE was observed (Figure 2(a)). The quantitative analysis of the PCR results confirm that ACAE treatment of 25 μg/mL resulted in significantly higher gene expression of RUNX2, OCN, and OPN, indicating increased osteogenic differentiation (Figure 2(b)). The results showed visibly darker and larger areas of Alizarin Red S

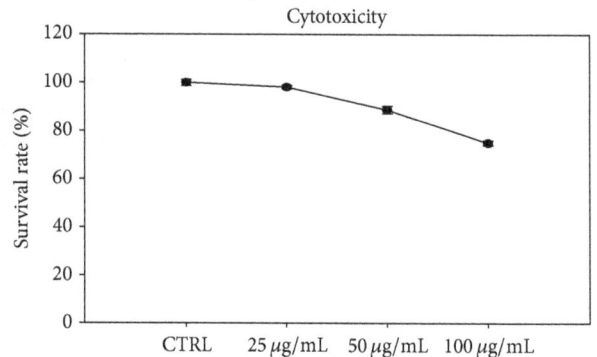

FIGURE 1: Cytotoxicity of ACAE on preosteoblasts. MTT assay was performed on preosteoblast cells after 24 h treatment with different concentrations of ACAE. Results are presented as percentages of cell viability. Representative results of 3 experiments demonstrated mean ± SD.

staining in the ACAE-treated culture relative to the control, which indicates more mineralization of extracellular matrix (Figure 2(c)). Quantitative analysis confirmed significantly higher staining in the preosteoblasts in the ACAE culture than in the control (Figure 2(d)). This supports our PCR data that ACAE promotes osteogenic differentiation in preosteoblasts *in vitro*.

3.3. Analysis of OPG and RANKL Ratio in Preosteoblasts with ACAE.
PCR was used to detect the degree of gene expression for the osteoclastogenic inhibitor OPG and RANKL which is essential to osteoclastogenesis, from a culture of preosteoblasts in α-MEM with 25 μg/mL ACAE to the control group without ACAE. Stronger expression of OPG and weaker expression of RANKL were observed when cultured with ACAE (Figure 3(a)). The quantitative analysis of the PCR results confirms that ACAE treatment resulted in significantly higher gene expression ratio of OPG to RANKL (Figure 3(b)). Results indicate that ACAE promotes the maintenance of the bone matrix through upregulation of OPG and downregulation of RANKL.

3.4. Bone Mineral Density Increased with ACAE Treatment.
BMD was measured on mice after their ovariectomy at 0 months before the test group began ACAE treatment. After four months, BMD was measured on the SHAM-operated along with the OVX-operated CTRL and ACAE group. SHAM-operated mice showed a decrease in BMD, but the OVX-operated CTRL group had a significantly amplified loss of BMD (see supplementary Figure 1 in Supplementary Material available online at http://dx.doi.org/10.1155/2016/2617868). After four months of ACAE treatment, the CTRL and ACAE groups were measured for bone mineral density (BMD) at the spine, knees (right and left), and femurs (right and left) using dual-energy X-ray absorptiometry. The average BMD scores of the six mice were subjected to quantitative analysis revealing that ACAE treatment resulted in significantly higher BMD than the control group in all sites tested in the OVX-SAMP8 mice (Figure 4).

(a)

(b)

(c)

(d)

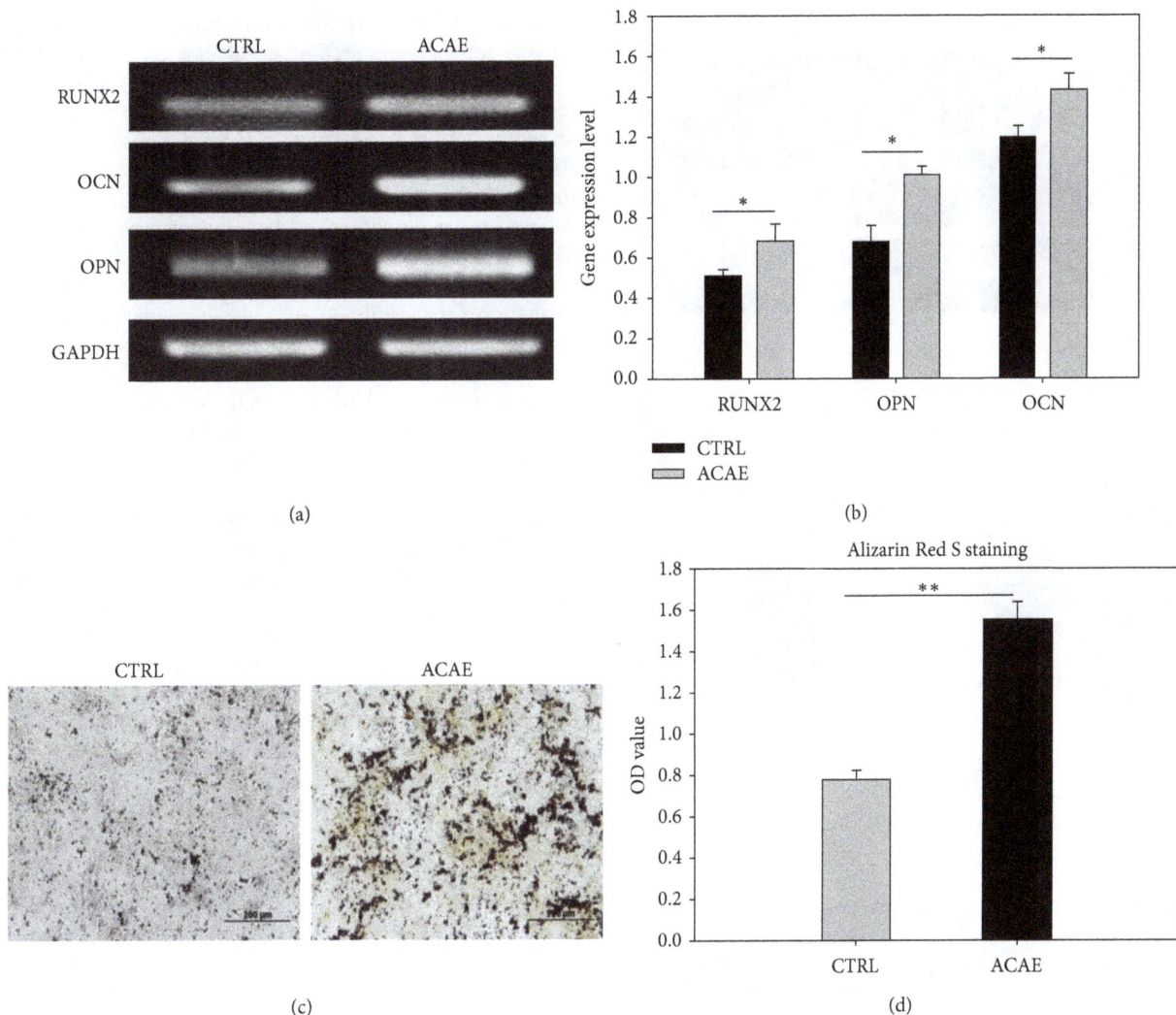

FIGURE 2: Analysis of *in vitro* osteoblastic differentiation of preosteoblasts treated with ACAE. (a) RT-PCR indicated the expression of osteogenic markers RUNX2, OCN, and OPN. (b) Quantitative analysis of the PCR results. (c) Alizarin Red S staining of preosteoblast mineralization. (d) Quantitative analysis of staining results. Representative results of 3 experiments demonstrated mean ± SD. $^*P < 0.05$; $^{**}P < 0.01$.

3.5. Analysis of Bone Quantity after ACAE Treatment. Photomicrographs using both 2D and 3D MicroCT displayed both higher percentage bone volume (PBV) and trabecular number (TBN) with ACAE. The arrows indicate areas of visibly higher bone volume in the MicroCT-2D (Figure 5(a)). Quantitative analysis of the photomicrographs showed a greatly increased PBV and TBN relative to the control group (Figure 5(b)). Histological slides showed higher ratios of trabecular bone in the femur and spine with ACAE relative to the control which showed more space (Figure 5(c)).

4. Discussion

The aim of this study was to determine the potential effects of *Antrodia camphorata* alcohol extracts (ACAE) in osteoporosis therapy. Our results suggest that ACAE could prevent bone loss and significantly induce bone recovery from osteoporosis by balancing bone remodeling. These findings provide the first reports of ACAE in bone regeneration and support it as a promising candidate for safe and effective osteoporosis therapy.

Antrodia camphorata (AC) has many previously explored medicinal properties in addition to newly explored potential in promoting osteoblast differentiation [18, 26]. In this study, we found that ACAE treatment of preosteoblasts (MC3T3-E1) was slightly toxic by MTT analysis while inducing osteoblastic differentiation. These findings support that not only is ACAE a promising cancer therapy but also it has the potential to promote osteogenesis in osteoporosis therapy. The potential of ACAE in osteogenesis was unknown and not yet investigated in previous studies; however, AC contains multiple components such as higher triterpenoids, polysaccharides (β-D Glucosan), ergosterol, and trace elements (calcium, phosphatase, germanium, and chitosan) [27], which

(a)

(b)

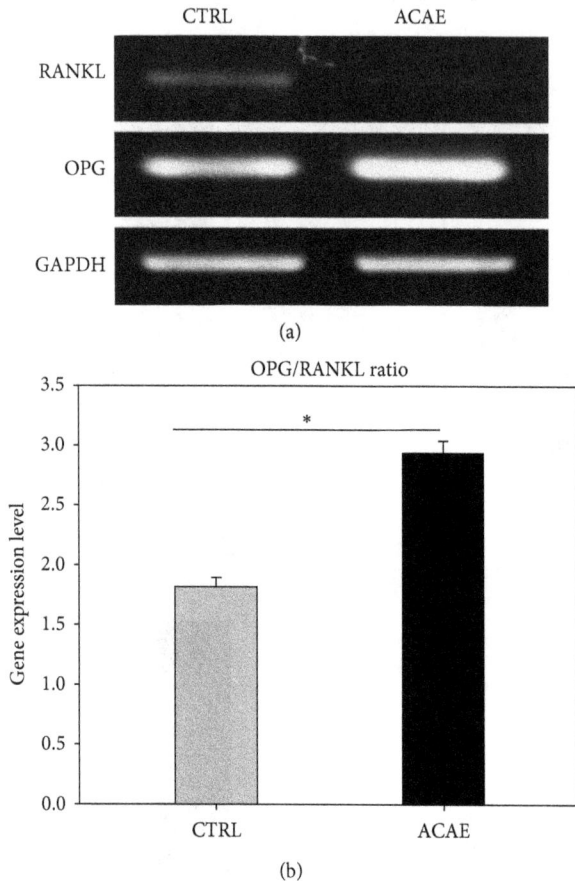

FIGURE 3: Analysis of osteogenic differentiation of preosteoblasts with ACAE. (a) RT-PCR indicated the expression of RANKL and OPG from a culture of preosteoblasts in α-MEM with 25 μg/mL ACAE and control (CTRL) group. (b) Quantitative analysis of PCR results. Representative results of 3 experiments demonstrated mean ± SD. $^{*}P < 0.05$ versus CTRL group.

are factors associated in the induction of osteogenic differentiation. Triterpenoids have been shown to exhibit significantly protective effects on bone remodeling regulation in osteoporosis therapy [28], while polysaccharides and polysaccharide-based scaffold promote osteogenesis [29], and ergosterol is a vitamin D precursor which is known to stimulate osteoblastic differentiation [30]. Furthermore, our RT-PCR analysis results demonstrated that ACAE treatment upregulated the gene expression of RUNX2, OPN, and OCN, along with strong mineralization of bone matrix observed by Alizarin Red S staining. Additionally, recent studies indicated that AC provides trace elements that contribute to bone health and showed that vitamin D and Ca deficiency increase the risk of osteoporosis and bone fractures [31, 32]. The above mentioned studies collectively support our finding that AC has the potential to induce osteogenesis in an osteoporotic animal model.

Current therapies widely depend on bisphosphonates to treat osteoporosis [33]. Although these drugs prevent

bone loss and decrease the risk of bone fractures in osteoporosis patients, there are many adverse reactions including upset stomach, erosion of the esophagus, flu-like symptoms, osteonecrosis of the jaw, intense musculoskeletal pain, atrial fibrillation, and atypical femur fractures [7]. Additionally, bisphosphonates carry warnings and contraindications for patients with reduced renal function, in contrast to AC which has demonstrated hepatoprotective qualities [34, 35]. Finally, bisphosphonates only mediate bone resorption through osteoclast inhibition without promoting bone formation [36], while ACAE has the potential to induce osteogenesis and could therefore greatly improve on current osteoporosis therapy. Our results demonstrated that ACAE could promote osteoblast differentiation and suppress osteoclastic differentiation by inhibiting RANKL expression and strongly increasing OPG expression in ACAE-treated OVX-SAMP8 mice in addition to improving bone density which collectively ameliorated osteoporosis in OVX-SAMP8 mice. Interestingly, this result is supported by previous finding that triterpenoids could inhibit osteoclast formation by reducing RANKL expression [37], suggesting that the triterpenoids in ACAE may be useful compounds for modulating bone resorption in osteoporosis therapy.

ACAE is an herbal medicine extract and is therefore a cocktail containing a multitude of components. The cellular responses to each pure compound as well as the mechanisms involved in producing therapeutic results have not been fully explored. Research on traditional herbal drugs is an important means to finding new drugs; however, their true properties may remain unknown even after studies have demonstrated their effectiveness [38]. Further examination of ACAE is warranted through the evaluation of its pure compounds. However, the ACAE cocktail was able to modulate osteogenesis in osteoporotic mice, and our results demonstrated that ACAE prevented bone loss and significantly increased percentage bone volume, trabecular bone number, and bone mineral density in OVX-SAMP8 mice. These findings and those of previous studies may be a product of synergistic activity that could promote osteogenesis in osteoporosis therapy. Although the key factors regulating the observed functional recovery are not fully characterized, the treatment potential may differ in every pure compound when used alone. We found that in vitro and in vivo results show promotion of osteogenesis and the potential to prevent osteoporosis by treatment with ACAE.

In this study we demonstrated that ACAE has the potential to maintain bone health through promotion of osteogenesis and the inhibition of bone digestion. The progression of cancer is linked to osteoporosis, and Martin et al. found that healthy bone could suppress bone metastasis. Maintaining bone volume and function could therefore reduce tumor invasion in breast cancer patients [39–41]. Subsequently, our results indicate that AC could potentially reduce bone metastasis in patients suffering from breast cancer and osteoporosis along with strongly inhibiting cancer growth, as shown in our previous study [18]. Our study supports the use of AC as an evidence-based complementary and alternative medicine for cancer therapy and osteoporosis in addition to other associated bone diseases through maintenance of bone health.

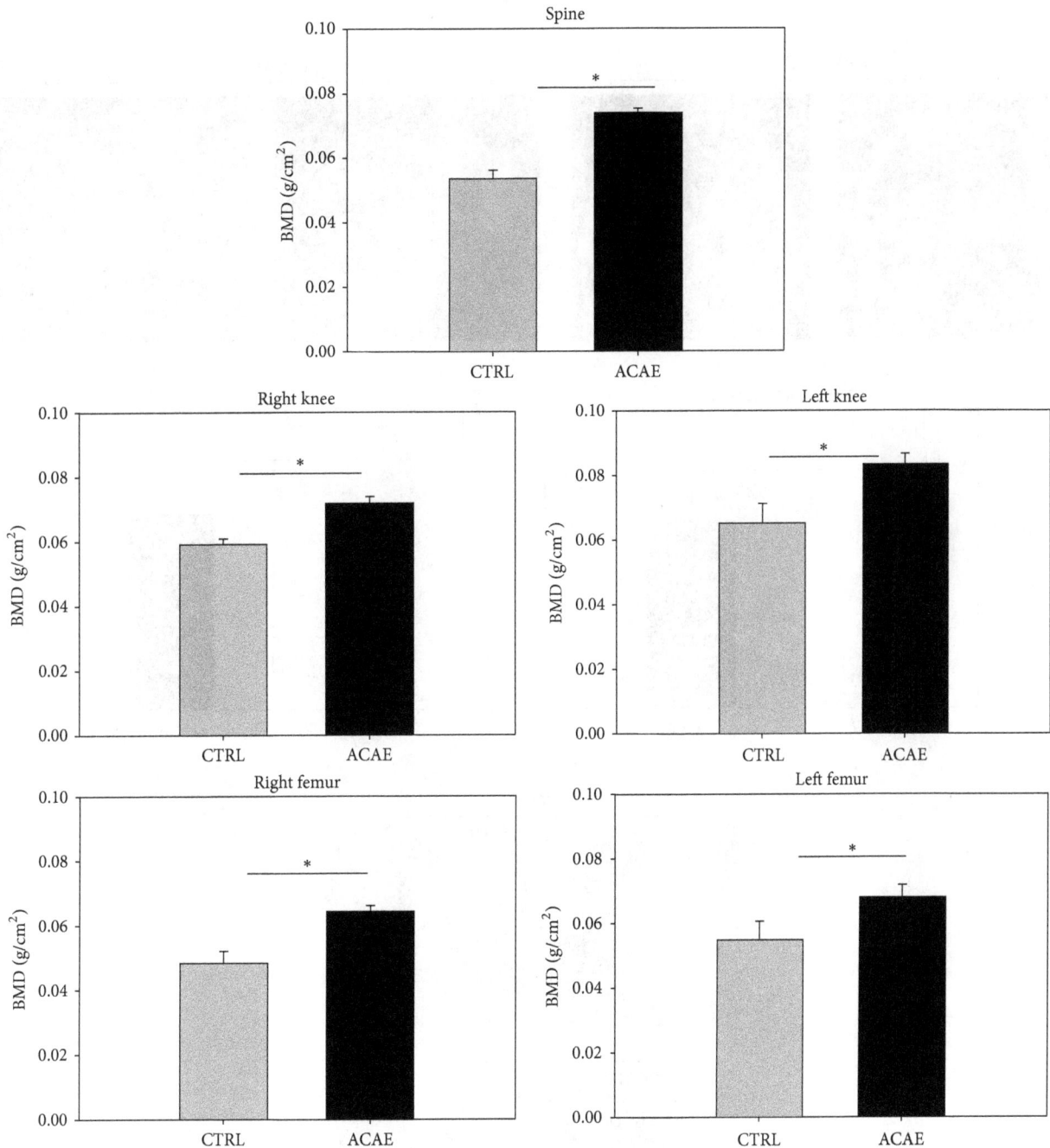

FIGURE 4: Bone mineral density with ACAE treatment. Bone mineral density (BMD) was measured by dual-energy X-ray absorptiometry for the spine, knees (right and left), and femurs (right and left). OVX-SAMP8 mice with ACAE treatment and CTRL group were measured at 4 months. Each bar represents the average from six animals. $^*P < 0.05$ versus CTRL group.

5. Conclusion

This study indicated ACAE promotion of osteogenesis *in vitro* in MC3T3-E1 preosteoblasts and *in vivo* in the OVX-SAMP8 osteoporotic mouse model in addition to inhibited RANKL relative to OPG (osteoclastogenesis). Our results demonstrated significant bone recovery and decreased bone loss that indicate improved bone remodeling balance and that ACAE could be a uniquely well-balanced treatment for osteoporosis.

Competing Interests

Hen-Yu Liu, Chiung-Fang Huang, Chun-hao Li, Ching-Yu Tsai, Wei-Hong Chen, Hong-Jian Wei, Ming-Fu Wang,

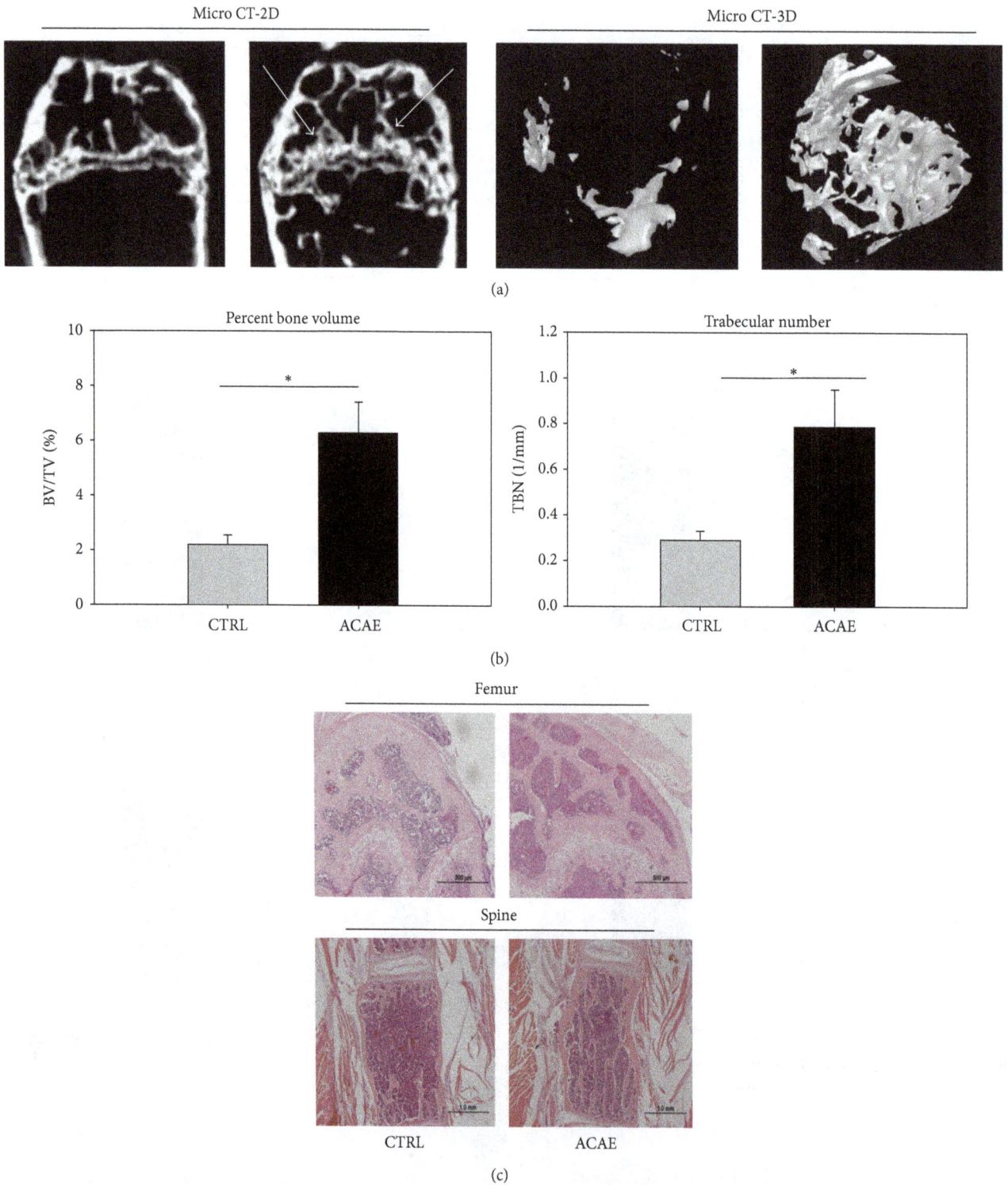

FIGURE 5: Analysis of bone quantity with photomicrographs. (a) 2D and 3D photomicrographs by MicroCT of femurs from OVX-SAMP8 mice with and without ACAE treatment. Arrows indicate areas of visibly higher bone volume in the MicroCT-2D. (b) Quantitative analysis of photomicrographs to determine percentage bone volume (PBV) and trabecular number (TBN). (c) Histological slides of the femur and spine with ACAE treatment and a control. Each bar represents the average from six animals. $^*P < 0.05$ versus CTRL group.

Yueh-Hsiung Kuo, Mei-Leng Cheong, and Win-Ping Deng declare that they have no conflict of interests with the mentioned trademarks or companies.

Authors' Contributions

Mei-Leng Cheong and Win-Ping Deng contributed equally to this work.

Acknowledgments

The authors thank the Taiwan Mouse Clinic (NSC 102-2325-B-001-042) which is funded by the National Research Program for Biopharmaceuticals (NRPB) at the National Science Council (NSC) of Taiwan for technical support in Bio-imaging (MicroCT) and histopathological analysis and CMU under the Aim for Top University Plan of the Ministry of Education, Taiwan, and Taiwan Ministry of Health and Welfare Clinical Trial and Research Center of Excellence (MOHW105-TDU-B-212-133019) and Research Center of Excellent (DOH 102-TD-B-111-004) for supporting this study. This research was also supported by the following grants and agencies: Ministry of Science and Technology (MOST 104-2221-E-038-016, MOST 103-2314-B-281-007 (M.-L. Cheong), and 104-2313-B-038-001), the Council of Agriculture, Executive Yuan (104 AS-16.3.1-ST-a8), and Stem Cell Research Center and Cancer Center, Taipei Medical University, Taipei, Taiwan. The authors also thank Well Shine Biotechnology Development Co. (Taipei, Taiwan), for providing for materials.

References

[1] C. J. Rosen and M. L. Bouxsein, "Mechanisms of disease: is osteoporosis the obesity of bone?" *Nature Clinical Practice Rheumatology*, vol. 2, no. 1, pp. 35–43, 2006.

[2] E. M. Lewiecki, "Osteoporosis," *Annals of Internal Medicine*, vol. 155, no. 1, p. ITC1-1, 2011.

[3] J. D. Adachi, G. Ioannidis, L. Pickard et al., "The association between osteoporotic fractures and health-related quality of life as measured by the Health Utilities Index in the Canadian Multicentre Osteoporosis Study (CaMos)," *Osteoporosis International*, vol. 14, no. 11, pp. 895–904, 2003.

[4] S. F. Hodgson, N. B. Watts, J. P. Bilezikian et al., "American Association of Clinical Endocrinologists medical guidelines for clinical practice for the prevention and treatment of postmenopausal osteoporosis: 2001 edition, with selected updates for 2003," *Endocrine Practice*, vol. 9, no. 6, pp. 544–564, 2003.

[5] M. C. Chapuy, R. Pamphile, E. Paris et al., "Combined calcium and vitamin D3 supplementation in elderly women: confirmation of reversal of secondary hyperparathyroidism and hip fracture risk: the Decalyos II study," *Osteoporosis International*, vol. 13, no. 3, pp. 257–264, 2002.

[6] R. P. Heaney, "Osteoporosis: Management and treatment strategies for orthopaedic surgeons," *The Journal of Bone & Joint Surgery—American Volume*, vol. 90, no. 11, pp. 2544–2545, 2008.

[7] R. E. Marx, Y. Sawatari, M. Fortin, and V. Broumand, "Bisphosphonate-induced exposed bone (osteonecrosis/ osteopetrosis) of the jaws: risk factors, recognition, prevention, and treatment," *Journal of Oral and Maxillofacial Surgery*, vol. 63, no. 11, pp. 1567–1575, 2005.

[8] A. Devine, I. M. Dick, S. S. Dhaliwal, R. Naheed, J. Beilby, and R. L. Prince, "Prediction of incident osteoporotic fractures in elderly women using the free estradiol index," *Osteoporosis International*, vol. 16, no. 2, pp. 216–221, 2005.

[9] M. J. Favus, "Bisphosphonates for osteoporosis," *The New England Journal of Medicine*, vol. 363, no. 21, pp. 2027–2035, 2010.

[10] W.-C. Lo, J.-F. Chiou, J. G. Gelovani et al., "Transplantation of embryonic fibroblasts treated with platelet-rich plasma induces osteogenesis in SAMP8 mice monitored by molecular imaging," *Journal of Nuclear Medicine*, vol. 50, no. 5, pp. 765–773, 2009.

[11] K. C. Hicok, T. V. Du Laney, Y. S. Zhou et al., "Human adipose-derived adult stem cells produce osteoid in vivo," *Tissue Engineering*, vol. 10, no. 3-4, pp. 371–380, 2004.

[12] Y. Zhou, Y. Ni, Y. Liu, B. Zeng, Y. Xu, and W. Ge, "The role of simvastatin in the osteogenesis of injectable tissue-engineered bone based on human adipose-derived stromal cells and platelet-rich plasma," *Biomaterials*, vol. 31, no. 20, pp. 5325–5335, 2010.

[13] E. Papadimitropoulos, G. Wells, B. Shea et al., "VIII: meta-analysis of the efficacy of vitamin D treatment in preventing osteoporosis in postmenopausal women," *Endocrine Reviews*, vol. 23, no. 4, pp. 560–569, 2002.

[14] D.-Z. Liu, H.-J. Liang, C.-H. Chen et al., "Comparative anti-inflammatory characterization of wild fruiting body, liquid-state fermentation, and solid-state culture of Taiwanofungus camphoratus in microglia and the mechanism of its action," *Journal of Ethnopharmacology*, vol. 113, no. 1, pp. 45–53, 2007.

[15] D.-Z. Liu, Y.-C. Liang, S.-Y. Lin et al., "Antihypertensive activities of a solid-state culture of *Taiwanofungus camphoratus* (Chang-Chih) in spontaneously hypertensive rats," *Bioscience, Biotechnology and Biochemistry*, vol. 71, no. 1, pp. 23–30, 2007.

[16] M. Geethangili and Y.-M. Tzeng, "Review of pharmacological effects of antrodia camphorata and its bioactive compounds," *Evidence-Based Complementary and Alternative Medicine*, vol. 2011, Article ID 212641, 17 pages, 2011.

[17] Y.-C. Hseu, F.-Y. Wu, J.-J. Wu et al., "Anti-inflammatory potential of *Antrodia Camphorata* through inhibition of iNOS, COX-2 and cytokines via the NF-κB pathway," *International Immunopharmacology*, vol. 5, no. 13-14, pp. 1914–1925, 2005.

[18] J.-F. Chiou, A. T. H. Wu, W.-T. Wang et al., "A preclinical evaluation of *Antrodia camphorata* alcohol extracts in the treatment of non-small cell lung cancer using non-invasive molecular imaging," *Evidence-Based Complementary and Alternative Medicine*, vol. 2011, Article ID 914561, 12 pages, 2011.

[19] C.-H. Huang, Y.-Y. Chang, C.-W. Liu et al., "Fruiting body of niuchangchih (antrodia camphorata) protects livers against chronic alcohol consumption damage," *Journal of Agricultural and Food Chemistry*, vol. 58, no. 6, pp. 3859–3866, 2010.

[20] J.-S. Deng, S.-S. Huang, T.-H. Lin et al., "Analgesic and anti-inflammatory bioactivities of eburicoic acid and dehydroeburicoic acid isolated from *Antrodia camphorata* on the inflammatory mediator expression in mice," *Journal of Agricultural and Food Chemistry*, vol. 61, no. 21, pp. 5064–5071, 2013.

[21] Y. W. Liu, K. H. Lu, C. T. Ho, and L. Y. Sheen, "Protective effects of *Antrodia cinnamomea* against liver injury," *Journal of Traditional and Complementary Medicine*, vol. 2, no. 4, pp. 284–294, 2012.

[22] M. F. Holick, "Vitamin D: importance in the prevention of cancers, type 1 diabetes, heart disease, and osteoporosis," *American Journal of Clinical Nutrition*, vol. 79, no. 3, pp. 362–371, 2004.

[23] L. C. Hofbauer, C. R. Dunstan, T. C. Spelsberg, B. L. Riggs, and S. Khosla, "Osteoprotegerin production by human osteoblast lineage cells is stimulated by vitamin D, bone morphogenetic protein-2, and cytokines," *Biochemical and Biophysical Research Communications*, vol. 250, no. 3, pp. 776–781, 1998.

[24] H. Kim, J.-H. Lee, and H. Suh, "Interaction of mesenchymal stem cells and osteoblasts for in vitro osteogenesis," *Yonsei Medical Journal*, vol. 44, no. 2, pp. 187–197, 2003.

[25] H.-Y. Liu, A. T. H. Wu, C.-Y. Tsai et al., "The balance between adipogenesis and osteogenesis in bone regeneration by platelet-rich plasma for age-related osteoporosis," *Biomaterials*, vol. 32, no. 28, pp. 6773–6780, 2011.

[26] M.-C. Lu, M. El-Shazly, T.-Y. Wu et al., "Recent research and development of *Antrodia cinnamomea*," *Pharmacology and Therapeutics*, vol. 139, no. 2, pp. 124–156, 2013.

[27] C.-C. Huang, M.-C. Hsu, W.-C. Huang, H.-R. Yang, and C.-C. Hou, "Triterpenoid-rich extract from antrodia camphorata improves physical fatigue and exercise performance in mice," *Evidence-Based Complementary and Alternative Medicine*, vol. 2012, Article ID 364741, 8 pages, 2012.

[28] J. X. Li, J. Liu, C. C. He et al., "Triterpenoids from Cimicifugae rhizoma, a novel class of inhibitors on bone resorption and ovariectomy-induced bone loss," *Maturitas*, vol. 58, no. 1, pp. 59–69, 2007.

[29] S. G. Kumbar, U. S. Toti, M. Deng et al., "Novel mechanically competent polysaccharide scaffolds for bone tissue engineering," *Biomedical Materials*, vol. 6, no. 6, Article ID 065005, 2011.

[30] C. Shui and A. M. Scutt, "Mouse embryo-derived NIH3T3 fibroblasts adopt an osteoblast-like phenotype when treated with 1α,25-dihydroxyvitamin D3 and dexamethasone in vitro," *Journal of Cellular Physiology*, vol. 193, no. 2, pp. 164–172, 2002.

[31] H. Y. Liu, M. C. Liu, M. F. Wang et al., "Potential osteoporosis recovery by deep sea water through bone regeneration in SAMP8 mice," *Evidence-Based Complementary and Alternative Medicine*, vol. 2013, Article ID 161976, 11 pages, 2013.

[32] T. O. Carpenter, S. J. Mackowiak, N. Troiano, and C. M. Gundberg, "Osteocalcin and its message: relationship to bone histology in magnesium-deprived rats," *American Journal of Physiology—Endocrinology and Metabolism*, vol. 263, no. 1, part 1, pp. E107–E114, 1992.

[33] R. Kunchur and A. N. Goss, "The oral health status of patients on oral bisphosphonates for osteoporosis," *Australian Dental Journal*, vol. 53, no. 4, pp. 354–357, 2008.

[34] G.-J. Huang, J.-S. Deng, S.-S. Huang et al., "Hepatoprotective effects of eburicoic acid and dehydroeburicoic acid from *Antrodia camphorata* in a mouse model of acute hepatic injury," *Food Chemistry*, vol. 141, no. 3, pp. 3020–3027, 2013.

[35] G.-J. Huang, J.-S. Deng, S.-S. Huang, Y.-Y. Shao, C.-C. Chen, and Y.-H. Kuo, "Protective effect of antrosterol from *Antrodia camphorata* submerged whole broth against carbon tetrachloride-induced acute liver injury in mice," *Food Chemistry*, vol. 132, no. 2, pp. 709–716, 2012.

[36] R. Keen, "Osteoporosis: strategies for prevention and management," *Best Practice and Research: Clinical Rheumatology*, vol. 21, no. 1, pp. 109–122, 2007.

[37] R. A. Fava, S. Elliott, L. Raymond et al., "The synthetic triterpenoid TP-222 inhibits RANKL stimulation of osteoclastogenesis and matrix metalloproteinase-9 expression," *Journal of Rheumatology*, vol. 34, no. 5, pp. 1058–1068, 2007.

[38] Z. Yan, H. Hua, Y. Xu, and L. P. Samaranayake, "Potent antifungal activity of pure compounds from traditional Chinese medicine extracts against six oral *Candida* species and the synergy with fluconazole against azole-resistant *Candida albicans*," *Evidence-Based Complementary and Alternative Medicine*, vol. 2012, Article ID 106583, 6 pages, 2012.

[39] E. Fontanges, A. Fontana, and P. Delmas, "Osteoporosis and breast cancer," *Joint Bone Spine*, vol. 71, no. 2, pp. 102–110, 2004.

[40] M. Gnant and P. Hadji, "Prevention of bone metastases and management of bone health in early breast cancer," *Breast Cancer Research*, vol. 12, no. 6, article 216, 2010.

[41] C. K. Martin, J. L. Werbeck, N. K. Thudi et al., "Zoledronic acid reduces bone loss and tumor growth in an orthotopic xenograft model of osteolytic oral squamous cell carcinoma," *Cancer Research*, vol. 70, no. 21, pp. 8607–8616, 2010.

15

Regional Influences on Chinese Medicine Education: Comparing Australia and Hong Kong

Caragh Brosnan,[1,2] Vincent C. H. Chung,[2,3] Anthony L. Zhang,[2,4] and Jon Adams[2]

[1]School of Humanities and Social Science, Faculty of Education and Arts, University of Newcastle, University Drive, Callaghan, NSW 2308, Australia
[2]Australian Research Centre in Complementary and Integrative Medicine, Faculty of Health, University of Technology Sydney, 15 Broadway, Ultimo, NSW 2007, Australia
[3]The Jockey Club School of Public Health and Primary Care, The Chinese University of Hong Kong, Prince of Wales Hospital, Shatin, New Territories, Hong Kong
[4]Health Sciences, RMIT University, P.O. Box 71, Bundoora, VIC 3083, Australia

Correspondence should be addressed to Caragh Brosnan; caragh.brosnan@newcastle.edu.au

Academic Editor: Hongcai Shang

High quality education programs are essential for preparing the next generation of Chinese medicine (CM) practitioners. Currently, training in CM occurs within differing health and education policy contexts. There has been little analysis of the factors influencing the form and status of CM education in different regions. Such a task is important for understanding how CM is evolving internationally and predicting future workforce characteristics. This paper compares the status of CM education in Australia and Hong Kong across a range of dimensions: historical and current positions in the national higher education system, regulatory context and relationship to the health system, and public and professional legitimacy. The analysis highlights the different ways in which CM education is developing in these settings, with Hong Kong providing somewhat greater access to clinical training opportunities for CM students. However, common trends and challenges shape CM education in both regions, including marginalisation from mainstream health professions, a small but established presence in universities, and an emphasis on biomedical research. Three factors stand out as significant for the evolution of CM education in Australia and Hong Kong and may have international implications: continuing biomedical dominance, increased competition between universities, and strengthened links with mainland China.

1. Introduction

As Chinese medicine (CM) has spread throughout the world, it has been absorbed, interpreted, and transformed within different national contexts [1–4]. A key channel through which such processes occur is in the training and education of CM practitioners and the intersection of CM training with broader national education systems. It is often via education that particular philosophies and practices come to predominate and are adopted by the next generation of practitioners. Critically analysing CM education in different national settings can therefore provide useful insights into how and why CM is evolving internationally. This discussion paper compares the status of CM education in Australia and Hong Kong in order to understand how these two contrasting national settings shape CM education and, in turn, the future CM workforce in each region.

CM practice in both Australia and Hong Kong is statutorily regulated. The Chinese Medicine Board of Australia (CMBA) and the Chinese Medicine Council of Hong Kong (CMCHK) are responsible for implementing regulations on CM practice, respectively, for the two regions. Obtaining licensure for practice from either regulatory body requires professional education in accredited programs. Unlike many other English-speaking jurisdictions, such programs are offered in public universities in both regions. The design of these 4–6-year programs invariably illustrates reference to the CM curriculum in mainland China, of which 60–70% of the content is focused on CM, and the remaining curriculum is focused upon biomedicine. In Hong Kong, the CM component is taught in Chinese, while the biomedicine component is often taught in English. In both Hong Kong and Australia, mandatory continuing medical education/continuing professional development (CME/CPD) for registered CM practitioners is in place and fulfilment of relevant requirements is necessary for revalidation. The majority of graduates from CM programs in both regions will practice in the private sector, providing outpatient services in either solo or group practice.

Despite these similarities, these programs operate in different cultural and health system contexts. In Hong Kong, the development of CM services has become a constitutional mandate after reunification of China. Limited outpatient CM services are provided in the tax-funded healthcare system and pilot programs on CM inpatient services within public hospital are in progress. While CM education has gained top-down legitimacy from the government, acceptance of CM graduates by conventional medical practitioners remains limited and there has been little interprofessional collaboration. In Australia, the only form of CM available through the public health system is acupuncture, where it is carried out by a medical doctor. Access to CM in Australia therefore involves out-of-pocket expenses, although costs may be subsidised by some private healthcare funds, with nearly 60% of the adult population having private health cover in Australia [5].

Given these similarities and differences, Australia and Hong Kong constitute excellent case studies for examining how wider historical and policy contexts may shape discussion and subsequent development of CM education in health systems where biomedicine dominates.

2. Materials and Methods

A small number of prior studies have examined the influence of culture and social structures on CM education in the United States [1, 3], United Kingdom [6], and Australia [7, 8]. However, there is a distinct lack of cross-national comparative research in this area, especially when considering the broader context of education in each country beyond specific degree programs. Here, we aim to broaden the analytic frame by taking stock of different influences on the form that CM education takes in two regions with distinct but overlapping regulatory contexts, organisational structures, and health system features.

Drawing on available literature, the paper first provides a brief overview of the historical position of CM in the Australian and Hong Kong education systems, before going on to examine CM's current position and the shifts taking place in higher education, the regulatory context and place of CM in the healthcare system, and the cultural legitimacy of CM in each region. Consideration is also given to the reasons for the similarities and differences in the status of CM education between Australia and Hong Kong. The paper then draws the key issues together to provide an overall assessment of the constraints and opportunities for developing CM education in the future in Australia and Hong Kong and considers the implications for other similar regions where

CM is taught. The conclusion highlights the importance and relevance of this research, especially in terms of future investigations into CM education worldwide.

3. Results

3.1. Historical Position of CM in the National Higher Education System. While the history of CM in Australia is vastly different to that of Hong Kong, historical events have nevertheless impacted CM's current position within the higher education systems of both countries.

3.1.1. Australia. Though still considered complementary or alternative to mainstream biomedicine, CM, including acupuncture and herbal medicine, has been well established in Australia since the gold rush era of the 1850s [2, 9]. Increased Asian migration to Australia in the late twentieth century was accompanied by a significant increase in CM use [9]. CM formal education has historically been skewed towards acupuncture, with the first (private) acupuncture colleges opening in the 1970s [10] (offering diplomas), prior to which some acupuncture training had been offered in chiropractic or naturopathic colleges [11]. Bachelor degree programs were established or transferred from colleges into four publicly funded universities from the early 1990s, with the first degree program covering both acupuncture and herbal medicine opening at the Royal Melbourne Institute of Technology (RMIT) in 1996 [10]. This move into the university system occurred well before the statutory regulation of CM practice in Australia and was seen as offering opportunities for greater access to research and teaching resources [7].

3.1.2. Hong Kong. As a tradition of China, CM has been used for centuries and it has been officially included in the healthcare system in mainland China since the 1950s [12]. With the government's consistent support, CM remains a key part of China's health service today [13]. Nevertheless, CM in Hong Kong has followed a very different path, due to Hong Kong's status as a British colony from 1841 to 1997. In the early colonial days, the local Chinese community considered CM as their main form of healthcare. Tung Wah Hospital was the first CM Hospital in Hong Kong, opening in the late nineteenth century. It made a significant contribution to the provision of basic healthcare in the Chinese population during that period [14]. However, following World War II, a tax-funded healthcare system was established with biomedicine being the exclusive type of healthcare and the role of CM largely sidelined to the private sector, often with CM practitioners working in solo practice. The colonial government regarded CM as part of the "Chinese cultural custom" instead of a formal healthcare modality [15]. Instead of the Secretariat for Health, CM came under the administrative purview of the Secretariat for Home Affairs [16].

The marginal status of CM was also reflected in legislation relating to healthcare. The colonial Medical Registration Ordinance specified that only biomedical clinicians were subject to regulation, and the practice of CM was considered to be out of scope [17]. Due to lack of regulation, tertiary education was not a prerequisite for practice in CM. Apprenticeships with family members or "masters" were the usual pathway to a CM career, often supplemented with lecture-based training provided by CM associations with mixed quality [18]. In the early 1990s, CM education first appeared in the School of Professional and Continuing Education, University of Hong Kong. However, despite its appearance in the tertiary education sector, CM remained marginalised. Only conventional clinicians were allowed to use the title "doctor," and this rule continues today even after regulation. Sharing clinics between biomedical and CM clinicians was prohibited and the latter had no rights in issuing death, sick leave, or health status assessment certificates and were forbidden to use any "biomedical" instruments like syringes and stethoscopes [19]. These regulations led to the creation of a formal medical system based only on biomedicine.

This situation changed with the reunification of Hong Kong and China on 1 July 1997, as the constitutional law of the then newly established Hong Kong Special Administrative Region (SAR) mandated the development of CM in the territory [20]. Under this policy initiative, Hong Kong Baptist University launched the full-time, five-year bachelor degree in CM in 1998: the first of its kind after reunification with China. Similar to Australia, the establishment of a School of Chinese Medicine within a public university was considered a milestone for research and learning in CM in postcolonial Hong Kong [21].

3.2. Current Higher Education Context and the Position of CM.
Differences exist between the current positions of CM in Australian higher education in comparison with Hong Kong, yet there are also similarities in terms of research and funding.

3.2.1. Australia. Despite having been represented within Australian universities for over two decades, Garvey [7] describes CM as just "one tiny fish in a very large tertiary education...pond" (p. 7). Indeed, only three of the 40 Australian universities currently teach CM (RMIT University, University of Technology Sydney, and University of Western Sydney). All now offer qualifications in both acupuncture and herbal medicine, and a range of four-/five-year bachelors and three-year (part-time) Masters programs are available. Entry requirements into these courses include an Australian Tertiary Admission Rank (ATAR) in the 70s–80s (out of 100), which is higher than the average ATAR of around 70 [22] and means CM university programs are more competitive to gain entrance to than nursing degrees, but less so than medicine. In addition to universities, 4-year CM bachelor degree programs are also offered at three private colleges (Endeavour College of Natural Health, Southern School of Natural Therapies, and Sydney Institute of Traditional Chinese Medicine).

National enrolment figures are not published regularly. A 2010 study reports 144 final year students across the (then) seven institutions [23] although national registration in 2012 may have seen these numbers expand. The profession itself is also relatively small, but growing, with just under 4500 practitioners registered in mid-2015 [24]. This compares to over 100,000 conventional medical doctors currently registered in Australia [25], representing a practitioner : population ratio of 1 : 232 for conventional medicine versus 1 : 5314 for CM.

As a minor player, CM is subject to shifts affecting the Australian higher education sector as a whole, including cuts in public funding and universities' increased reliance on student fees and external research grants. Currently under discussion in Australia are policy changes that would see universities permitted to charge uncapped fees for courses and increased public funding for private education providers. CM is unusual among complementary medicine and other disciplines in Australia in that CM degrees are already offered both by universities and by private colleges. The proposed deregulation of university funding in Australia would see increased competition for students from private colleges, which may be able to undercut universities' fees, potentially impacting CM's position in the university sector. The case of naturopathy is informative here: it gradually disappeared from Australian universities after new funding schemes for private education were introduced in 2006 [26].

At an international level, the opening of higher education markets and a new emphasis on competitive ranking systems have affected CM alongside all other university disciplines [27]. Recent global competition centres on research funding and outputs and within universities disciplines are increasingly evaluated against these metrics, with natural and medical science disciplines typically coming out on top [28]. In Australian universities, complementary medicine disciplines have struggled to keep pace with this research environment, although among them CM has had the greatest success, with a number of competitive public research grants awarded in CM in the past decade [29]. However, CM research is not necessarily recognised as such in the national research assessment exercise, the "Excellence in Research for Australia" (ERA). Within the ERA, there is a single category for "complementary and alternative medicine" as a research field, and many of the CM studies conducted are counted within the "clinical sciences" or "pharmacology and pharmaceutical sciences" categories, thereby masking the actual research strength of CM in Australia. This merging of CM with other disciplines may also reflect a trend towards the biomedicalisation of CM. Indeed, funding is typically awarded for research that fits within a biomedical paradigm, focussing on molecular biology or employing randomised-control trials [7]. Such funding success may represent a double-edged sword for CM, with some commentators raising concerns over the fate of CM's traditional concepts which are not easily included in such research frameworks [7].

Funds from the Chinese Government and Chinese pharmaceutical companies have also provided important resources for CM research in Australia, and many universities and private colleges are affiliated with Chinese institutions [30]. The relationship between research and education in CM within Australia is not straightforward however, and recent years have seen substantial research funding for complementary medicine directed towards universities or university centres that do not necessarily teach it, for example, the establishment of the Zhendong Australia-China Centre for Molecular Traditional Chinese Medicine, University of Adelaide, and the Australian Research Centre in Complementary and Integrative Medicine (ARCCIM), University of Technology Sydney. While some of these centres promote collaborations between research and clinical practice/practitioners, the potential increased privatisation of higher education in Australia may result in a deeper split between complementary medicine research and teaching.

3.2.2. Hong Kong. In Hong Kong, it has been 17 years since the first batch of full-time students enrolled in an undergraduate CM program offered by a public university. While there are three Schools of Chinese Medicine in the territory (Chinese University of Hong Kong, Hong Kong Baptist University, and University of Hong Kong), the scale of CM undergraduate education has remained small, with total new enrolment of about 100 per year [31]. Entry requirements from high school are similar to those for nursing degrees and lower than those for medicine [32–34]. The curriculum at all institutions was designed according to the accreditation requirement from the CMCHK, covering Chinese herbal medicine, acupuncture, and bone setting [35]. The degree programs have now extended to 6 years. Despite such small intakes, the CM workforce is not small as many practitioners have been able to obtain registration via grandfathering processes. By 2015, there were 6,898 registered Chinese medicine practitioners on the CMCHK list [36]. This translates to a CM-practitioner-to-population ratio of 1 : 1053, significantly higher than in Australia. The conventional doctor : population ratio is 1 : 541 [37], but since CM only constitutes about 20% of all outpatient care provision in Hong Kong [38], there is a slight oversupply of CM practitioners.

This risk of oversupply is exaggerated by an increasing number of candidates sitting for the CMCHK licensing examinations. On top of local CM students, graduates from 31 recognized CM universities in mainland China are eligible to sit the examination and become registered CM practitioners in Hong Kong if they pass all requirements. Every year, more than one thousand Hong Kong high school graduates are admitted to mainland CM universities and the number is increasing. It is likely that they will return to Hong Kong and sit for the licensing examination [39]. Mainland CM universities are now in direct competition with the local CM programs for enrolment. The Hong Kong program is slightly disadvantaged as it is one year longer than the 5-year course provided across mainland China, and the fees are at least 4 times higher [40]. Another threat to the local CM programs is the relatively lower government funding as compared to other clinical subjects like conventional medicine and dentistry. Although all these programs are six years in length, public funding for CM is two times less, causing staff shortages in the local schools of CM [31].

With regard to research, schools of CM in Hong Kong face similar challenges to their Australian counterparts in maintaining competitiveness. A dedicated CM theme was established under the Hong Kong Health and Medical Research Fund in 2002, encouraging health services research and clinical trials on CM. However, with a cap of HKD$ 1

million (AUD$ 185,000) per project, only trials of modest size can be performed [41]. Another difficulty is that a very stringent requirement is set by the Department of Health on the use of Chinese herbal medicine in clinical trial settings. At the time of writing, there is only one Chinese herbal product approved for human trial, despite the fact that such herbs are widely used in the community already. Despite the government's attempt to develop Chinese medicine in an "evidence based" approach, the largest share of research funding is often granted to laboratory based research that does not inform clinical practice directly. Such funding is often channelled to departments that have no involvement in CM teaching. While the three Schools of Chinese Medicine were performing satisfactorily in the last research assessment exercise, it is uncertain how this may impact educational outcomes, as pedagogical research is minimal in all three schools. Policy directions on CM research and teaching in Hong Kong appear to be developed in an uncoordinated fashion and are not entirely concordant with the government's initiative in building an evidence base for CM practice [42].

3.3. Regulatory Context and Place in the Healthcare System. Similarities in the path towards statutory regulation of CM in Australia and Hong Kong reflect their British colonial histories, while CM's current regulatory status is indicative of government policies regarding both CM and biomedicine.

3.3.1. Australia. In 2000, the State of Victoria, Australia, became the first western state in the world to establish statutory regulation of CM [10], which included the introduction of minimum education standards for the first time. This was followed in 2012 by the inclusion of CM in Australia's National Registration and Accreditation Scheme, where it joined 13 other health professions. This process led to the application of national education and competency standards to CM practitioners, including the requirement of a recognised degree qualification in CM to be able to register and practice. The degree programs themselves must be accredited by the CMBA in order for their graduates to be eligible for registration and each CM degree program is currently undergoing or has recently undergone this new accreditation process for the first time, placing a significant administrative and financial burden on CM education providers. Accreditation standards have been developed and tailored specifically for CM degree programs and include detailed requirements relating to the theory and practice of acupuncture and herbal medicine, basic understanding of Chinese language, and mastery of the Pin Yin system, as well as basic scientific competencies and more generic health professional learning outcomes relating to ethical conduct, communication, risk management, and so on [43].

Despite having joined the list of registered professions, CM practitioners remain largely excluded from publicly funded healthcare and hospitals in Australia and most CM practitioners operate as private businesspeople in the community. Rather than being integrated into the health system, CM students receive most of their clinical training in a single university- or college-based clinic, limiting their exposure to both clinical populations and presentations. Although it is common for Australian-based CM students to also complete a placement in China, the therapies, conditions, and clinical settings predominant in the Chinese health system do not necessarily apply to practice in Australia. Unlike many other health professions (e.g., medicine, pharmacy, and psychology), there are currently no formal supervisory or training pathways for CM graduates in Australia, aside from standard CPD requirements.

Interestingly, the Australian Government has recently signalled its support of CM through the signing of a letter of understanding with the Chinese Government in June 2015 (in conjunction with a new free trade agreement) agreeing to promote cooperation between the two countries around CM research and the recognition of qualifications [44] and the sustained Australian Government policy of increasing Australia's links to Asia may reap benefits for CM education.

3.3.2. Hong Kong.
Though now reunified with China, Hong Kong's regulatory situation for CM is very similar to Australia and continues to reflect the region's British colonial heritage. Despite statutory regulation and CM program accreditation, CM practitioners remain a "parallel" profession to conventional medical doctors as well as other healthcare professionals. While all CM programs include biomedicine components, exposure to CM in medical, nursing, and allied health education remains very limited. Interprofessional learning is yet to be scaled up, although, at undergraduate level, Schools of Chinese Medicine are providing basic CM education to medical, nursing, and pharmacy students. At postgraduate level, local universities also collaborated with the Hospital Authority in organising a CM training course for practising healthcare professionals. Since CM is not provided in all publicly funded hospitals and clinics, teamwork across CM and conventional medicine is rare. Currently, there is no formal mechanism for facilitating interprofessional referral between CM and conventional medical clinicians, and no publicly funded hospitals currently accept referral from private CM practitioners. Given the limited interaction between CM and biomedical clinicians, the two professions are considered "parallel": in the public sector, CM practitioners are not subordinate to conventional clinicians, as CM provision is often provided in stand-alone clinics with very limited interprofessional referral mechanisms; and, in the private sector, there is no mechanism for interprofessional teamwork and therefore subordination does not exist.

The government has provided partial subsidy (20%) to CM outpatient services, which are comanaged in a tripartite mode by the schools of CM, nongovernmental organizations, and the Hospital Authority (the public healthcare service provider) on a predominantly self-financed basis. The first tripartite CM clinic was established in 2003 and currently there are 18 in the territory [45]. Patients' out-of-pocket payments are the main source of funding although quotas of fee waivers are reserved for those with financial difficulties. These tripartite clinics must balance between maintaining financial sustainability and serving as clinical training sites for CM students. They are also the main employer for local CM graduates, providing a structured training program over

a three-year contract. While the contribution of tripartite clinics to training junior CM practitioner should be recognized, training quality may be compromised due to financial pressure [46].

CM hospitals in mainland China are alternative sites for clinical training for Hong Kong CM students. There, CM students' final year internship often takes place in environments where both CM and biomedical treatments are prescribed by the same clinician. However, as with Australian-based CM students, knowledge and skills gained from an integrative inpatient environment in China are not directly applicable to Hong Kong CM students' future role as a primary care clinician providing CM-only treatments in Hong Kong [47].

In Hong Kong, CME is mandatory for CM practice license revalidation but it is often viewed negatively by local CM graduates and repetition of undergraduate content in CME is common as such content is often geared to less well trained practitioners who previously received grandfathering licenses [21].

3.4. Public and Professional Legitimacy.
While there are differences in terms of public use and acceptance of CM in Australia and Hong Kong, issues regarding its legitimacy within public medicine and tertiary institutions exist in both countries and primarily stem from the relationship between CM and biomedicine.

3.4.1. Australia.
Accompanying the uneven government support of CM practice and education in Australia are varying levels of acceptance among the public and other health professions. Acupuncture and Chinese herbal medicine are relatively commonly used, with 9.2% and 7% (resp.) of national survey respondents reporting usage in the previous 12 months [48]. However, CM is argued to lack a strong presence in Australia [7] as well as an identifiable peak professional body [30]. In terms of CM education, Garvey [7] has suggested that because regulated and accredited CM training remains a relatively new concept in Australia, the discipline will continue to be treated with scepticism by proponents of biomedicine and will need to "prove" its legitimacy as a healthcare practice.

Indeed, the same year in which CM was included in the national registration system saw a significant backlash against the teaching of complementary medicine in Australian universities. This campaign was led by the Friends of Science in Medicine, a lobby group primarily composed of academic doctors and scientists, who argued through the news media that complementary medicine, including CM, was "pseudoscience" that should not be taught in publicly funded universities [49]. Representatives of universities teaching CM and other types of complementary medicine responded to the campaign predominantly by asserting that such degree programs are in fact based on bioscientific foundations [49]. What this (ongoing) debate suggests is that the legitimacy of CM within Australian universities does hinge on its integration of bioscientific approaches.

3.4.2. Hong Kong.
While current support for CM education and service within the public sector is limited, usage of

CM among the Hong Kong population is high with more than 60% of the general public having ever consulted a CM practitioner [50]. One territory-wide survey suggested that the prevalence of consulting a CM practitioner in the past year is around 20%. Within this 20%, 17% sought care from both CM and biomedicine clinicians and 3% only consulted CM practitioners [38]. The current Chief Executive of Hong Kong has shown strong support for the further advancement of CM in an "evidence based" manner, and in 2013 a Chinese Medicine Development Committee was established with the Secretary for Food and Health as Chairman [51]. Following recommendations from the Chinese Medicine Development Committee, three main policy initiatives have been announced in 2015 [52]. The first will be the establishment of a testing centre for Chinese medicines directly managed by the Department of Health and with a goal of setting up reference standards on safety, quality, and testing methods of Chinese herbal medicines. This centre will provide upstream assurance on the safe use of herbs. The other two policies are more service oriented. A site is reserved for the establishment of a new CM hospital in the territory, to provide inpatient care as well as teaching support. This is an entirely new initiative for the Hong Kong health system.

In order to explore feasible modes of operation, the third policy of piloting integrative Chinese biomedical clinical services in public hospitals was launched. Three pilot integrative care projects on cancer palliative care, low back pain, and stroke rehabilitation were launched and evaluation results will inform regulation and mode of operation of the future CM hospital. In these pilots, the CM treatments for all three conditions are mainly based on protocols that were designed by reviewing existing evidence and consensus between CM and biomedicine experts. Prescription flexibility of CM practitioners is limited and the essential feature of individualized treatment in CM is partly compromised. These three policy initiatives seem to suggest that the "biomedical standardization" of CM practice is key for acceptance in a healthcare environment dominated by conventional medicine. Unlike in Australia where CM's legitimacy is being directly challenged, in Hong Kong, the patterns tend to favour the assimilation of CM with a gatekeeping role for conventional medical clinicians and pharmacists. Recently, the Hong Kong Government has issued a call for Expressions of Interest from organizations that are keen to participate in the future operation of the Chinese medicine hospital [53]. These opinions may shape possible operational models and impact the interprofessional relationship between Chinese and conventional clinicians.

4. Discussion

The comparison of the factors impacting CM education in Hong Kong and Australia has revealed some striking similarities between the two regions, as well as important differences, highlighting the role of history, culture, and politics in the evolution of CM. CM was integrated into the formal tertiary education sector much earlier in Australia than in Hong Kong, first via private colleges and later also via universities. However, the reunification with China acted as a catalyst for the development of CM education in Hong Kong, and CM now has a comparatively larger presence in the university sector there, with three out of eight public universities teaching CM, compared to less than 10 per cent of universities in Australia. Postgraduate clinical training pathways are much better established in Hong Kong via the publicly funded CM clinics, while no such programs exist in Australia where CM remains truly excluded from the public healthcare system. However, rates of CM usage in Hong Kong are only two to three times higher than in Australia, while the practitioner : population ratio is five times higher, making oversupply of CM practitioners a greater problem in Hong Kong, where conventional medicine also predominates.

Beyond these differences, three key interrelated issues seem to stand out as being significant for the status of CM education in both Australia and Hong Kong. These key factors also potentially have ramifications for CM education in other regions outside mainland China. The first is the impact of ongoing biomedical dominance within healthcare systems. In both Hong Kong and Australia, this has limited the CM clinical training opportunities available at undergraduate and postgraduate levels and curbed the development of interprofessional education, now recognised as crucial in other health disciplines [54]. This situation is, in turn, likely to perpetuate CM's marginalisation, as other health practitioners' understanding of CM and ability to refer to CM practitioners will remain limited. Furthermore, the relatively low profile of CM in these regions, compared to conventional medicine, means that the scale of CM education has remained small, being represented in only 3 universities apiece in Australia and Hong Kong. As a university discipline, CM lacks the critical mass within these regions that is needed to develop a strong professional field, through holding local conferences, establishing cross-institutional collaborations, and so on.

This leads on to the second key issue we have identified, which is the impact that the global competition between universities (for students, status, and research funding) is having on CM education and may have in the future. University schools of CM in Hong Kong compete for students with the more affordable mainland universities, while Australian CM university departments compete with private colleges, and both compete with other disciplines for resources within their own institutions. As CM student numbers are not large in either Hong Kong or Australia, any fluctuations in enrolments caused by policy changes or increased competition would render these university programs vulnerable. In Australia, it is unlikely that new university programs will open in the near future, when universities teaching complementary medicine are under the scrutiny of sceptic groups that target universities' reputations [49]. Private college degree programs in Australia must go through a similar accreditation process as in universities, yet colleges are less likely to have access to the same research facilities and high-tech biomedical teaching equipment available in universities. A move towards greater private provision therefore may impact how CM is learned as well as the potential relationship between CM teaching and research.

Research provides another important source of income for universities, but, in both Hong Kong and Australia, research funding for CM is limited and not always funnelled into the same schools that actually teach CM. The research funding that is available for CM is typically directed mostly to basic science or clinical research involving standardised protocols. In general, research fitting a biomedical model attracts the largest funds and produces the most outputs for universities [28]. This factor, coupled with ongoing pressure for CM to "prove" its legitimacy within a context in which biomedicine dominates, means that within universities CM is likely to continue to become biomedicalised, at least when it comes to research, that is, tested through methods that do not necessarily allow for traditional knowledge or individualised approaches to be incorporated. Whether this biomedicalisation extends to how CM is taught within degree programs depends in part on how the relationship between teaching and research evolves, but a lack of alignment between the two domains is unlikely to be tenable in an environment where the scientific basis of CM degrees is under scrutiny. This points to an urgent need to evaluate the balance between research and education in the tertiary CM education sector.

A third important observation is that the relationship with mainland China exerts a significant influence on CM and CM education in both Australia and Hong Kong. This is interesting given that CM has been observed to have changed and adapted to the various transnational settings in which it is found [3, 55] and, in the case of Australia, the extensive period in which it has been established in local universities. Still, for both Australian and Hong Kong students, mainland China remains a common clinical training destination. This is despite the more restricted scope of practice and position in the health system for CM in these regions compared to the mainland. However, in Hong Kong, the recent policy developments and establishment of a CM hospital signify increased alignment with the status of CM in mainland China. For Australia, China already provides a useful source of CM research funding, and the new formal agreement between the two countries around CM means such investments are likely to continue. This may help to consolidate CM's position in Australian universities, although, as discussed, strengthened research programs will not necessarily impact the position of taught courses.

5. Conclusion

This cross-regional comparison has proved fruitful for identifying factors currently influencing the status of CM education, those that lie within and those that transcend national boundaries. The research has highlighted similarities and differences in CM education in Australia and Hong Kong in terms of history, current context and position, regulatory context and place in healthcare systems, and public and professional legitimacy. Further, the paper identifies issues of significance which have the potential to influence CM education in other regions, such as the impact of continued biomedical dominance within healthcare systems, and the increasing level of global competition between universities. Additionally, the relationship *between* nations has

been identified as an important factor. While this currently revolves around links between mainland China and other regions, the global movement of the CM workforce may see connections developing between other regions in relation to CM and CM education. The growing worldwide popularity of CM and the associated demand for quality education programs underscores the relevance of this paper and highlights the necessity for future research into how the developments identified here might further impact the evolution of CM education.

Competing Interests

The authors declare that they have no competing interests.

Acknowledgments

The authors thank Dr. Jan McLeod who assisted with background research for this paper. Caragh Brosnan is funded by an Australian Research Council Discovery Early Career Researcher Award (DE140100097). Jon Adams is supported by an Australian Research Council Professorial Future Fellowship.

References

[1] H. Flesch, "A foot in both worlds: education and the transformation of chinese medicine in the united states," *Medical Anthropology: Cross Cultural Studies in Health and Illness*, vol. 32, no. 1, pp. 8–24, 2013.

[2] P. Martyr, *Paradise of Quacks: An Alternative History of Medicine in Australia*, Macleay Press, Sydney, Australia, 2002.

[3] S. Pritzker, *Living Translation: Language and the Search for Resonance in U.S. Chinese Medicine*, Berghahn, New York, NY, USA, 2014.

[4] V. Scheid, *Chinese Medicine in Contemporary China: Plurality and Synthesis*, Duke University Press, Durham, UK, 2002.

[5] Australian Bureau of Statistics, "4364.0.55.002-Australian Health Survey: Health Service Usage and Health Related Actions, 2011-12," 2013, http://www.abs.gov.au/ausstats/abs@.nsf/Lookup/4364.0.55.002main+features12011-12#.

[6] A. Givati, "Performing 'pragmatic holism': professionalisation and the holistic discourse of non-medically qualified acupuncturists and homeopaths in the United Kingdom," *Health*, vol. 19, no. 1, pp. 34–50, 2015.

[7] M. Garvey, "The transmission of Chinese medicine in Australia," *PORTAL Journal of Multidisciplinary International Studies*, vol. 8, no. 2, pp. 1–13, 2011.

[8] A. O'Neill, *Enemies Within & Without: Educating Chiropractors, Osteopaths and Traditional Acupuncturists*, La Trobe University Press, Bundoora, Australia, 1994.

[9] C. C. Xue and D. Story, "Chinese medicine in Australia," *Asia-Pacific Biotech News*, vol. 8, no. 23, pp. 1252–1256, 2004.

[10] C. C. Xue, Q. Wu, W. Y. Zhou, W. H. Yang, and D. F. Story, "Comparison of Chinese medicine education and training in China and Australia," *Annals of the Academy of Medicine Singapore*, vol. 35, no. 11, pp. 775–779, 2006.

[11] Parliament of Victoria, *Report from the Osteopathy, Chiropractic and Naturopathy Committee: Together with Appendices*,

C. H. Rixon Government Printer, Melbourne, Australia, 1975, http://www.parliament.vic.gov.au/papers/govpub/VPARL1974-76NoD27.pdf.

[12] S. M. Griffiths, V. C. H. Chung, and J. L. Tang, "Integrating traditional Chinese medicine: Experiences from China," *Australasian Medical Journal*, vol. 3, no. 7, pp. 385–396, 2010.

[13] V. C. H. Chung, P. H. X. Ma, H. H. X. Wang et al., "Integrating traditional Chinese medicine services in community health centers: insights into utilization patterns in the pearl river region of China," *Evidence-Based Complementary and Alternative Medicine*, vol. 2013, Article ID 426360, 8 pages, 2013.

[14] E. Sinn, *Power and Charity: The Early History of the Tung Wah Hospital*, Oxford University Press, Hong Kong, 1989.

[15] M. Topley, *Chinese and Western Medicine in Hong Kong: Some Social and Cultural Determinants of Variation, Interaction and Change*, US Government Printing Office, Washington, DC, USA, 1975.

[16] R. P. L. Lee, "Perceptions and uses of Chinese medicine among the Chinese in Hong Kong," *Culture, Medicine and Psychiatry*, vol. 4, no. 4, pp. 345–375, 1980.

[17] R. P. L. Lee, "Chinese and western health care systems: professional stratification in a modernizing society," in *Social Life and Development in Hong Kong*, A. Y. C. King and R. P. L. Lee, Eds., pp. 255–273, Chinese University Press, Hong Kong, 1st edition, 1981.

[18] Y. G. Xie, *History of Traditional Chinese Medicine in Hong Kong*, San Lian Book Shop, Hong Kong, 1998.

[19] L. Koo, "Chinese medicine in colonial Hong Kong (Part I): principles, usage, and status vis-a-vis Western medicine," *Asia Pacific Biotech News*, vol. 1, pp. 682–684, 1998.

[20] S. Griffiths and V. Chung, "Development and regulation of traditional Chinese medicine practitioners in Hong Kong," *Perspectives in Public Health*, vol. 129, no. 2, pp. 64–67, 2009.

[21] V. C. H. Chung, M. P. M. Law, S. Y. S. Wong, S. W. Mercer, and S. M. Griffiths, "Postgraduate education for Chinese medicine practitioners: a Hong Kong perspective," *BMC Medical Education*, vol. 9, article 10, 2009.

[22] University Admissions Centre, Australian Tertiary Admissions Rank, April 2016, http://www.uac.edu.au/atar/.

[23] A. Moore, R. Canaway, and K. A. O'Brien, "Chinese medicine students' preparedness for clinical practice: an Australian survey," *The Journal of Alternative and Complementary Medicine*, vol. 16, no. 7, pp. 733–743, 2010.

[24] Chinese Medicine Board of Australia, *Chinese Medicine Health Practitioner Registrant Data: June 2015*, 2015.

[25] Medical Board of Australia, *Medical Practitioner Registrant Data: June 2015*, 2015.

[26] J. Wardle, A. Steel, and J. Adams, "A review of tensions and risks in naturopathic education and training in Australia: a need for regulation," *Journal of Alternative and Complementary Medicine*, vol. 18, no. 4, pp. 363–370, 2012.

[27] R. Münch, *Academic Capitalism: Universities in the Global Struggle for Excellence*, Routledge, London, UK, 2014.

[28] F. Collyer, "The production of scholarly knowledge in the global market arena: university ranking systems, prestige and power," *Critical Studies in Education*, vol. 54, no. 3, pp. 245–259, 2013.

[29] J. Wardle and J. Adams, "Are the CAM professions engaging in high-level health and medical research? Trends in publicly funded complementary medicine research grants in Australia," *Complementary Therapies in Medicine*, vol. 21, no. 6, pp. 746–749, 2013.

[30] A. Bensoussan and S. P. Myers, *Towards a Safer Choice: The Practice of Traditional Chinese Medicine in Australia*, NSW Faculty of Health, University of Western Sydney Macarthur, Campbelltown, Australia, 1996.

[31] Y. Tam, Opinion on Chinese Medicine Education in Hong Kong. Takungpao, Hong Kong, December 2013, http://health.takungpao.com.hk/q/2013/1220/2119759.html.

[32] Chinese University of Hong Kong, Bachelor of Chinese Medicine, 2016, http://www.scm.cuhk.edu.hk/en-GB/programs/bachelor-of-chinese-medicine/bachelor-of-chinese-medicine.

[33] University of Hong Kong, Admissions requirements. School of Chinese Medicine, 2016, http://www.scm.hku.hk/english-undergrad-page-12.html.

[34] Hong Kong Baptist University, Bachelor of Chinese Medicine and Bachelor of Science (Hons) in Biomedical Science, 2016, http://scm.hkbu.edu.hk/en/education/undergraduate_programmes/bachelor_of_chinese_medicine_and_bachelor_of_scien/index.html.

[35] Chinese Medicine Council of Hong Kong, Regulation of Chinese Medicine Practitioners, Licensing Examination, 2015, http://www.cmchk.org.hk/cmp/eng/#main_rcmp02.htm.

[36] Chinese Medicine Council of Hong Kong, *List of Registered Chinese Medicine Practitioners*, 2015, http://www.cmchk.org.hk/cmp/eng/#main_rdoctor_choice.htm.

[37] Department of Health, Health Facts of Hong Kong, 2015, http://www.dh.gov.hk/english/statistics/statistics_hs/files/Health_Statistics_pamphlet_E.pdf.

[38] V. C. H. Chung, C. H. Lau, E. K. Yeoh, and S. M. Griffiths, "Age, chronic non-communicable disease and choice of traditional Chinese and western medicine outpatient services in a Chinese population," *BMC Health Services Research*, vol. 9, article 207, 2009.

[39] X. Huang, *Are the Graduands of Chinese Medicine in Hong Kong a Result of Academic Resources Misallocation*, Mingpao, Hong Kong, 2014, http://news.mingpao.com/pns/web_tc/article/20140426/s00012/1398450557704.

[40] Z. Lin, The Challenges and Strategies of Chinese Medicine Education under the New Academic Structure in Hong Kong. Takungpao, Hong Kong, August 2012, http://www.mcmia.org/download/TCM_TaiKungPao/2012/2012.08.24.pdf.

[41] Food and Health Bureau, About Health and Medical Research Fund (HMRF), 2014, https://rfs2.fhb.gov.hk/english/funds/funds_hmrf/funds_hmrf_abt/funds_hmrf_abt.html.

[42] Food and Health Bureau, Chinese Medicine Development Committee, 2013, http://www.fhb.gov.hk/en/committees/cmdc/cmdc.html.

[43] Chinese Medicne Board of Australia, *Accreditation Standards: Chinese Medicine*, AHPRA, Melbourne, Australia, 2013, http://www.chinesemedicineboard.gov.au/Accreditation.aspx.

[44] A. Robb and G. Hucheng, *Side Letter on Traditional Chinese Medicine*, Department of Foreign Affairs and Trade, Commonwealth Government of Australia, Canberra, Australia, 2015.

[45] Hospital Authority, Introduction to HA Chinese Medicine Service, 2015, http://www.ha.org.hk/chinesemedicine/intro.asp?lan=en.

[46] Y. Tam, "Opinion on Chinese Medicine Education in Hong Kong (2). Takungpao," January 2014, http://news.takungpao.com.hk/paper/q/2014/0103/2149213.html.

[47] Z. Lin, *Government is in Honor Bound to Assist in Chinese Medicine Education in Hong Kong*, Takungpao, Hong Kong, 2011, http://www.mcmia.org/download/TCM_TaiKungPao/2011/20111209.pdf.

[48] C. C. L. Xue, A. L. Zhang, V. Lin, C. Da Costa, and D. F. Story, "Complementary and alternative medicine use in Australia: a national population-based survey," *Journal of Alternative and Complementary Medicine*, vol. 13, no. 6, pp. 643–650, 2007.

[49] C. Brosnan, "'Quackery' in the academy? professional knowledge, autonomy and the debate over complementary medicine degrees," *Sociology*, vol. 49, no. 6, pp. 1047–1064, 2015.

[50] Census and Statistics Department, Thematic Household Survey Report No. 50 2013, http://www.censtatd.gov.hk/fd.jsp?file=B11302502013XXXXB0100.pdf&product_id=B1130201&lang=1.

[51] Food and Health Bureau, Press Release of Establishment of Chinese Medicine Development Committee, 2013, http://www.info.gov.hk/gia/general/201301/17/P201301170520.htm.

[52] Food and Health Bureau, Legislative Council Panel on Health Services 2015 Policy Address Policy Initiatives of the Food Health Bureau (Extract on development of Chinese medicine) 2015, http://www.fhb.gov.hk/en/committees/cmdc/extract_2015_4.html.

[53] Hong Kong Government, "Government invites expression of interest for development of Chinese medicine hospital," Press release, January 2016, http://www.info.gov.hk/gia/general/201601/15/P201601150397.htm.

[54] S. Reeves, M. Tassone, K. Parker, S. J. Wagner, and B. Simmons, "Interprofessional education: an overview of key developments in the past three decades," *Work*, vol. 41, no. 3, pp. 233–245, 2012.

[55] M. Zhan, *Other-Worldly: Making Chinese Medicine through Transnational Frames*, Duke University Press, Durham, NC, USA, 2009.

16

Transcriptomics Analysis of *Candida albicans* Treated with Huanglian Jiedu Decoction Using RNA-seq

Qianqian Yang,[1,2] **Lei Gao,**[3] **Maocan Tao,**[1] **Zhe Chen,**[1] **Xiaohong Yang,**[1] **and Yi Cao**[1]

[1]*Zhejiang Hospital of Traditional Chinese Medicine, Zhejiang Chinese Medical University, 54 Youdian Road, Hangzhou 310006, China*
[2]*College of Agronomy and Plant Protection, Qingdao Agricultural University, Qingdao 266109, China*
[3]*Shandong Provincial Research Center for Bioinformatic Engineering and Technique, School of Life Sciences, Shandong University of Technology, 266 West Cunxi Road, Zibo 255049, China*

Correspondence should be addressed to Yi Cao; caoyi1965@163.com

Academic Editor: Letizia Angiolella

Candida albicans is the major invasive fungal pathogen of humans, causing diseases ranging from superficial mucosal infections to disseminated, systemic infections that are often life-threatening. Resistance of *C. albicans* to antifungal agents and limited antifungal agents has potentially serious implications for management of infections. As a famous multiherb prescription in China, Huanglian Jiedu Decoction (HLJJD, *Orengedokuto* in Japan) is efficient against *Trichophyton mentagrophytes* and *C. albicans*. But the antifungal mechanism of HLJDD remains unclear. In this study, by using RNA-seq technique, we performed a transcriptomics analysis of gene expression changes for *C. albicans* under the treatment of HLJDD. A total of 6057 predicted protein-encoding genes were identified. By gene expression analysis, we obtained a total of 735 differentially expressed genes (DEGs), including 700 upregulated genes and 35 downregulated genes. Genes encoding multidrug transporters such as ABC transporter and MFS transporter were identified to be significantly upregulated. Meanwhile, by pathway enrichment analysis, we identified 26 significant pathways, in which pathways of DNA replication and transporter activity were mainly involved. These results might provide insights for the inhibition mechanism of HLJDD against *C. albicans*.

1. Introduction

Candida albicans is the most prevalent opportunistic fungal pathogen implicated in superficial mucosal infections as well as invasive disseminated infections, especially in immunocompromised patients [1, 2]. *C. albicans* infections are usually treated with antifungal agents, such as azoles, echinocandins, and polyene drugs. Limited by the number of available antifungal targets, the antifungal agents still remain restricted. The azoles are the most widely used drugs for treating pathogenic fungal infections. Sterol 14α-demethylase (ERG11) is an ancestral activity of the cytochrome P450 superfamily, which is required for ergosterol biosynthesis in fungi and cholesterol biosynthesis in mammals [3]. As a key enzyme of sterol biosynthesis, Erg11 is the main target for therapeutic azole antifungal drugs [4, 5].

Widespread overuse of azole drugs for decades has led to the occurrence of drug-resistant isolates [6–8]. The prolonged

and repeated treatment of OPC (oropharyngeal candidiasis) in AIDS patients has resulted in an increasing frequency of therapy failures caused by the emergence of fluconazole-resistant *C. albicans* strains. In one study, the levels of fluconazole resistance of a series of 17 clinical isolates taken from a single HIV-infected patient who was treated with azoles over 2 years increased over 200-fold [9]. In recent years, the incidence of azole-resistant strains of *C. albicans* has increased, especially the rapid emergence of fluconazole-resistant strains. In the vast majority of countries, far less than 10% of *C. albicans* strains isolated from 1997 to 2001 are resistant to fluconazole [10]. But recent study in China showed that the rate of fluconazole resistance in *C. albicans* was almost 14.1% [11]. In USA, compared with 2008, the proportion of cases identified from 2008 to 2013 from Georgia and Maryland with fluconazole resistance decreased (GA: 8.0% to 7.1%, −10%; MD: 6.6% to 4.9%, −25%), but the proportion of cases with an isolate resistant to an echinocandin increased (GA: 1.2% to 2.9%, +147%; MD: 2.0% to 3.5%, +77%) [12]. So far, several resistance mechanisms of *C. albicans* have been well characterized: alterations in the sterol biosynthesis pathway, mutations in the *ERG11* gene encoding the drug target enzyme, overexpression of the *ERG11* gene, and overexpression of genes encoding efflux pumps [13]. Resistance of *C. albicans* to antifungal agents and limited antifungal agents has potentially serious implications for management of infections.

As a famous multiherb prescription in China, Huanglian Jiedu Decoction (HLJJD, *Orengedokuto* in Japan) is an aqueous extract of 4 herbal materials, *Coptidis Rhizoma*, *Scutellariae Radix*, *Phellodendri Cortex*, and *Gardeniae Fructus* with the ratio of 3 : 2 : 2 : 3. HLJJD was first mentioned in the book *Wai-Tai-Mi-Yao* compiled by Wang Tao in the Tang dynasty (about 752 AD), and it has been widely used in the clinical practice in China and officially listed in the Chinese Pharmacopoeia [14]. HLJJD has been widely used in the treatment of gastrointestinal disorders, inflammation and cardiovascular diseases, and Alzheimer's disease in China [15–17]. Modern pharmacological research also demonstrated multiple biological activities of HLJDD: decreasing levels of plasma glucose and blood lipid in type 2 diabetes mellitus [18, 19]; increasing the cerebral blood flow, inhibiting the platelet aggregation; reducing hypertension and altering the gene expression profiles of spontaneous hypertensive rats [20–23]; reducing hepatic triglyceride accumulation, restraining the preadipocyte differentiation and lipid accumulation, inhibiting the lipid peroxidation, and preventing atherosclerosis [15, 24–26]. Anti-inflammatory effects of HLJDD were also investigated in some papers [18, 27–29]. Moreover, in *Mugil cephalus*, 1% modified HLJDD feeding for 28 days may be an optimal dose to prevent *Lactococcus garvieae* infection and could be used in aquaculture industries. In in vitro study, the modified HLJDD also activated the plasma bactericidal activities [30].

Each herb of HLJDD contains many chemical components. Some papers had reported the content determinations of components contained in HLJDD [31, 32]. HLJDD contains multiple bioactive secondary metabolites, mainly including alkaloids from *Coptidis Rhizoma* and *Phellodendri Cortex*, flavonoids from *Scutellariae Radix*, and terpenes from *Gardeniae Fructus*. There are 4 typical compounds from HLJDD: geniposide, baicalin, berberine, and baicalein [27]. Further study showed that the combination of fluconazole and baicalein or berberine produced potently synergistic action in vitro, while baicalein and berberine showed weak antifungal activity when they were tested alone [33, 34]. Our preliminary work showed that HLJDD is efficient against *Trichophyton mentagrophytes* and *C. albicans* [35]. HLJDD showed its impressive antifungal effect by multitarget and multichannel actions, due to the multiple components. For that reason, the use of HLJDD may be more beneficial to human health in fungal infection treatment as diverse mechanisms showed complementary effects between herbs. But the antifungal mechanism of HLJDD remains unclear.

RNA-seq (deep-sequencing of cDNA) has been used successfully to identify and quantify gene expression at a genome scale level under different conditions or in different cell types. Moreover, it is significantly more sensitive than microarray hybridization approaches [36]. This approach has already been used in *C. albicans* to generate a high-resolution map of the *C. albicans* transcriptome under several different environmental conditions [37]. The effect of berberine chloride on *Microsporum canis* infection was analyzed by the construction of a transcriptome of the *M. canis* cellular responses upon berberine treatment [38]. Therefore, in this study, by using RNA-seq technique, we performed a large-scale analysis of gene expression changes when *C. albicans* was exposed to HLJDD, to better understand how HLJDD inhibits the growth of *C. albicans*.

2. Materials and Methods

2.1. Strain and Culture Conditions. The *C. albicans* strain used in this study is SC5314 [39]. *C. albicans* strains were routinely grown on YPD (1% yeast extract, 2% peptone, and 2% glucose) medium.

2.2. Preparation of the Extract of HLJDD. The herbal medicines of modified HLJDD were dried at 40°C for 24 h and then pulverized to powder using a mechanical blender. 0.5%, 1%, and 2% w/w of the powder was prepared and boiled for 30 min with 200 mL of deionized water, and the aqueous extracts were filtered through Whatman number 1 filter paper. The HLJDD residues were also boiled with another 200 mL of deionized water.

2.3. Determination of Sensitivity of the SC5314 Strain to HLJDD. Antifungal susceptibility testing was performed by using the CLSI M27-A3 microbroth dilution method [40]. MICs were determined after growth at 30°C for 24 h for HLJDD. MICs were read as the lowest drug concentration producing a prominent decrease in turbidity translating to 100% growth reduction compared with the drug-free control.

2.4. Total RNA Extraction. To identify genes in the early response of *C. albicans* to HLJDD, we treated the isolate with HLJDD at 20 mg/mL, the lowest drug concentration producing a prominent decrease in turbidity translating to 100% growth reduction compared with the drug-free control determined above. To extract total RNA, the cells of SC5314 were inoculated into YPD medium and cultured at 30°C overnight. Before SC5314 were harvested for RNA extraction, the culture was treated with HLJDD at 20 mg/mL for 3 h. The untreated culture was used as the control. Total RNA was isolated according to the protocol described by Alison et al. [41].

2.5. RNA Sequencing and Assembling. Three independent experiments were performed for the study of either control *C. albicans* or *C. albicans* with HLJDD treatment. Shear cDNA into 300–500 bp fragments using ultrasonic apparatus (Fisher) and purify it with Ampure beads (Agencourt, America). Library of all the samples was constructed according to the procedure of NEBNext® UltraTM RNA Library Prep Kit for Illumina (NEB, America). Sequencing library was checked with Onedrop quantitation, 2% agarose gel electrophoresis detection, and high sensitivity of DNA chip detection. Paired-end sequencing of cDNA was carried out with Illumina Hiseq TM2000. Raw data was filtered by removing reads with adaptor sequences, as well as low quality reads. Then, clean reads were obtained and mapped to reference sequences using SOAP (2.21) [42].

2.6. Gene Prediction and Annotation. Trinity software was used to assemble the clean reads into contigs and BLAST (2.2.23) was used to do gene prediction. Predicted sequences (*e*-value < 1.0*e* − 05) were annotated with information from GenBank NR, GO, and KEGG using BLAST2GO (2.2.5). GO classification was conducted using WEGO [43].

2.7. Analysis of Differential Expressed Genes. The expression level for each gene is determined by the numbers of reads uniquely mapped to the specific gene and the total number of uniquely mapped reads in the sample. The gene expression level is calculated by using RPKM (Reads Per kb per Million reads) method [36]. Then, NOI seq method was applied to screen differentially expressed genes between two groups, with the threshold of significance as fold change of RPKM ≥ 3 and Probability ≥ 0.8 [44].

2.8. Enrichment Analysis of GO and KEGG Pathways. Enrichment analysis was performed by hypergeometric test to find significantly enriched GO terms and KEGG pathways in DEGs. False discovery rate (FDR) of pathways was calculated. The threshold of significance of pathways was set as FDR < 0.05.

2.9. Real-Time Quantitative Reverse Transcription- (qRT-) PCR. To evaluate the validation of RNA-seq results, we conducted quantitative real-time (RT) PCR assays for determination of expression of 8 genes. Gene expression levels were calculated using the $2^{-\Delta\Delta Ct}$ method [45]. For each sample, PCR amplifications with primer pair actin-F and actin-R for the quantification of expression of actin gene were performed as a reference. The experiment was repeated 3 times.

3. Results

3.1. RNA Sequencing and Gene Prediction. Approximately 12,000,000 raw reads were obtained from each sample. After filtering by quality, about 96% clean reads were mapped. Summary of mapping result was shown in Table 1. Using the longest sequence of a subgroup as the unigene as the reference sequence, we got 6057 predicted protein-encoding genes totally. The data have been submitted to NCBI under BioProject accession number PRJNA314910.

3.2. Identification and Verification of Differentially Expressed Genes. By using the threshold of significance as fold change of RPKM ≥ 3 and Probability ≥ 0.8, we obtained a total of 735 differentially expressed genes (DEGs), including 700 upregulated genes and 35 downregulated genes (Supporting Information Table S1 in Supplementary Material available online at http://dx.doi.org/10.1155/2016/3198249). The 20

TABLE 1: Summary of reads in *C. albicans* with or without HLJDD treatment.

Sample	Total reads	Total mapped reads	Mapping percentage
Ca_CK_1	12,377,083	11,840,278	95.66%
Ca_CK_2	11,758,367	11,313,372	96.22%
Ca_CK_3	12,283,182	11,830,964	96.32%
Ca_HT_1	12,406,841	11,924,995	96.12%
Ca_HT_2	11,803,831	11,338,558	96.06%
Ca_HT_3	12,212,721	11,727,140	96.02%

most upregulated genes in response to HLJDD are listed in Table 2.

A total of 8 genes including 7 upregulated and 1 downregulated gene from DGE libraries were selected for real-time PCR analysis to validate the DGE data. The results showed that 8 genes were demonstrated to have a consistent change for both DGE and real-time PCR while actin genes had no significant difference in real-time PCR (Supporting Information Table S2).

3.3. Effects of HLJDD Treatment on the Genes Involved in Sterol Biosynthesis. As the most widely used antifungal drugs, azoles can block fungal sterol biosynthesis pathway. Thus, effects of HLJDD on the genes involved in sterol biosynthesis were analyzed in detail. Expression of 23 genes involved in sterol biosynthesis was detected in the RNA-seq analysis, and expression of 8 genes showed a more than 2-fold increase after *C. albicans* was treated with HLJDD; only the genes encoding sterol 24-C-methyltransferase (*ERG6*) and C-8 sterol isomerase (*ERG2*) were upregulated by more than 3 times (Table 3). None of these 23 genes was downregulated significantly (Probability > 0.8) by HLJJD.

3.4. Effects of HLJDD Treatment on the Genes Encoding Multidrug Transporters. In *C. albicans*, upregulation of multidrug transporter genes is one of the well-documented mechanisms of resistance to azole antifungal agents [9, 46–48]. Two families of multidrug transporters, the ABC (ATP-binding cassette) transporter family (Cdr1p and Cdr2p) and the major facilitator superfamily (MFS, CaMdr1p), have been shown to be involved in resistance to azole antifungal agents [47, 48]. Thus, we also paid attention to the multidrug transporter genes. In genome sequences of *C. albicans*, a total of 36 genes are annotated as multidrug transporters. In this study, expression of 32 genes was detected by the RNA-seq, and 7 genes were identified to be significantly upregulated more than 3 times by HLJDD treatment (Table 4), including *CDR2* (*Candida* Drug Resistance) from the family of ABC transporters. Cdr2 has been shown as the principal mediators of resistance to azoles due to transport phenomena [47, 48].

3.5. Enrichment Analysis of GO and KEGG Pathways. GO and KEGG assignments were used to classify the genes in the response of *C. albicans* to HLJDD. By GO classification analysis, the percentage and distribution of top-level GO terms were portrayed in the 3 categories: (A) cellular component; (B) molecular function, and (C) biological process

TABLE 2: The 20 most upregulated genes in response to HLJDD treatment.

Standard or systematic name in CGD	ID in GenBank	Annotation	Size	$\log_2$ ratio	Probability
C7_01060W_A	XP_720301.1	Hypothetical protein	142 aa	11.25	0.81
C5_04240C_A	XP_721977.1	Hypothetical protein	103 aa	11.21	0.80
C1_03880C_A	XP_711956.1	Hypothetical protein	120 aa	9.85	0.95
C7_01130C_A	XP_712469.1	Hypothetical protein	146 aa	9.42	0.92
PGA39	EEQ43586.1	Predicted protein	288 aa	9.32	0.85
C1_12040W_A	XP_716393.1	Hypothetical protein	143 aa	9.31	0.92
CR_01870C_A	XP_718251.1	Hypothetical protein	196 aa	8.90	0.85
CR_04980C_A	XP_711981.1	Hypothetical protein	193 aa	8.87	0.92
LIP10	XP_723508	Secretory lipase 10	465 aa	8.85	0.81
C3_01010W_A	XP_718606.1	Hypothetical protein	102 aa	8.67	0.90
C4_06150C_A	EEQ44911.1	Tat binding protein 1-interacting	175 aa	8.27	0.99
C7_03900W_A	XP_715240.1	Hypothetical protein	109 aa	7.96	0.94
CR_07970C_A	XP_714226.1	Hypothetical protein	119 aa	7.91	0.81
CR_06990W_A	XP_712676.1	Transcription activator	865 aa	7.84	0.88
C5_02090W_A	EEQ43139.1	Predicted protein	100 aa	7.84	0.84
SPO22	XP_718811.1	Meiosis specific protein	566 aa	7.73	0.96
CR_07550C_A	XP_710398.1	Hypothetical protein	101 aa	7.72	0.82
C3_02250C_A	XP_721699.1	Hypothetical protein	162 aa	7.71	0.85
C7_01060W_A	XP_718305.1	Hypothetical protein	111 aa	7.70	0.89

(Figure 1). A high percentage of genes were assigned to "cell," "cell part," "binding," "catalytic," "cellular process," and "metabolic process" (Figure 1).

By enrichment analysis, with FDR < 0.05, 23 significant GO terms and 3 significant KEGG pathways were identified (Supporting Information Table S3). These significant pathways were mainly associated with DNA replication and transporter activity. The maps with highest unigene representation were meiosis (cal04113; 23 unigenes), followed by cell cycle (cal04111; 23 unigenes), and DNA replication (cal03030; 11 unigenes).

4. Discussion

C. albicans is the most prevalent opportunistic fungal pathogen causing superficial to systemic infections in immunocompromised individuals [1, 2]. The concomitant use of drugs and the lack of available drugs frequently result in the occurrence of drug-resistant isolates and strains display multidrug resistance (MDR). In search of novel fungicides, efficiency of medicinal plants against fungi has been reported, but studies on their underlying mechanisms are very few [49]. In this study, we explored a famous multiherb prescription in China, Huanglian Jiedu Decoction (HLJJD, Orengedokuto in Japan), for its antifungal potential. Our preliminary work showed that HLJDD is efficient against Trichophyton mentagrophytes and C. albicans [35]. HLJDD showed its impressive antifungal effect by multitarget and multichannel actions, but studies on the underlying mechanisms are very few. To determine the antifungal mechanism of HLJDD against C. albicans, we performed a large-scale analysis of gene expression changes when C. albicans was exposed to HLJDD, to better understand how HLJDD inhibits the growth of C. albicans. Due to the multiple components of HLJDD, it is most likely that the antifungal effect is multitarget and multichannel actions. KEGG analysis suggested that 3 cellular functions were affected in C. albicans upon HLJDD treatment, including meiosis, cell cycle, and DNA replication. Most genes (56 genes) involved in the 3 cellular functions were upregulated excepted for 1 gene, potential hexose transporter (XP_719596.1). Among these genes, Spo22 (also called Zip4) (XP_718811.1) was upregulated obviously upon HLJDD treatment. Zip4/Spo22 was shown to be a central protein of the SICs (synapsis initiation complexes), from which the polymerization of the transverse filament proceeds. In S. cerevisiae, Zip4/Spo22 was identified as a member of the ZMM group of proteins that also includes Zip1, Zip2, Zip3, Msh4, Msh5, and Mer3 which together control the formation of class I COs [50–52]. In Arabidopsis thaliana, Zip4/Spo22 function in class I CO formation is conserved with budding yeast. However, mutation in AtZIP4 does not prevent synapsis, showing that both aspects of the Zip4 function (i.e., class I CO maturation and synapsis) can be uncoupled [51].

Azoles are the most widely used antifungal drugs, which target on cytochrome P450 lanosterol 14α-demethylase encoded by the ERG11 gene. In Fusarium graminearum, using a deep serial analysis of gene expression (DeepSAGE) sequencing approach, the transcriptional response of F. graminearum to tebuconazole (a widely used azole fungicide) was profiled. Expression of 23 genes involved in sterol biosynthesis was detected in the DeepSAGE analysis, and expression of 9 genes showed a more than 5-fold increase after the fungus was treated with tebuconazole. None of these 23 genes was downregulated by more than 5 times by tebuconazole [53]. Thus, effects of HLJDD on the genes involved in sterol

TABLE 3: Response to HLJDD of the genes involved in ergosterol biosynthesis.

Standard or systematic name in CGD	ID in GenBank	Annotation	$\log_2$ ratio	Probability
ERG1	XP_711894.1	Squalene monooxygenase	2.13	0.95
ERG2	XP_718886.1	C-8 sterol isomerase	3.23	0.94
ERG3	XP_713577.1	C-5 sterol desaturase	1.84	0.94
ERG4	XP_717662.1	Sterol C-24 (28) reductase	−0.34	0.65
ERG5	XP_716933.1	Cytochrome P450 61	2.02	0.97
ERG6	XP_721588.1	Sterol 24-C-methyltransferase	3.33	0.97
ERG7	XP_722471.1	2,3-Oxidosqualene-lanosterol cyclase	−0.23	0.38
ERG8	XP_722678.1	Phosphomevalonate kinase	−0.01	0.03
ERG9	XP_714460.1	Squalene synthetase	−0.60	0.77
ERG10	XP_710124.1	Acetyl-CoA acetyltransferase IA	0.96	0.91
ERG11	XP_716761.1	Cytochrome P450 51	2.02	0.97
ERG12	XP_723305.1	Mevalonate kinase	0.97	0.85
ERG13	XP_716446.1	Hydroxymethylglutaryl-CoA synthase	2.30	0.97
MVD1/ERG19	XP_718960.1	Diphosphomevalonate decarboxylase	0.04	0.12
ERG24	XP_710205.1	Delta(14)-sterol reductase	2.53	0.93
ERG25	XP_713420.1	C-4 methylsterol oxidase	1.31	0.91
	XP_722703.1	C-4 methylsterol oxidase	1.02	0.92
ERG26	XP_715564.1	C-3 sterol dehydrogenase/C-4 decarboxylase	0.23	0.39
ERG27	XP_717865.1	3-Keto sterol reductase	1.67	0.90
ERG28	XP_717865.1	Hypothetical protein	0.38	0.68
HMG1	XP_713636.1	Hydroxymethylglutaryl-CoA reductase	2.36	0.96
IDI1	XP_720295.1	Isopentenyl-diphosphate delta-isomerase	−0.09	0.24
CYB5	XP_720295.1	Cytochrome b5	−0.27	0.62

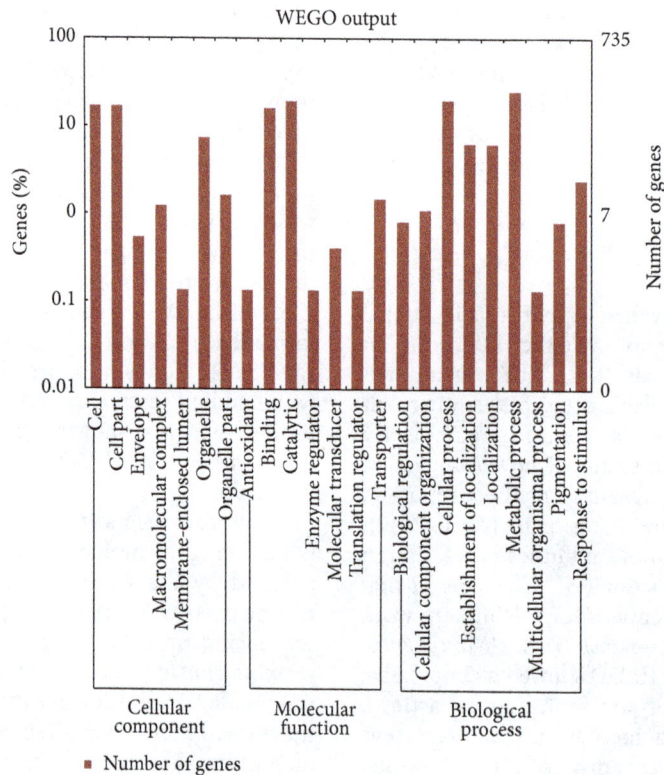

FIGURE 1: Functional categories of genes in *C. albicans* in response to HLJDD.

TABLE 4: Response to HLJDD of the genes involved in multidrug resistance of C. albicans.

Standard or systematic name in CGD	ID in GenBank	Annotation	$\log_2$ ratio	Probability
CDR1	XP_723062.1	Multidrug resistance protein CDR1	2.42	0.99
CDR2	XP_723022.1	Multidrug resistance ABC transporter	**5.32**	0.99
CDR3	XP_441615.1	N terminal 2/3 of opaque-specific ABC transporter	0.75	0.67
CDR4	XP_717543.1	Potential ABC transporter	-2.49	0.99
ATM1	XP_712090.1	Potential mitochondrial ABC transporter similar to S. cerevisiae ATM1	0.79	0.76
HST6	XP_716101.1	Potential ABC transporter similar to S. cerevisiae STE6	**5.44**	0.88
MDL1	XP_718280.1	Potential ABC transporter similar to S. cerevisiae mitochondrial inner membrane MDL1	0.81	0.79
MLT1	XP_717637.1	Vacuolar multidrug resistance ABC transporter	1.75	0.93
MDR1	XP_719165.1	Major Facilitator Transporter	0.63	0.77
CR_04620C_A	XP_717510.1	MFS transporter, DHA1 family, multidrug resistance protein	**4.46**	0.91
SGE1	XP_715705.1	Potential MFS-MDR transporter	1.31	0.84
C1_10710C_A	XP_714012.1	MFS transporter, DHA2 family, multidrug resistance protein	**5.1**	0.90
C3_03070W_A	XP_720131.1	MFS transporter, DHA2 family, multidrug resistance protein	0.47	0.66
NAG4	XP_712435.1	MFS transporter, DHA1 family, multidrug resistance protein	**5.83**	0.77
TPO4	XP_717426.1	MFS transporter, DHA1 family, multidrug resistance protein	2.34	0.95
C6_01870C_A	XP_716705.1	MFS transporter, DHA1 family, multidrug resistance protein	2.59	0.94
NAG3	XP_712434.1	MFS transporter, DHA1 family, multidrug resistance protein	2.8	0.85
C1_10200C_A	XP_723572.1	MFS transporter, DHA1 family, multidrug resistance protein	1.23	0.91
C2_02570W_A	EEQ45693.1	MFS transporter, DHA1 family, multidrug resistance protein	1.34	0.78
TPO3	XP_723233.1	MFS transporter, DHA1 family, multidrug resistance protein	-0.95	0.85
HOL1	XP_721489.1	MFS transporter, DHA1 family, multidrug resistance protein	2.0	0.85
CR_01340W_A	XP_718285.1	MFS transporter, DHA1 family, multidrug resistance protein	**3.93**	0.93
HOL4	XP_712971.1	MFS transporter, DHA1 family, multidrug resistance protein	0.88	0.81
C3_03440C_A	XP_720169.1	Potential drug or polyamine transporter	3.44	0.95
TPO2	XP_715197.1	Potential drug or polyamine transporter	2.31	0.82
QDR3	XP_714342.1	Potential multidrug resistance transporter	2.33	0.87
C2_00540W_A	XP_719644.1	Potential MATE family drug/sodium antiporter	-0.28	0.56
C7_03590C_A	EEQ47129.1	Multidrug resistance protein, MATE family	0.16	0.26
C1_00830W_A	XP_718985.1	Potential MATE family drug/sodium antiporter	0.44	0.34
CR_10640W_A	XP_719407.1	Multidrug resistance protein, MATE family	**3.15**	0.96
QDR2	XP_714698.1	Potential quinidine/multidrug transporter	1.63	0.94
FLU1	XP_721413.1	Multidrug efflux transporter	1.76	0.91

biosynthesis were analyzed in detail. Expression of 23 genes involved in sterol biosynthesis was detected in the RNA-seq analysis, and expression of 8 genes showed a more than 2-fold increase after the fungus was treated with HLJDD, only the genes encoding sterol 24-C-methyltransferase (ERG6) and C-8 sterol isomerase (ERG2) were upregulated by more than 3 times (Table 3). None of these 23 genes was downregulated significantly (Probability > 0.8) by HLJJD. These results indicate that HLJDD might also affect sterol biosynthesis of C. albicans.

Overexpression of multidrug resistance efflux transporter genes in several fungi was found to be correlated with azole resistance [54]. In C. albicans, a number of efflux transporter genes have been cloned and characterized. Two families of multidrug transporters, the ABC (ATP-binding cassette) transporter family (Cdr1p and Cdr2p) and the major facilitator superfamily (MFS, CaMdr1p), have been shown to be involved in resistance to azole antifungal agents [47, 48]. Expression of 32 genes out of 36 genes annotated as multidrug transporters in genome sequences of C. albicans was detected by the RNA-seq sequencing. Expression of 13 genes was upregulated by more than 2 times by HLJDD; meanwhile, only 2 genes were significantly downregulated including CDR4. In addition, expression of only 4 genes was upregulated by more than 3 times by HLJDD, including CDR2, which plays an important role in azole resistance (Table 4). The upregulated expression of these genes may be related to efflux of HLJJD, which provides supporting evidence to previous studies on expression level.

Previous study examined changes in the gene expression profile of C. albicans following exposure to representatives of the 4 currently available classes of antifungal agents, the azoles (ketoconazole), polyenes (amphotericin B), echinocandins (caspofungin), and nucleotide analogs (5-flucytosine). And the data showed that none of the differentially regulated genes found exhibited similar changes in expression for all 4 classes of drugs. Thus, the response of C. albicans to different drugs seems to be highly specific [55]. Ketoconazole exposure increased the expression of genes involved in lipid, fatty acid, sterol metabolism, and several genes associated with azole resistance, including CDR1 and CDR2 [56]. It is surprising that HLJDD increased the expression of genes involved in sterol metabolism and azole resistance (CDR1 and CDR2). Considering the similarity of expression changing pattern, it is possible that HLJDD affects sterol metabolism. And further experiments are required to confirm this hypothesis.

5. Conclusions

In conclusion, we performed a transcriptomics analysis of gene expression changes for C. albicans under treatment of HLJDD using RNA-seq technique. Overall, a total of 6057 predicted protein-encoding genes were identified. Further gene expression analysis revealed a total of 735 differentially expressed genes (DEGs), including 700 upregulated genes and 35 downregulated genes. Intensive bioinformatics analysis identified 26 significant pathways, and DNA replication and transporter activity were mainly involved.

In addition, genes encoding multidrug transporters such as ABC transporter and MFS transporter were identified to be significantly upregulated. Overall, the results from this study might provide insights in understanding of the mechanisms for the response of C. albicans to HLJJD. Furthermore, this work demonstrates the potential utility of the RNA-seq technique in antifungal studies.

Competing Interests

The authors declare that they have no competing interests.

Authors' Contributions

Qianqian Yang and Lei Gao equally contributed to this work.

Acknowledgments

The research was supported by the National Science Foundation (81173271 and 31540034), Zhejiang Provincial Natural Science Foundation (LQ14C010005), and Open Project Program of Key Laboratory of Mental Health, Institute of Psychology, Chinese Academy of Sciences (KLMH2014G03).

References

[1] C. E. B. Linares, S. R. Giacomelli, S. H. Alves, M. R. C. Schetinger, D. Altenhofen, and V. M. Morsch, "Fluconazole and amphotericin-B resistance are associated with increased catalase and superoxide dismutase activity in Candida albicans and Candida dubliniensis," Revista da Sociedade Brasileira de Medicina Tropical, vol. 46, no. 6, pp. 752–758, 2013.

[2] L. Zhang, K. Yan, Y. Zhang et al., "High-throughput synergy screening identifies microbial metabolites as combination agents for the treatment of fungal infections," Proceedings of the National Academy of Sciences of the United States of America, vol. 104, no. 11, pp. 4606–4611, 2007.

[3] S. L. Kelly, D. C. Lamb, C. J. Jackson, A. G. S. Warrilow, and D. E. Kelly, "The biodiversity of microbial cytochromes P450," Advances in Microbial Physiology, vol. 47, pp. 131–186, 2003.

[4] J. E. Parker, M. Merkamm, N. J. Manning, D. Pompon, S. L. Kelly, and D. E. Kelly, "Differential azole antifungal efficacies contrasted using a Saccharomyces cerevisiae strain humanized for sterol 14α-demethylase at the homologous locus," Antimicrobial Agents and Chemotherapy, vol. 52, no. 10, pp. 3597–3603, 2008.

[5] A. G. S. Warrilow, C. M. Martel, J. E. Parker et al., "Azole binding properties of Candida albicans sterol 14-α demethylase (CaCYP51)," Antimicrobial Agents and Chemotherapy, vol. 54, no. 10, pp. 4235–4245, 2010.

[6] P. J. Gallagher, D. E. Bennett, M. C. Henman et al., "Reduced azole susceptibility of oral isolates of Candida albicans from HIV-positive patients and a derivative exhibiting colony morphology variation," Journal of General Microbiology, vol. 138, no. 9, pp. 1901–1911, 1992.

[7] S. Redding, J. Smith, G. Farinacci et al., "Resistance of Candida albicans to fluconazole during treatment of oropharyngeal candidiasis in a patient with AIDS: documentation by in vitro susceptibility testing and DNA subtype analysis," Clinical Infectious Diseases, vol. 18, no. 2, pp. 240–242, 1994.

[8] T. C. White, K. A. Marr, and R. A. Bowden, "Clinical, cellular, and molecular factors that contribute to antifungal drug resistance," *Clinical Microbiology Reviews*, vol. 11, no. 2, pp. 382–402, 1998.

[9] T. C. White, "Increased mRNA levels of *ERG16*, *CDR*, and *MDR1* correlate, with increases in azole resistance in *Candida albicans* isolates from a patient infected with human immunodeficiency virus," *Antimicrobial Agents and Chemotherapy*, vol. 41, no. 7, pp. 1482–1487, 1997.

[10] K. C. Hazen, E. J. Baron, A. L. Colombo et al., "Comparison of the susceptibilities of *Candida* spp. to fluconazole and voriconazole in a 4-year global evaluation using disk diffusion," *Journal of Clinical Microbiology*, vol. 41, no. 12, pp. 5623–5632, 2003.

[11] W. Liu, J. Tan, J. Sun et al., "Invasive candidiasis in intensive care units in China: in vitro antifungal susceptibility in the China-SCAN study," *The Journal of Antimicrobial Chemotherapy*, vol. 69, no. 1, pp. 162–167, 2014.

[12] A. A. Cleveland, L. H. Harrison, M. M. Farley et al., "Declining incidence of candidemia and the shifting epidemiology of *Candida* resistance in two US metropolitan areas, 2008–2013: results from population-based surveillance," *PLoS ONE*, vol. 10, no. 3, Article ID e0120452, 2015.

[13] J. Morschhäuser, "The genetic basis of fluconazole resistance development in *Candida albicans*," *Biochimica et Biophysica Acta*, vol. 1587, no. 2-3, pp. 240–248, 2002.

[14] R. R. Coifman and G. Weiss, *Analyse Harmonique Non-Commutative sur Certains Espaces Homogenes*, vol. 242 of *Lecture Notes in Mathematics*, Springer, Berlin, Germany, 2010.

[15] Y. Ohta, T. Kobayashi, K. Nishida, E. Sasaki, and I. Ishiguro, "Preventive effect of Oren-gedoku-to (Huanglian-Jie-Du-Tang) extract on the development of stress-induced acute gastric mucosal lesions in rats," *Journal of Ethnopharmacology*, vol. 67, no. 3, pp. 377–384, 1999.

[16] L. M. Wang and S. Mineshita, "Preventive effects of Unsei-in and Oren-gedoku-to, Chinese traditional medicines, against rat paw oedema and abdominal constriction in mice," *Journal of Pharmacy and Pharmacology*, vol. 48, no. 3, pp. 327–331, 1996.

[17] Y. H. Hu, P. Jiang, S. P. Wang et al., "Plasma pharmacochemistry based approach to screening potential bioactive components in Huang-Lian-Jie-Du-Tang using high performance liquid chromatography coupled with mass spectrometric detection," *Journal of Ethnopharmacology*, vol. 141, no. 2, pp. 728–735, 2012.

[18] X.-J. Zhang, Y.-X. Deng, Q.-Z. Shi, M.-Y. He, B. Chen, and X.-M. Qiu, "Hypolipidemic effect of the Chinese polyherbal Huanglian Jiedu decoction in type 2 diabetic rats and its possible mechanism," *Phytomedicine*, vol. 21, no. 5, pp. 615–623, 2014.

[19] Y.-L. Yu, S.-S. Lu, S. Yu et al., "Huang-Lian-Jie-Du-Decoction modulates glucagon-like peptide-1 secretion in diabetic rats," *Journal of Ethnopharmacology*, vol. 124, no. 3, pp. 444–449, 2009.

[20] G.-H. Yue, S.-Y. Zhuo, M. Xia, Z. Zhang, Y.-W. Gao, and Y. Luo, "Effect of Huanglian Jiedu Decoction on thoracic aorta gene expression in spontaneous hypertensive rats," *Evidence-Based Complementary and Alternative Medicine*, vol. 2014, Article ID 565784, 9 pages, 2014.

[21] X. Fu, Z. Xu, Y. He, and H. Chi, "Protective function of Huanglian Jiedu Tang on rats after focal cerebral ischemic reperfusion and its influence on caspase-3 expression," *Modern Journal of Integrated Traditional Chinese and Western Medicine*, vol. 18, no. 14, pp. 1598–1599, 2009.

[22] Y. S. Hwang, C. Y. Shin, Y. Huh, and J. H. Ryu, "Hwangryun-Hae-Dok-tang (Huanglian-Jie-Du-Tang) extract and its constituents reduce ischemia-reperfusion brain injury and neutrophil infiltration in rats," *Life Sciences*, vol. 71, no. 18, pp. 2105–2117, 2002.

[23] Q. Zhang, Y.-L. Ye, Y.-X. Yan et al., "Protective effects of Huanglian-Jiedu-Tang on chronic brain injury after focal cerebral ischemia in mice," *Journal of Zhejiang University Medical sciences*, vol. 38, no. 1, pp. 75–80, 2009.

[24] T. Hayashi, Y. Ohta, S. Inagaki, and N. Harada, "Inhibitory action of Oren-gedoku-to extract on enzymatic lipid peroxidation in rat liver microsomes," *Biological and Pharmaceutical Bulletin*, vol. 24, no. 10, pp. 1165–1170, 2001.

[25] N. Ikarashi, M. Tajima, K. Suzuki et al., "Inhibition of preadipocyte differentiation and lipid accumulation by orenge-dokuto treatment of 3T3-L1 cultures," *Phytotherapy Research*, vol. 26, no. 1, pp. 91–100, 2012.

[26] N. Sekiya, M. Kainuma, H. Hikiami et al., "Oren-gedoku-to and Keishi-bukuryo-gan-ryo inhibit the progression of atherosclerosis in diet-induced hypercholesterolemic rabbits," *Biological and Pharmaceutical Bulletin*, vol. 28, no. 2, pp. 294–298, 2005.

[27] J. Lu, J.-S. Wang, and L.-Y. Kong, "Anti-inflammatory effects of Huang-Lian-Jie-Du decoction, its two fractions and four typical compounds," *Journal of Ethnopharmacology*, vol. 134, no. 3, pp. 911–918, 2011.

[28] M. Fukutake, N. Miura, M. Yamamoto et al., "Suppressive effect of the herbal medicine Oren-gedoku-to on cyclooxygenase-2 activity and azoxymethane-induced aberrant crypt foci development in rats," *Cancer Letters*, vol. 157, no. 1, pp. 9–14, 2000.

[29] H. Zeng, S. Dou, J. Zhao et al., "The inhibitory activities of the components of Huang-Lian-Jie-Du-Tang (HLJDT) on eicosanoid generation via lipoxygenase pathway," *Journal of Ethnopharmacology*, vol. 135, no. 2, pp. 561–568, 2011.

[30] W. M. Choi, C. L. Lam, W. Y. Mo et al., "Effects of the modified Huanglian Jiedu decoction on the disease resistance in grey mullet (*Mugil cephalus*) to *Lactococcus garvieae*," *Marine Pollution Bulletin*, vol. 85, no. 2, pp. 816–823, 2014.

[31] L. Liu, S. Yu, and L. Xie, "Simultaneous determination of geniposide and 4 flavonoids in the traditional Chinese medicinal preparation Huanglian Jiedu decoction by HPLC with programmed wavelength UV detection," *Chinese Journal of Pharmaceutical Analysis*, vol. 28, no. 2, pp. 182–186, 2008.

[32] Q. Li, L. Wang, R. Dai, and K. Bi, "Determination of berberine hydrochloride in coptis decoction by HPLC," *Northwest Pharmaceutical Journal*, vol. 19, pp. 51–52, 2004.

[33] S. Huang, Y. Y. Cao, B. D. Dai et al., "In vitro synergism of fluconazole and Baicalein against clinical isolates of *Candida albicans* resistant to fluconazole," *Biological and Pharmaceutical Bulletin*, vol. 31, no. 12, pp. 2234–2236, 2008.

[34] H. Quan, Y.-Y. Cao, Z. Xu et al., "Potent in vitro synergism of fluconazole and berberine chloride against clinical isolates of *Candida albicans* resistant to fluconazole," *Antimicrobial Agents and Chemotherapy*, vol. 50, no. 3, pp. 1096–1099, 2006.

[35] M. Tao, X. Xia, and Y. Cao, "In vitro antifungal effect of coptidis decoction for detoxification or combined with western medicine," *Chinese Archives of Traditional Chinese Medicine*, vol. 27, no. 3, pp. 585–587, 2009.

[36] Z. Wang, M. Gerstein, and M. Snyder, "RNA-Seq: a revolutionary tool for transcriptomics," *Nature Reviews Genetics*, vol. 10, no. 1, pp. 57–63, 2009.

[37] V. M. Bruno, Z. Wang, S. L. Marjani et al., "Comprehensive annotation of the transcriptome of the human fungal pathogen

Candida albicans using RNA-seq," *Genome Research*, vol. 20, no. 10, pp. 1451–1458, 2010.

[38] C.-W. Xiao, Q.-A. Ji, Q. Wei, Y. Liu, L.-J. Pan, and G.-L. Bao, "Digital gene expression analysis of *Microsporum canis* exposed to berberine chloride," *PLoS ONE*, vol. 10, no. 4, Article ID e0124265, 2015.

[39] A. M. Gillum, E. Y. H. Tsay, and D. R. Kirsch, "Isolation of the *Candida albicans* gene for orotidine-5′-phosphate decarboxylase by complementation of *S. cerevisiae* ura3 and *E. coli* pyrF mutations," *Molecular and General Genetics*, vol. 198, no. 1, pp. 179–182, 1984.

[40] Standards NCfCL, *Reference Method for Broth Dilution Antifungal Susceptibility Testing of Yeasts: Approved Standard*, National Committee for Clinical Laboratory Standards, 2002.

[41] A. Alison, D. E. Gottschling, and C. A. Kaiser, *Methods in Yeast Genetics*, Cold Spring Harbor Laboratory Press, New York, NY, USA, 1998.

[42] R. Li, C. Yu, Y. Li et al., "SOAP2: an improved ultrafast tool for short read alignment," *Bioinformatics*, vol. 25, no. 15, pp. 1966–1967, 2009.

[43] J. Ye, L. Fang, H. Zheng et al., "WEGO: a web tool for plotting GO annotations," *Nucleic Acids Research*, vol. 34, pp. W293–W297, 2006.

[44] S. Tarazona, F. García-Alcalde, J. Dopazo, A. Ferrer, and A. Conesa, "Differential expression in RNA-seq: a matter of depth," *Genome Research*, vol. 21, no. 12, pp. 2213–2223, 2011.

[45] K. J. Livak and T. D. Schmittgen, "Analysis of relative gene expression data using real-time quantitative PCR and the $2^{-\Delta\Delta C_T}$ method," *Methods*, vol. 25, no. 4, pp. 402–408, 2001.

[46] S. Perea, J. L. López-Ribot, B. L. Wickes et al., "Molecular mechanisms of fluconazole resistance in *Candida dubliniensis* isolates from human immunodeficiency virus-infected patients with oropharyngeal candidiasis," *Antimicrobial Agents and Chemotherapy*, vol. 46, no. 6, pp. 1695–1703, 2002.

[47] D. Sanglard, F. Ischer, M. Monod, and J. Bille, "Cloning of *Candida albicans* genes conferring resistance to azole antifungal agents: characterization of CDR2, a new multidrug ABC transporter gene," *Microbiology*, vol. 143, no. 2, pp. 405–416, 1997.

[48] D. Sanglard, K. Kuchler, F. Ischer, J.-L. Pagani, M. Monod, and J. Bille, "Mechanisms of resistance to azole antifungal agents in *Candida albicans* isolates from AIDS patients involve specific multidrug transporters," *Antimicrobial Agents and Chemotherapy*, vol. 39, no. 11, pp. 2378–2386, 1995.

[49] C. W. Xiao, Q. A. Ji, Z. I. Rajput, Q. Wei, Y. Liu, and G. L. Bao, "Antifungal efficacy of *Phellodendron amurense* ethanol extract against *Trichophyton mentagrophytes* in rabbits," *Pakistan Veterinary Journal*, vol. 34, no. 2, pp. 219–223, 2014.

[50] M. C. Whitby, "Making crossovers during meiosis," *Biochemical Society Transactions*, vol. 33, no. 6, pp. 1451–1455, 2005.

[51] L. Chelysheva, G. Gendrot, D. Vezon, M.-P. Doutriaux, R. Mercier, and M. Grelon, "Zip4/Spo22 is required for class ICO formation but not for synapsis completion in *Arabidopsis thaliana*," *PLoS Genetics*, vol. 3, no. 5, pp. 802–813, 2007.

[52] J. Perry, N. Kleckner, and G. V. Börner, "Bioinformatic analyses implicate the collaborating meiotic crossover/chiasma proteins Zip2, Zip3, and Spo22/Zip4 in ubiquitin labeling," *Proceedings of the National Academy of Sciences of the United States of America*, vol. 102, no. 49, pp. 17594–17599, 2005.

[53] X. Liu, J. Jiang, J. Shao, Y. Yin, and Z. Ma, "Gene transcription profiling of *Fusarium graminearum* treated with an azole fungicide tebuconazole," *Applied Microbiology and Biotechnology*, vol. 85, no. 4, pp. 1105–1114, 2010.

[54] A. Lupetti, R. Danesi, M. Campa, M. D. Tacca, and S. Kelly, "Molecular basis of resistance to azole antifungals," *Trends in Molecular Medicine*, vol. 8, no. 2, pp. 76–81, 2002.

[55] T. T. Liu, R. E. B. Lee, K. S. Barker et al., "Genome-wide expression profiling of the response to azole, polyene, echinocandin, and pyrimidine antifungal agents in *Candida albicans*," *Antimicrobial Agents and Chemotherapy*, vol. 49, no. 6, pp. 2226–2236, 2005.

[56] M. D. De Backer, T. Ilyina, X.-J. Ma, S. Vandoninck, W. H. M. L. Luyten, and H. V. Bossche, "Genomic profiling of the response of *Candida albicans* to itraconazole treatment using a DNA microarray," *Antimicrobial Agents and Chemotherapy*, vol. 45, no. 6, pp. 1660–1670, 2001.

17

Cortex phellodendri Extract Relaxes Airway Smooth Muscle

Qiu-Ju Jiang,[1] Weiwei Chen,[1] Hong Dan,[2] Li Tan,[1] He Zhu,[1] Guangzhong Yang,[3] Jinhua Shen,[1] Yong-Bo Peng,[1] Ping Zhao,[1] Lu Xue,[1] Meng-Fei Yu,[1] Liqun Ma,[1] Xiao-Tang Si,[1] Zhuo Wang,[4] Jiapei Dai,[4] Gangjian Qin,[5] Chunbin Zou,[6] and Qing-Hua Liu[1]

[1]*Institute for Medical Biology & Hubei Provincial Key Laboratory for Protection and Application of Special Plants in Wuling Area of China, College of Life Sciences, South-Central University for Nationalities, Wuhan 430074, China*
[2]*Key Laboratory of Chinese Medicine Resource and Compound Prescription, Hubei University of Chinese Medicine, Wuhan 430065, China*
[3]*College of Pharmacy, South-Central University for Nationalities, Wuhan 430074, China*
[4]*Wuhan Institute for Neuroscience and Engineering, South-Central University for Nationalities, Wuhan 430074, China*
[5]*Department of Medicine-Cardiology, Feinberg Cardiovascular Research Institute, Northwestern University Feinberg School of Medicine, Chicago, IL 60611, USA*
[6]*Acute Lung Injury Center of Excellence, Division of Pulmonary, Allergy, and Critical Care Medicine, Department of Medicine, University of Pittsburgh School of Medicine, Pittsburgh, PA 15213, USA*

Correspondence should be addressed to Qing-Hua Liu; liu258q@yahoo.com

Academic Editor: Alexandre de Paula Rogerio

Cortex phellodendri is used to reduce fever and remove dampness and toxin. Berberine is an active ingredient of *C. phellodendri*. Berberine from *Argemone ochroleuca* can relax airway smooth muscle (ASM); however, whether the nonberberine component of *C. phellodendri* has similar relaxant action was unclear. An n-butyl alcohol extract of *C. phellodendri* (NBAECP, nonberberine component) was prepared, which completely inhibits high K^+- and acetylcholine- (ACH-) induced precontraction of airway smooth muscle in tracheal rings and lung slices from control and asthmatic mice, respectively. The contraction induced by high K^+ was also blocked by nifedipine, a selective blocker of L-type Ca^{2+} channels. The ACH-induced contraction was partially inhibited by nifedipine and pyrazole 3, an inhibitor of TRPC3 and STIM/Orai channels. Taken together, our data demonstrate that NBAECP can relax ASM by inhibiting L-type Ca^{2+} channels and TRPC3 and/or STIM/Orai channels, suggesting that NBAECP could be developed to a new drug for relieving bronchospasm.

1. Introduction

Asthma is a common chronic respiratory disease [1]. Excessive airway obstruction is a cardinal symptom that results from the contraction of airway smooth muscle (ASM). In this study, we attempted to develop an effective and safe drug from bitter Chinese herbs to inhibit ASM contraction.

Cortex phellodendri, called Huang Bai in Chinese, which tasted bitter, is the dried bark of *Phellodendron chinense* Schneid. or *Phellodendron amurense* Rupr., which belongs to the group of Rutaceae arbor plants. It is bitter in flavor and cold in nature, categorized in kidney, urinary bladder, and large intestine meridians. The traditional functions are to

clear heat, dry dampness, purge fire, and remove toxicity. It is one of fundamental traditional Chinese medicines. Previous study reported that *C. phellodendri* has many physiological activities, including antioxidant [2, 3], anti-inflammatory [4–6], antiulcer [7], and immune-stimulating properties [8], as well as neuroprotection and inhibition of coronavirus replication [9, 10]. Moreover, *C. phellodendri* combining with other herbs can reduce complications of corticosteroid-resistant asthma [11]. Berberine is one active ingredient of *C. phellodendri*; berberine from *Argemone ochroleuca* was demonstrated to have a relaxant effect in guinea-pig ASM [12]. However, whether the nonberberine component has similar relaxant action has not been investigated.

In the present study, we found that an n-butyl alcohol extract of *C. phellodendri* (NBAECP, nonberberine component) exerted inhibitory action on ASM contraction, and the underlying mechanism was also investigated.

2. Materials and Methods

2.1. C. phellodendri Extraction. C. phellodendri, bark of *Phellodendron chinensis* Schneid. (Rutaceae), were collected in Sichuan Province, China, and were authenticated by Professor Dr. Ding-Rong Wan of our university. A voucher specimen (SCUN201310010) is deposited at the Herbarium of College of Pharmacy, South-Central University for Nationalities, China.

Air-dried *C. phellodendri* (1 Kg) was milled into powder and immersed into 70% ethanol (5 L) for 24 h. The components in the mixture were extracted by hot reflux and were centrifuged. The supernatant was collected and evaporated to dryness under reduced pressure using a rotary evaporator to remove ethanol and get residues, which were immersed in a 2% HCl solution (1000 mL). The yellow precipitates (mainly berberine) were removed and the supernatants were consecutively extracted with petroleum ether, chloroform, ethyl acetate, and n-butyl alcohol. The n-butyl alcohol extract was further evaporated under reduced pressure, and the extraction yield was 1.5% of the raw material dry weight. The dried n-butyl alcohol extract of *C. phellodendri* (NBAECP) was dissolved in 3% DMSO for the experiments.

2.2. Reagents. Nifedipine, acetylcholine chloride (ACH), and pyrazole 3 (Pyr 3) were purchased from Sigma Chemical Co. (St. Louis, MO, USA); DMEM was purchased from Gibco BRL Co. (Invitrogen Life Technologies, Carlsbad, CA, USA). Other chemicals were purchased from Sinopharm Chemical Reagent Co. (Shanghai, China).

2.3. Animals. Sexually mature male BALB/c mice were purchased from the Hubei Provincial Center for Disease Control and Prevention (Wuhan, China). The mice were housed at room temperature (20–25°C) and constant humidity (50–60%) under a 12 h light-dark cycle in an SPF grade animal facility. The experiments on animals were approved by the Animal Care and Ethics Committee of the South-Central University for Nationalities and conformed to the guidelines of the Institutional Animal Care and Use Committee of the South-Central University for Nationalities (QHL-6, 12-10-2013).

2.4. Experimental Asthma Model in Mice. Asthmatic mice were prepared as described previously [13]. Briefly, mice were sensitized by intraperitoneal injection administration of 0.2 mL of 0.9% saline solution containing 0.6 mg OVA and 0.4 mg of adjuvant aluminum hydroxide on days 1 and 8; then, the mice were challenged from days 15 through 19 by daily intranasal instillation of 50 μL of OVA solution (3 mg/mL). Control mice were sensitized and challenged by identical vehicle media.

2.5. Tracheal ASM Contraction Measurement. Mouse ASM contraction was measured as previously described [14]. Adult male BALB/c mice were sacrificed by an intraperitoneal injection of sodium pentobarbital (150 mg/kg), and their tracheae were isolated and quickly transferred to ice cold PSS (composition in mM: NaCl 135, KCl 5, MgCl$_2$ 1, CaCl$_2$ 2, HEPES 10, glucose 10, pH 7.4). The connective tissue was removed, and tracheal rings (~5 mm) were cut from the bottom of the tracheae. Each ring was mounted with a preload of 0.5 g in an organ bath with a 10 mL capacity containing PSS bubbled with 95% O$_2$ and 5% CO$_2$ at 37°C. The rings were equilibrated for 60 min, precontracted with high K$^+$ (80 mM) or ACH (10^{-4} M), washed, and rested for a total of 3 times. The experiments were performed following an additional 30 min rest.

2.6. Bronchial ASM Contraction Measurement. Lung slices were prepared according to a previous report [15]. Lung slices were placed in a chamber and were held with a small nylon mesh. Perfusion was maintained in Hanks' balanced salt solution (HBSS) at a rate of ~800 μL/min. HBSS was supplemented with 20 mM HEPES buffer (composition in mM: NaCl 137.93, KCl 5.33, NaHCO$_3$ 4.17, CaCl$_2$ 1.26, MgCl$_2$ 0.493, MgSO$_4$ 0.407, KH$_2$PO 0.4414, Na$_2$HPO4 0.338, and D-glucose 5.56) and adjusted to a pH of 7.4. Images of lung slices under 10x objective were acquired at the rate of 30 frames/min using an LSM 700 laser confocal microscope (Carl Zeiss, Goettingen, Germany). The cross-sectional area of the bronchial lumen was measured using Zen 2010 software (Carl Zeiss, Goettingen, Germany). The experiments were performed at room temperature.

2.7. Data Analysis. The results are expressed as the mean ± SEM. Comparisons of 2 groups were performed using Student's *t*-test. Differences with $P < 0.05$ were considered significant.

3. Results

3.1. NBAECP Inhibits High K$^+$-Induced Tracheal Smooth Muscle Contraction. To observe the effect of NBAECP on the contraction of airway smooth muscle (ASM), the tracheal rings (TRs) from healthy mice (i.e., controls) were contracted using high K$^+$. Following the increase in the K$^+$ concentration from 10 to 80 mM, the TRs exhibited dose-dependent contraction (Figure 1(a)). Upon the contraction reaching the maximum (at 80 mM K$^+$), NBAECP was added. The contraction was inhibited in a dose-dependent manner. An identical experiment was also performed in a TR from an asthmatic model mouse, and similar results were observed (Figure 1(b)). NBAECP-induced relaxation in both control and asthmatic TRs was analyzed, and the values of half maximal inhibitory concentration (IC$_{50}$) were calculated (Figure 1(c)). There were no significant differences between the two traces and the values of IC$_{50}$. These results indicated that NBAECP could inhibit agonist-induced sustained contraction of control and asthmatic ASM.

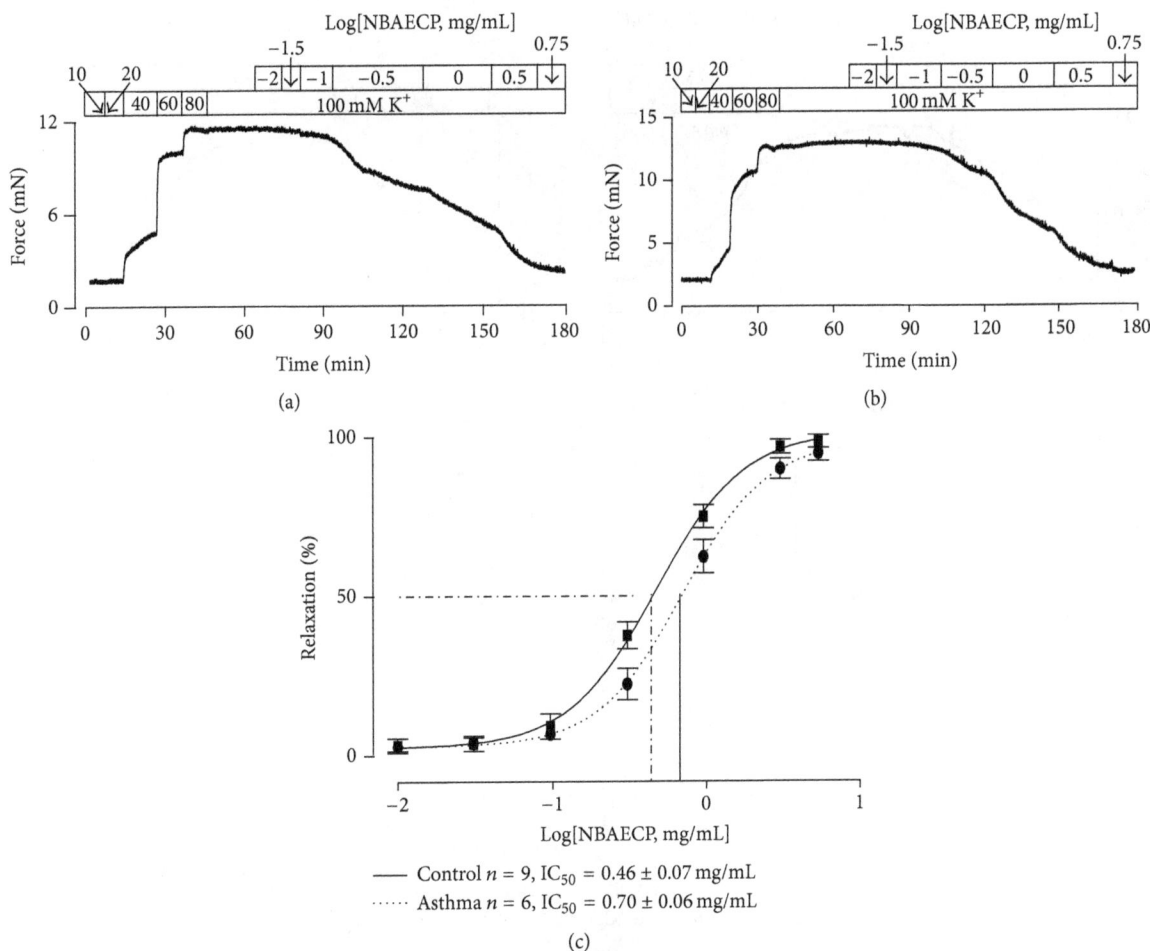

FIGURE 1: NBAECP inhibits high K^+-induced contraction in TRs. (a) High K^+ triggered contractions in a healthy (i.e., control) TR, which reached the maximum at 80 mM K^+. Following cumulative additions of NBAECP, the sustained contraction was totally blocked. (b) An identical experiment was performed using an asthmatic TR, and a similar result was observed. (c) Dose-relaxation relationships of NBAECP from 9 control and 6 asthmatic TRs. The IC_{50} of NBAECP was $48.9 \pm 1.5 \, \mu g/mL$ ($n = 9$) in control TRs and $73.1 \pm 1.6 \, \mu g/mL$ ($n = 6$) in asthmatic TRs. These data demonstrated that NBAECP could block high K^+-induced precontraction in control and asthmatic tracheal smooth muscle.

3.2. NBAECP Blocks ACH-Induced Tracheal Smooth Muscle Contraction.

To know whether NBAECP is capable of inhibiting another agonist-induced precontraction in ASM, healthy TRs were contracted using ACH. Upon the contraction reaching the maximum, NBAECP was added (Figure 2(a)). Similar dose-dependent relaxation responses occurred. Moreover, these responses existed in asthmatic TRs (Figure 2(b)). The dose-relaxation relationships and IC_{50} values of NBAECP were analyzed (Figure 2(c)), and they did not show differences between the control and asthmatic TRs. These experiments demonstrated that NBAECP could also inhibit ACH-induced precontraction in control and asthmatic ASM.

Were these relaxation responses also mediated by L-type Ca^{2+} channels? To answer this question, TRs from healthy and asthmatic mice were precontracted with ACH, and $10 \, \mu M$ nifedipine, a selective blocker of voltage-dependent L-type Ca^{2+} channels (VDCCs), was then added (Figures

3(a) and 3(b)). Following the addition of nifedipine, the contractions were partially inhibited. The resistant components were further blocked by NBAECP. The inhibitions induced by nifedipine and NBAECP were not different between the control and asthmatic TRs (Figure 3(c)).

To further investigate the underlying mechanism of NBAECP-induced relaxation of the nifedipine-resistant component, TRs were incubated with $10 \, \mu M$ nifedipine for 10 min and contracted using ACH, and we then observed the action of Pyr 3 (an inhibitor of TRPC3 and STIM/Orai channels). The results showed that Pyr 3 induced partial relaxation, and the remaining contractions were completely blocked by NBAECP (Figures 4(a) and 4(b)); however, Pyr 3-induced relaxation in asthmatic TRs was markedly greater than in the controls (Figure 4(c)).

Taken together, these results indicated that NBAECP-induced relaxation responses were mediated by L-type Ca^{2+}, TRPC3, and/or STIM/Orai channels.

(a)

(b)

— Control $n = 7$, $IC_{50} = 0.23 \pm 0.15$ mg/mL
...... Asthma $n = 6$, $IC_{50} = 0.13 + 0.02$ mg/mL

(c)

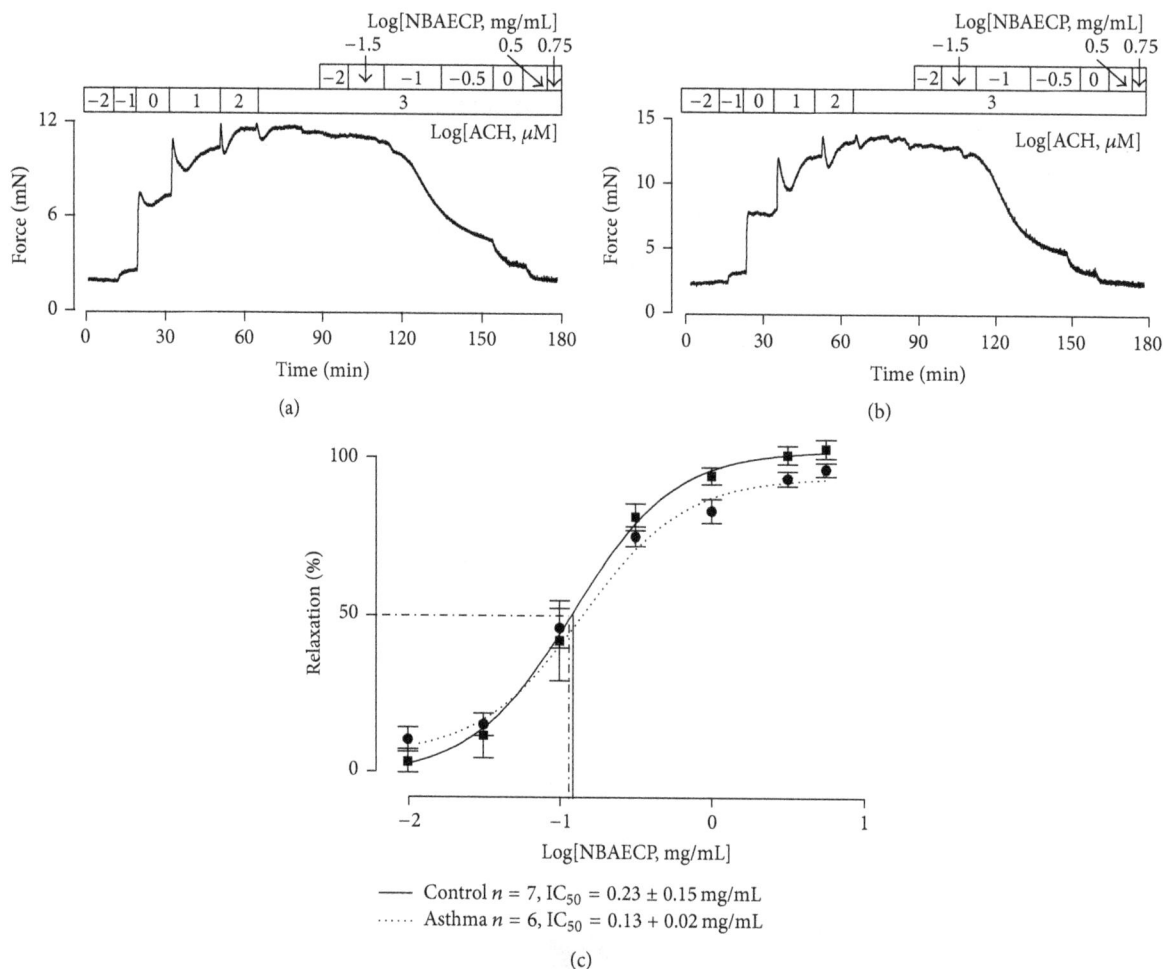

FIGURE 2: NBAECP inhibits ACH-induced precontraction in TRs. (a) Following cumulative addition of ACH, a TR reached a sustained contraction, which was inhibited following cumulative application of NBAECP. (b) A similar experiment was performed in asthmatic TR. (c) The summary results of NBAECP-induced relaxation in 7 control and 6 asthmatic TRs. The IC_{50} of NBAECP was 12.2 ± 1.3 μg/mL in control TRs and 12.8 ± 1.2 μg/mL in asthmatic TRs. These results indicated that NBAECP could block ACH-induced sustained contractions in control and asthmatic tracheal smooth muscle.

3.3. NBAECP Inhibits Bronchial Smooth Muscle Contraction.

To define whether NBAECP has similar relaxant action on bronchial smooth muscle, lung slices were cut, and the cross-sectional area of the airway lumen was measured. The area of the airway lumen from healthy mice markedly decreased following application of 100 μM ACH; however, it was restored upon addition of 3.16 mg/mL NBAECP (Figure 5(a)). Identical experiments were conducted in lung slices from asthmatic mice, and similar phenomena were observed (Figure 5(b)). The summary data are shown in Figure 5(c). These results indicated that NBAECP had similar relaxant action on bronchial smooth muscle.

4. Discussion

In the present study, our data demonstrate that NBAECP can inhibit L-type Ca^{2+} channels, blocking high K^+-induced contractions in healthy and asthmatic airway smooth muscle and additionally inhibiting TRPC3 and/or STIM/Orai channels

to reduce ACH-induced contractions in both types of airway smooth muscle. These results indicate that NBAECP could be a new bronchodilator for the treatment of asthma.

The purpose of this study was to find bronchodilators among Chinese medicines. We extracted a component (NBAECP, nonberberine active ingredient) from C. phellodendri. To investigate whether NBAECP has relaxant action, we used high K^+ and ACH to contract airway smooth muscle and then observed the effect of NBAECP. NBAECP totally relaxed high K^+-induced precontractions (Figure 1). High K^+ could induce membrane depolarization, resulting in the activation of voltage-dependent L-type Ca^{2+} channels (VDCCs) [16]. The channels then mediated Ca^{2+} influx, resulting in intracellular Ca^{2+} concentration increases, leading to muscle contraction. Nifedipine, a selective blocker of VDCCs, completely blocked high K^+-induced contractions. This phenomenon was observed in our previous study [14, 17]. These results indicated that high K^+-induced contractions completely depended on L-type Ca^{2+} channel-mediated Ca^{2+}

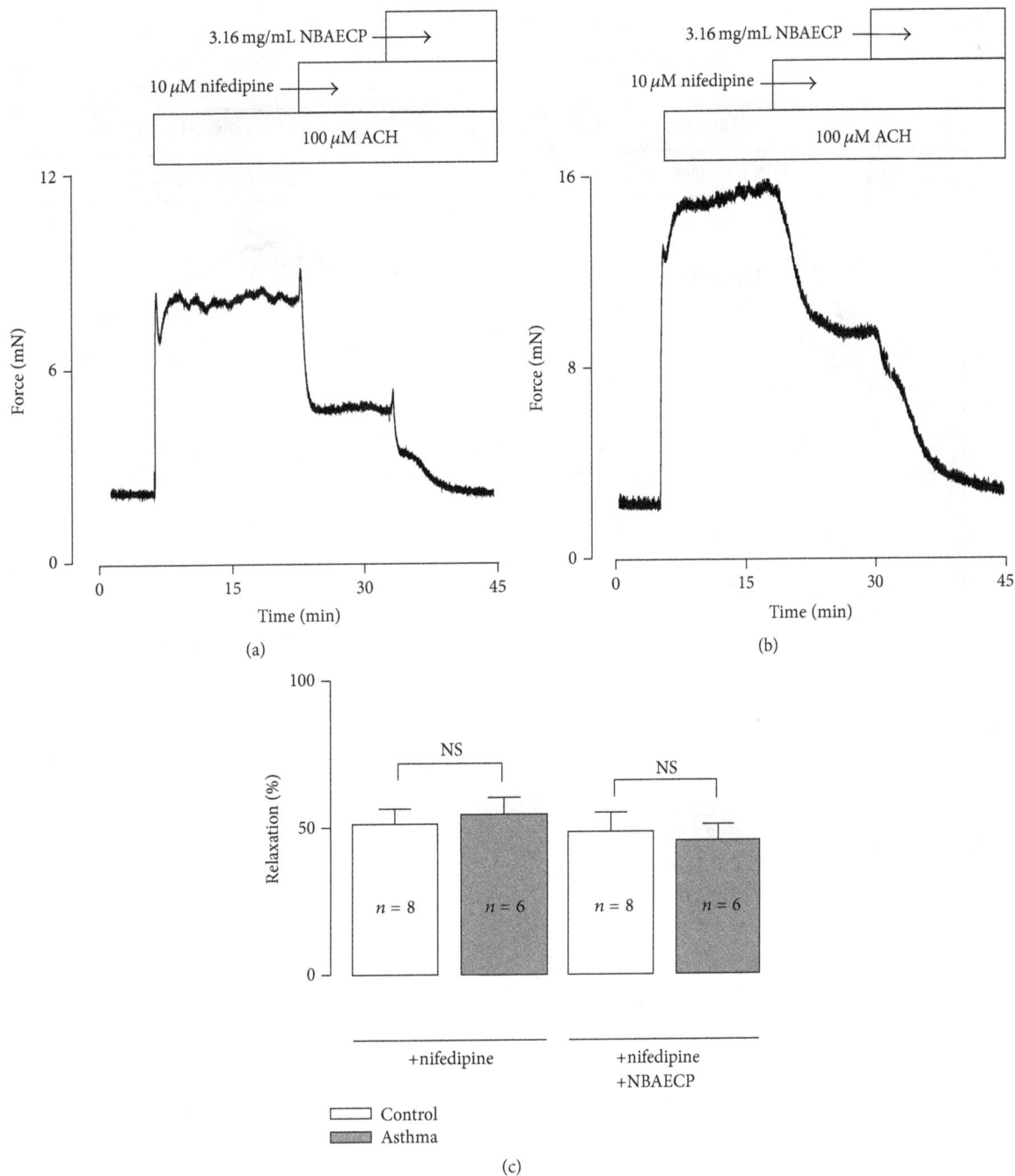

FIGURE 3: Nifedipine partially inhibits ACH-caused contraction. (a) ACH ($100\,\mu$M) induced a sustained contraction in a control TR, which was partially inhibited by nifedipine ($10\,\mu$M). The remaining contract was further blocked by NBAECP ($3.16\,$mg/mL). (b) An identical experiment was performed in an asthmatic TR. (c) The summary data from 8 control and 6 asthmatic TRs. $^{NS}P > 0.05$. These data demonstrated that activation of L-type Ca^{2+} channels played a role in ACH-induced contraction, and NBAECP could inhibit nifedipine-resistant channels, resulting in total relaxation.

influx. Thus, NBAECP-induced complete inhibition of high K^+-induced contraction due to NBAECP resulted in the inhibition of L-type Ca^{2+} channels, thus terminating Ca^{2+} influx. However, the inhibitory mechanism of NBAECP on L-type Ca^{2+} channels must be further investigated.

Airway smooth muscle expresses the muscarinic (M) receptor family, which includes 5 subtypes (M1–M5) [18].

Among them, G protein-coupled M3 plays a more important role in the contraction of airway smooth muscle [19]. Stimulation of M3 by agonists results in intracellular Ca^{2+} release from the sarcoplasmic reticulum (SR) via the PLC-IP3-IP3R pathway [20]. This leads to intracellular Ca^{2+} concentrations increasing and further triggering airway smooth muscle contraction. However, this pathway only mediates

(a)

(b)

(c)

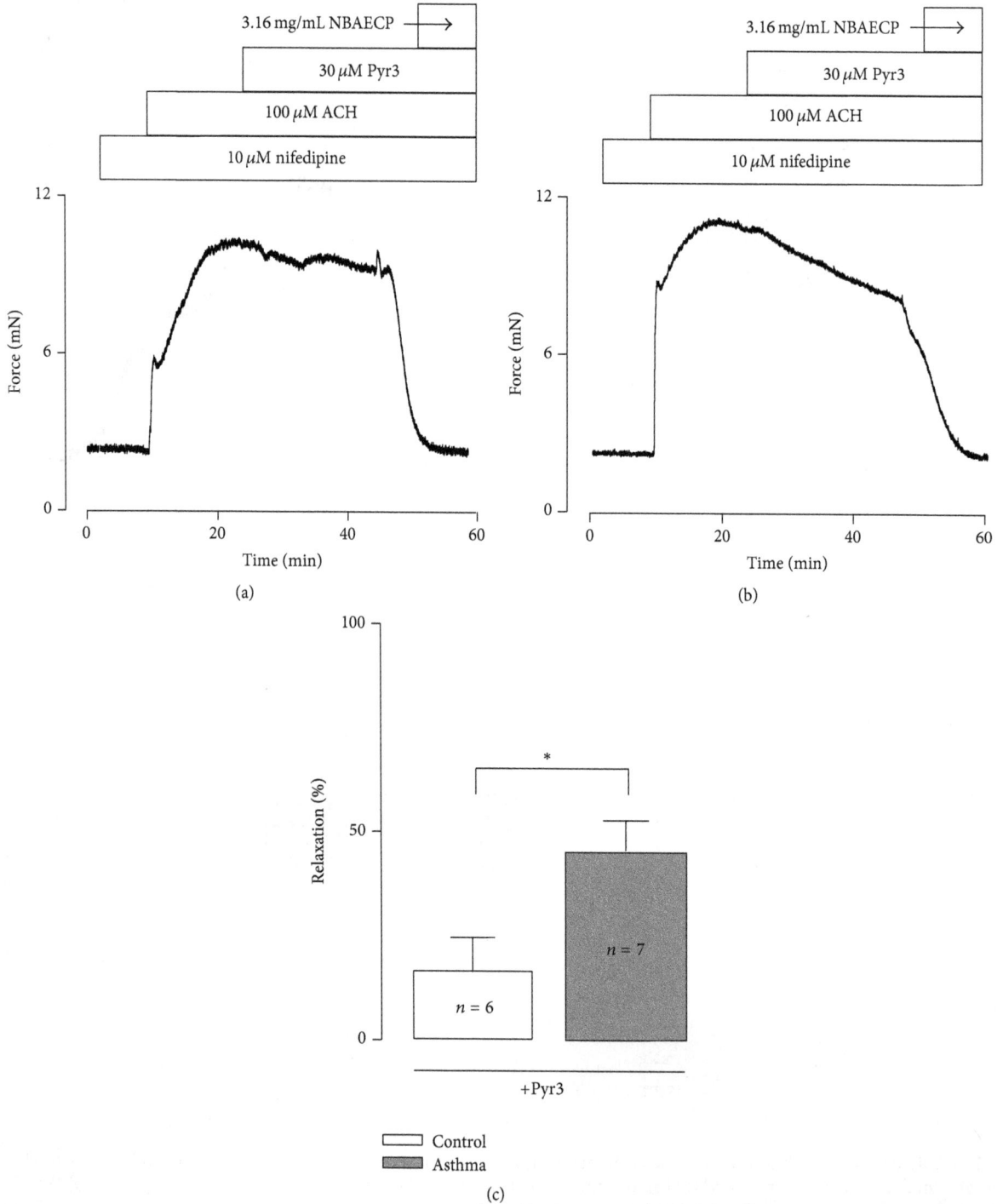

FIGURE 4: Pyr 3 partially inhibits ACH-induced contraction. (a) In the presence of nifedipine (10 μM), ACH-induced sustained contraction was partially inhibited by Pyr 3 (a blocker of TRPC3 and STIM/Orai channels) and then was completely blocked by NBAECP. (b) The same experiment was performed in an asthmatic TR. (c) Summary results from 6 control and 7 asthmatic TRs. *$P < 0.05$. These results indicated that activation of TRPC3 and/or STIM/Orai channels participated in ACH-induced contraction, and these channels were inhibited by NBAECP, thus resulting in relaxation.

transient contractions [21], while the sustained contraction depends on Ca^{2+} influx from the extracellular side and/or Ca^{2+} sensitization [22, 23]. Hence, the M3 agonist ACH-induced sustained contraction in airway smooth muscle (Figure 2) was probably due to Ca^{2+} influx. Previous reports have demonstrated that L-type Ca^{2+} channels play roles in ACH-induced airway smooth muscle contraction [24]. These findings were further confirmed in this study, in which

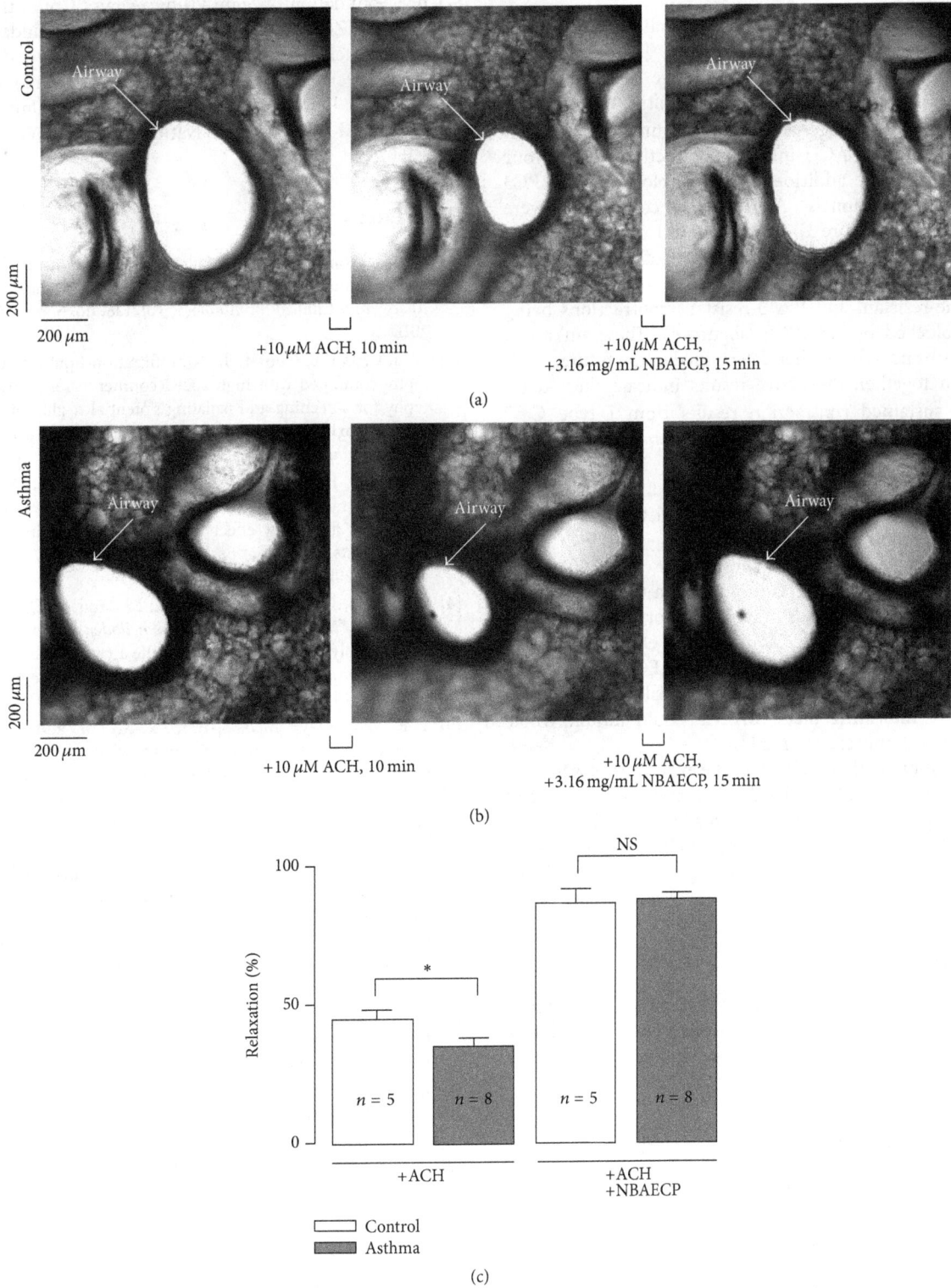

FIGURE 5: NBAECP inhibits bronchial smooth muscle contraction. (a) The intrapulmonary airway in a lung slice from a control mouse (left) following addition of ACH (10 μM for 10 min): the cross-section area of the airway lumen decreased (middle); then upon application of NBAECP (3.16 mg/mL for 15 min), the cross-section area of the airway lumen increased (right). (b) Similar measurements in an asthmatic lung slice. (c) Summary data from 8 slices/8 control mice and 5 slices/5 asthmatic mice. $^{*}P < 0.05$, $^{NS}P > 0.05$. These experiments demonstrated that NBAECP could inhibit ACH-induced contraction in bronchial smooth muscle.

nifedipine partially inhibited ACH-induced contraction in TRs (Figure 3).

Moreover, TRPC3 and/or STIM/Orai channels also play roles in ACH-induced contractions [14, 25]. TRPC3 and STIM/Orai channels are nonselective cation channels (NSCCs) that can mediate Ca^{2+} influx, resulting in intracellular Ca^{2+} increase to trigger airway smooth muscle contraction and contributing to ACH-induced contractions [26]. In our data, following the addition of Pyr 3 (blocker of TRPC3 and STIM/Orai channels), ACH-induced contractions were partly inhibited (Figure 3). In addition to L-type Ca^{2+} channels and two types of NSCCs, there are still other mechanisms that mediate ACH-induced contraction on the basis of nifedipine-resistant and Pyr 3-resistant contractions being further blocked by NBAECP (Figure 4). These unknown mechanisms must be further determined in the future.

Taken together, the above results indicate that ACH-induced sustained contraction results from L-type Ca^{2+} channels- and TRPC3 and/or STIM/Orai channels-mediated Ca^{2+} influx and unknown mechanisms. Thus, NBAECP-induced inhibition could be partially due to NBAECP inhibiting these channels. However, the detailed inhibitory mechanism requires further investigation.

Although the above data showed that NBAECP could inhibit agonist-induced precontractions in tracheal smooth muscle, whether it has similar inhibitory functions on bronchial smooth muscle is uncertain. Our experiments conducted in lung slices showed that NBAECP was also able to inhibit precontraction in small bronchial smooth muscle (Figure 5), indicating that NBAECP could inhibit whole airway smooth muscle contraction.

In addition, in this study, all of the experiments were performed in both healthy and asthmatic smooth muscles, and similar responses were observed. This finding indicates that NBAECP has similar inhibitory roles in both types of ASM, suggesting that NBAECP could be a potent bronchodilator for asthmatics.

5. Conclusions

NBAECP can inhibit agonist-induced sustained contractions of healthy and asthmatic airway smooth muscle by inhibiting several types of ion channels. These findings indicate that NBAECP could be a new inhibitor of asthma attacks.

Competing Interests

The authors declare no conflict of interests.

Authors' Contributions

Qiu-Ju Jiang, Weiwei Chen, and Hong Dan contributed equally to this work.

Acknowledgments

This work was supported by the National Natural Science Foundation of China (31571200, 31140087, and 30971514 to Qing-Hua Liu and 81400015 to Weiwei Chen), the Natural Science Foundation of State Ethnic Affairs Commission of China (14ZNZ021 to Liqun Ma), the Open Foundation of Hubei Provincial Key Laboratory for Protection and Application of Special Plants in Wuling Area of China, and the Fundamental Research Funds for the Central Universities, South-Central University for Nationalities (CZW15012 and CZW15025).

References

[1] D. J. Jackson, A. Sykes, P. Mallia, and S. L. Johnston, "Asthma exacerbations: origin, effect, and prevention," *The Journal of Allergy and Clinical Immunology*, vol. 128, no. 6, pp. 1165–1174, 2011.

[2] S. Li, C. Liu, L. Guo et al., "Ultrafiltration liquid chromatography combined with high-speed countercurrent chromatography for screening and isolating potential α-glucosidase and xanthine oxidase inhibitors from *Cortex Phellodendri*," *Journal of Separation Science*, vol. 37, no. 18, pp. 2504–2512, 2014.

[3] Y.-M. Lee, H. Kim, E.-K. Hong, B.-H. Kang, and S.-J. Kim, "Water extract of 1:1 mixture of *Phellodendron cortex* and *Aralia cortex* has inhibitory effects on oxidative stress in kidney of diabetic rats," *Journal of Ethnopharmacology*, vol. 73, no. 3, pp. 429–436, 2000.

[4] Y.-F. Mao, Y.-Q. Li, L. Zong, X.-M. You, F.-Q. Lin, and L. Jiang, "Methanol extract of *Phellodendri cortex* alleviates lipopolysaccharide-induced acute airway inflammation in mice," *Immunopharmacology and Immunotoxicology*, vol. 32, no. 1, pp. 110–115, 2010.

[5] Y.-F. Xian, Q.-Q. Mao, S.-P. Ip, Z.-X. Lin, and C.-T. Che, "Comparison on the anti-inflammatory effect of Cortex Phellodendri Chinensis and Cortex Phellodendri Amurensis in 12-O-tetradecanoyl-phorbol-13-acetate- induced ear edema in mice," *Journal of Ethnopharmacology*, vol. 137, no. 3, pp. 1425–1430, 2011.

[6] G. Chen, K.-K. Li, C.-H. Fung et al., "Er-Miao-San, a traditional herbal formula containing Rhizoma Atractylodis and Cortex Phellodendri inhibits inflammatory mediators in LPS-stimulated RAW264.7 macrophages through inhibition of NF-κB pathway and MAPKs activation," *Journal of Ethnopharmacology*, vol. 154, no. 3, pp. 711–718, 2014.

[7] T. Uchiyama, H. Kamikawa, and Z. Ogita, "Anti-ulcer effect of extract from phellodendri cortex," *Yakugaku Zasshi*, vol. 109, no. 9, pp. 672–676, 1989.

[8] J.-I. Park, J.-K. Shim, J.-W. Do et al., "Immune-stimulating properties of polysaccharides from Phellodendri cortex (Hwang-bek)," *Glycoconjugate Journal*, vol. 16, no. 3, pp. 247–252, 1999.

[9] H. W. Jung, G.-Z. Jin, S. Y. Kim, Y. S. Kim, and Y.-K. Park, "Neuroprotective effect of methanol extract of Phellodendri Cortex against 1-methyl-4-phenylpyridinium (MPP+)-induced apoptosis in PC-12 cells," *Cell Biology International*, vol. 33, no. 9, pp. 957–963, 2009.

[10] H.-Y. Kim, H.-S. Shin, H. Park et al., "In vitro inhibition of coronavirus replications by the traditionally used medicinal herbal extracts, Cimicifuga rhizoma, Meliae cortex, Coptidis rhizoma, and Phellodendron cortex," *Journal of Clinical Virology*, vol. 41, no. 2, pp. 122–128, 2008.

[11] Z. Xie, C. Wen, J. Sun, and Y. Fan, "Clinical retrospective study on the characteristics of pattern of syndromes and traditional Chinese medicines in different using phases of glucocorticoid

in treating bronchial asthma," *Journal of Zhejiang University of Traditional Chinese Medicine*, vol. 35, no. 1, pp. 21–22, 30, 2011.

[12] M. E. Sánchez-Mendoza, C. Castillo-Henkel, and A. Navarrete, "Relaxant action mechanism of berberine identified as the active principle of *Argemone ochroleuca* Sweet in guinea-pig tracheal smooth muscle," *Journal of Pharmacy and Pharmacology*, vol. 60, no. 2, pp. 229–236, 2008.

[13] Q.-R. Tuo, Y.-F. Ma, W. Chen et al., "Reactive oxygen species induce a Ca^{2+}-spark increase in sensitized murine airway smooth muscle cells," *Biochemical and Biophysical Research Communications*, vol. 434, no. 3, pp. 498–502, 2013.

[14] L. Tan, W. Chen, M.-Y. Wei et al., "Relaxant action of *Plumula Nelumbinis* extract on mouse airway smooth muscle," *Evidence-Based Complementary and Alternative Medicine*, vol. 2015, Article ID 523640, 10 pages, 2015.

[15] Y. Bai and M. J. Sanderson, "Airway smooth muscle relaxation results from a reduction in the frequency of Ca^{2+} oscillations induced by a cAMP-mediated inhibition of the IP_3 receptor," *Respiratory Research*, vol. 7, article 34, 2006.

[16] T. Kirschstein, M. Rehberg, R. Bajorat, T. Tokay, K. Porath, and R. Köhling, "High K^+-induced contraction requires depolarization-induced Ca^{2+} release from internal stores in rat gut smooth muscle," *Acta Pharmacologica Sinica*, vol. 30, no. 8, pp. 1123–1131, 2009.

[17] W.-B. Sai, M.-F. Yu, M.-Y. Wei et al., "Bitter tastants induce relaxation of rat thoracic aorta precontracted with high K^+," *Clinical and Experimental Pharmacology and Physiology*, vol. 41, no. 4, pp. 301–308, 2014.

[18] M. Ishii and Y. Kurachi, "Muscarinic acetylcholine receptors," *Current Pharmaceutical Design*, vol. 12, no. 28, pp. 3573–3581, 2006.

[19] A. F. Roffel, C. R. S. Elzinga, and J. Zaagsma, "Muscarinic M3 receptors mediate contraction of human central and peripheral airway smooth muscle," *Pulmonary Pharmacology*, vol. 3, no. 1, pp. 47–51, 1990.

[20] Y.-H. Liu, S.-Z. Wu, G. Wang, N.-W. Huang, and C.-T. Liu, "A long-acting β2-adrenergic agonist increases the expression of muscarine cholinergic subtype-3 receptors by activating the β2-adrenoceptor cyclic adenosine monophosphate signaling pathway in airway smooth muscle cells," *Molecular Medicine Reports*, vol. 11, no. 6, pp. 4121–4128, 2015.

[21] S. Mukherjee, J. Trice, P. Shinde, R. E. Willis, T. A. Pressley, and J. F. Perez-Zoghbi, "Ca^{2+} oscillations, Ca^{2+} sensitization, and contraction activated by protein kinase C in small airway smooth muscle," *The Journal of General Physiology*, vol. 141, no. 2, pp. 165–178, 2013.

[22] L. Tang, T. M. Gamal El-Din, J. Payandeh et al., "Structural basis for Ca^{2+} selectivity of a voltage-gated calcium channel," *Nature*, vol. 505, no. 7481, pp. 56–61, 2014.

[23] S. H. Young, O. Rey, and E. Rozengurt, "Intracellular Ca^{2+} oscillations generated via the extracellular Ca^{2+}-sensing receptor (CaSR) in response to extracellular Ca^{2+} or 1-phenylalanine: impact of the highly conservative mutation Ser170Thr," *Biochemical and Biophysical Research Communications*, vol. 467, no. 1, pp. 1–6, 2015.

[24] M.-Y. Wei, L. Xue, L. Tan et al., "Involvement of large-conductance Ca^{2+}-activated K^+ channels in chloroquine-induced force alterations in pre-contracted airway smooth muscle," *PLoS ONE*, vol. 10, no. 3, Article ID e0121566, 2015.

[25] T. Zhang, X.-J. Luo, W.-B. Sai et al., "Non-selective cation channels mediate chloroquine-induced relaxation in precontracted

mouse airway smooth muscle," *PLoS ONE*, vol. 9, no. 7, Article ID e101578, 2014.

[26] T. Song, Q. Hao, Y. M. Zheng, Q. H. Liu, and Y. X. Wang, "Inositol 1,4,5-trisphosphate activates TRPC3 channels to cause extracellular Ca^{2+} influx in airway smooth muscle cells," *American Journal of Physiology—Lung Cellular and Molecular Physiology*, vol. 309, no. 12, pp. L1455–L1466, 2015.

18

Danshen (*Salvia miltiorrhiza*) Compounds Improve the Biochemical Indices of the Patients with Coronary Heart Disease

Boyan Liu,[1] Yanhui Du,[1] Lixin Cong,[1] Xiaoying Jia,[2] and Ge Yang[1]

[1]*Department of Geriatrics, Affiliated Hospital, Changchun University of Traditional Chinese Medicine, Changchun 130000, China*
[2]*Department of Neurology, Jilin Province People's Hospital, Changchun 130000, China*

Correspondence should be addressed to Ge Yang; yangge338@163.com

Academic Editor: Roja Rahimi

Danshen was able to reduce the risk of the patients with coronary heart disease (CHD), but the mechanism is still widely unknown. Biochemical indices (lipid profile, markers of renal and liver function, and homocysteine (Hcy)) are closely associated with CHD risk. We aimed to investigate whether the medicine reduces CHD risk by improving these biochemical indices. The patients received 10 Danshen pills (27 mg/pill) in Dashen group, while the control patients received placebo pills, three times daily. The duration of follow-up was three months. The serum biochemical indices were measured, including lipid profiles (LDL cholesterol (LDL-C), HDL-C, total cholesterol (TC), triglycerides (TG), apolipoprotein (Apo) A, ApoB, ApoE, and lipoprotein (a) (Lp(a))); markers of liver function (gamma-glutamyl transpeptidase (GGT), total bilirubin (TBil), indirect bilirubin (IBil), and direct bilirubin (DBil)); marker of renal function (uric acid (UA)) and Hcy. After three-month follow-up, Danshen treatment reduced the levels of TG, TC, LDL-C, Lp(a), GGT, DBil, UA, and Hcy ($P < 0.05$). In contrast, the treatment increased the levels of HDL-C, ApoA, ApoB, ApoE, TBil, and IBil ($P < 0.05$). *Conclusion.* Danshen can reduce the CHD risk by improving the biochemical indices of CHD patients.

1. Introduction

Coronary heart disease (CHD) is the leading cause of death in the world [1, 2]. The number of CHD patients will reach 82 million in 2020 [2]. CHD still cannot be cured and present treatment prevents symptom development and reduces the incidences of heart attacks. CHD therapy mainly includes exercise-based cardiac rehabilitation [3], the changes of the dietary patterns (stopping alcohol consumption) [4], and medication [5] as well as aortic valve replacement and coronary-artery bypass graft surgery [6]. Therefore, due to the lack of effective therapy, it is necessary to discover new treatments for preventing CHD risk.

Traditional Chinese medicine (TCM) has a profound history and has been practiced in many diseases. It is an approach to exploring new medicine and mechanism for CHD therapy [7]. Danshen (*Salvia miltiorrhiza*), a form of TCM, is often applied in the therapy for coronary heart disease [8, 9]. The results of a number of publications pointed

to antioxidant [10, 11], anti-inflammatory [12], protective [13], or antiplatelet [14] properties of Danshen and its active compounds. A salvianolic acid B (SaB), an important bioactive ingredient in the root of Danshen, is being suggested to be responsible for its antioxidant property [10]. Other active water-soluble compounds, such as protocatechuic aldehyde (PAl), 3,4-dihydroxyphenyl lactic acid (DLA), and SaB with peroxides scavenging activities, were able to prevent the expression of adhesion molecules in vascular endothelium and inhibit vascular damage and the components such as tanshinone IIA and tanshinone IIB can inhibit the activity of NADPH oxidase and the aggregation of platelet [11]. This may explain the medicine usage for treating various microcirculatory disturbances. Anti-inflammatory properties of major ingredients SaB, tanshinone IIA (Tansh), and protocatechuic acid preventing the expression of adhesive molecules, cytokines, chemokines, and platelet P-selectin were also observed [12]. Furthermore, low-concentration Danshen was able to protect human umbilical vein endothelial cells

(HUVECs) and improve their functions [13]. Its main components, rosmarinic acid, lithospermic acid, SaB, salvianolic acid C (SaC), D (SaD), and and H/I (SaHI), have also antiplatelet potential [14].

It is well known that the changes in the levels of a number of biochemical parameters are directly or indirectly associated with the risk of occurrence of CHD. Firstly, low-density lipoprotein cholesterol (LDL-C) is an important risk factor for CHD and the concentration should be well controlled for reducing the incidences of CHD [15], while the concentration of high-density lipoprotein cholesterol (HDL-C) is strongly and inversely associated with CHD risk [16]. A correlation with the occurrence with this disease was also observed with the changes in levels of total cholesterol (TC) and triglycerides (TG) [17, 18] as well as in the case of apolipoproteins A (ApoA), B (ApoB), E (ApoE) and lipoprotein (a) (Lp(a)) genes expression profile changes [19–22]. The markers of liver function such as γ-glutamyl transpeptidase (GGT) [23], total bilirubin (TBil) [24], indirect bilirubin (IBil), and direct bilirubin (DBil) [25] are also related to CHD risk. Furthermore, serum level of uric acid, one of markers of renal function [26, 27], can also reflect the severity of CHD [28]. Moreover, the high concentration of homocysteine (Hcy) concentration is regarded as a risk factor for cardiovascular disease [29, 30].

Several clinical trials showed also positive effects in the field of above-mentioned parameters, including improvement of the lipid patterns of hyperlipidemic patients [31] and protective properties in the patients with liver [32] or renal injury [33]. We hypothesized that Danshen may be able to reduce the incidences of CHD by improving these biochemical indices (lipid profile, markers of renal and liver function, and Hcy) of CHD patients. Therefore, placebo-controlled, prospective, and randomized study was conducted to investigate the effects of the medicine on biochemical indices of CHD patients and explore the possible mechanisms of its functions.

2. Methods

2.1. Patients. Before the study, all protocols were approved by the human ethical committee of Affiliated Hospital of Changchun University of Traditional Chinese Medicine. The study was conducted according to the principles of the Declaration of Helsinki [34]. All patients signed the informed consents before being enrolled in this study. From March 2011 to June 2012, 432 CHD patients attended our hospital. A total of 126 patients met following inclusion criteria and were considered for enrollment in the study.

2.2. Inclusion Criteria. Inclusion criteria were given according to guidelines for the management of patients with myocardial infarction [35–37]. All patients should have one of the following clinical symptoms: (1) unstable angina; (2) ST-elevation myocardial infarction (STEMI) and non-STEMI; (3) patients undergoing coronary-artery bypass grafting (CABG) surgery; (4) patients undergoing undergone percutaneous coronary intervention (PCI); patients undergoing coronary-artery stent; (5) CHD determined by angiography.

2.3. Exclusion Criteria. Exclusion criteria were determined according to previous reports [38–40]. The following exclusion criteria were used: (1) pregnancy and lactation; (2) renal failure with a creatinine level > 3 mg/dL; (3) multiple myeloma; (4) history of hypersensitivity; (5) cardiogenic shock or left ventricular ejection fraction < 40%; (6) patients undergoing heart transplants; (7) patients undergoing cardiac resynchronization therapy (CRT); (8) having implantable defibrillators (ICD); (9) difficult communication and other reasons.

2.4. Groups. Danshen compounds were extracted by ethanol and the quality was controlled according to the standard designed by China State Food and Drug Administration (http://www.sda.gov.cn/WS01/CL1236/114286.html). The main contents of ethanol extracts are tanshinone IIA, cryptotanshinone, tanshinone I [41], rosmarinic acid, and salvianolic acid B [42]. Danshen pills were the extracts of *S. miltiorrhiza* and provided as 27 mg/pill by Tianjin Tasly Group Co., Ltd (Tianjin, China). Danshen pill is composed of 0.28% tanshinone IIA, 0.21% cryptotanshinone, 0.04% tanshinone I, 1.2% rosmarinic acid, 5.8% salvianolic acid B, and most starch. After the selection of inclusion and exclusion criteria, final 126 patients were evenly and randomly assigned into two groups: Danshen group and control group. Each person was assigned to one group using an electronic spreadsheet with the indicated number. To avoid the blinding of this study, three-month run-in period was added. During the period, all patients were treated as usual. Meanwhile, to keep the stable results, the changes of lifestyle and daily food calorie intake were discouraged. CHD patients in both groups had in-person visits or telephone contact in each week. The biochemical indices were maintained constant between two groups after 3-month run-in period and then entered treatment period with Danshen.

After three-month run-in period, the patients received 10 Danshen pills/time in Dashen group [43], while the control patients received placebo pills, three times daily. Meanwhile, all patients receive the normal therapy as in run-in period and the changes of lifestyle and daily food calorie intake were discouraged. CHD patients in both groups had in-person visits or telephone contact in each week. The duration of follow-up was 3 months.

2.5. The Measurement of Biochemical Indices. Blood sample was obtained from the antecubital vein of each patient on the day of enrollment, after 3-month run-in period, and 3-month administration of Danshen or placebo. Serum was separated from peripheral venous blood (4 mL) after centrifuge at 4°C at 3000 rpm for 10 min. The biochemical indices were measured, including lipid profiles (LDL-C, TC, TG, HDL-C, ApoA, ApoB, ApoE, and Lp(a)), markers of liver function (GGT, TBil, IBil, and DBil), marker of renal function (UA), and a risk factor for cardiovascular disease (Hcy).

All kits were commercially available. Low-density lipoprotein cholesterol (LDL-C) BioAssay ELISA Kit (Human), Cat. number 196116, was from Beijing Huamei Scientific (Beijing, China). High-density lipoprotein cholesterol, HDL-C, ELISA Kit, Cat. number CSB-E08954h, was from Cusabio

Biotech Co., Ltd (Wuhan, China). Human total cholesterol (TC) ELISA Kit, Cat. number QY-E00062, was from Qayee Bio-Technology Co., Ltd (Shanghai, China). Human TG (Triglyceride) ELISA Kit, Cat. number E-EL-H5437, was from Elabscience Biotechnology Co., Ltd (Beijing, China). Lipoprotein A (ApoA) Human ELISA Kit, Cat. Number ab108878, Apolipoprotein B (ApoB) Human ELISA kit, Cat. number ab108807, and Apolipoprotein E (ApoE) Human ELISA Kit, Cat. number ab108813, were from Abcam Trading (Shanghai) Company, Ltd (Shanghai, China). ELISA Kit for Lipoprotein (a), Lp(a), Cat. number SEA842Hu, was from Wuhan USCN Business Co., Ltd (Wuhan, China). Human gamma-glutamyl transpeptidase, GGT ELISA Kit, Cat. number E1375h, was from Everlight Biotech (Taipei, Taiwan). Total Bilirubin, Human, ELISA Kit, Cat. number E01T0143, was from ARP American Research Products, Inc (Waltham, MA, USA). Bilirubin (Total and Direct) Colorimetric Assay Kit, Cat. number K553-100, was from BioVision, Inc (Milpitas, CA, USA). Uric Acid Assay Kit, Cat. number KA1651, was from Anova Corporation (Taipei, Taiwan). Human Homocysteine (HCY) ELISA Kit, Cat. number, was from Flarebio Biotech (Wuhan, China).

Just as in a run-in period, in order to avoid the variations in biochemical indices because of normal therapy, the changes of daily food calorie intake, and lifestyle, all these changes were discouraged in three-month treatment period. After three-month follow-up, serum biochemical indices were measured on all available data. These variables still include serum lipid profiles (LDL-C, HDL-C, TC, TG, ApoA, ApoB, ApoE, and Lp(a)); serum markers of liver function, GGT, TBil, IBil, and DBil; serum marker of renal function, UA, and CHD risk factor, Hcy.

2.6. Statistical Analysis. A total of 126 patients (63 in each group) provided 90% power to detect the difference between two groups with an alpha level set at 0.05. All data were presented as mean values ± SD. Chi-squared test and t-test were applied. Analysis of variance was used to compare the serum levels of lipids at baseline and after 3-month treatment period in each group. $P < 0.05$ (2-tailed) will be regarded as statistically significant. The analysis was conducted by using SPSS version 20.0 (IBM corporation; Chicago, IL, USA).

3. Results

3.1. Baseline Characters of CHD Patients. A total of 432 patients attended our hospital from March 2011 to June 2012. Of these patients, 306 CHD patients were excluded after selection with inclusion and exclusion criteria (Figure 1). Before administration of Danshen, 3-month run-in period was performed to make sure that there was no significant change in biochemical indices, although some of these patients are still taking the medicine for CHD therapy. Thus, 126 patients were selected and were randomly assigned to two groups: the Danshen group ($n = 63$) and the control group ($n = 63$). After another 3-month follow-up, 61 and 62 CHD patients finished the study in Danshen and control groups, respectively.

There was no significant difference for the clinical and procedural characteristics between Danshen and control groups (Table 1) ($P > 0.05$), including age, sex, risk element, clinical presentation, preprocedural laboratory results, and medication. There were 26 (41.3%) and 24 (38.1%) males in Danshen and control groups, respectively. The age of all CHD patients ranged from 60.2 to 73.5 years. Most CHD patients had unstable angina with 37 cases (58.7%) in Danshen group and 34 cases (54.0%) in control group. More than half number of patients was overweight according to BMI values (overweight = BMI of 25–29.9) in both groups [44]. Hypertension was an obvious symptom with 48 cases (76.2%) in Danshen group and 50 cases (79.4%) in control group.

3.2. Biochemical Indices at Baseline. Serum biochemical indices were analyzed on all available data, to primarily identify these variables associated with CHD risk. These variables include serum lipid profiles (LDL-C, HDL-C, TC, TG, ApoA, ApoB, ApoE, and Lp(a)); serum markers of liver function, GGT, TBil, IBil, and DBil; serum marker of renal function, UA and CHD risk factor, and Hcy. All serum biochemical indices between Danshen and control groups were statistically insignificant ($P > 0.05$) (Table 2).

3.3. Biochemical Indices after 3-Month Run-In Period. In order to avoid the variations in biochemical indices because of normal therapy, the changes of daily food calorie intake, and lifestyle, it is necessary to add three-month run-in period to make sure of the variations. Meanwhile, all these changes were discouraged. After three-month run-in period, serum biochemical indices were measured on all available data, which are associated with CHD risk. These variables still include serum lipid profiles (LDL-C, HDL-C, TC, TG, ApoA, ApoB, ApoE, and Lp(a)); serum markers of liver function, GGT, TBil, IBil, and DBil; serum marker of renal function, UA and CHD risk factor, and Hcy. The results also showed that there was no significantly statistical difference for these serum biochemical indices between Danshen and control groups after three-month run-in period (Table 3) ($P > 0.05$).

3.4. Analysis of Biochemical Indices after Three-Month Administration of Danshen. After three-month follow-up, two persons dropped out from Danshen group and one patient dropped out from control group. Thus, 61 and 62 patients finished the trial in Danshen and control groups (Figure 1), respectively. Danshen treatment reduced the levels of TG, TC, LDL-C, Lp(a), GGT, DBil, UA, and Hcy from median values (mg/dL) 114, 190, 113, 32, 3.3 (IU/dL), 0.4, 5.1, and 2.3 (Table 3) to media values (mg/dL) 101, 155, 98, 8, 1.6 (IU/dL), 0.2, 4.5, and 14 (Table 4), respectively ($P < 0.05$). In contrast, Danshen treatment increased the levels of HDL-C, ApoA, ApoB, ApoE, TBil, and IBil from median values (mg/dL) 55, 98, 76, 7.0, 0.5, and 0.5 (Table 3) to median values (mg/dL) 62, 119, 93, 8.7, 0.8, and 0.6 (Table 4), respectively ($P < 0.05$). Meanwhile, there were significantly statistical differences for these biochemical indices between Danshen and control groups after three-month follow-up (Table 4) ($P < 0.05$). Comparatively, there was no significantly statistical difference

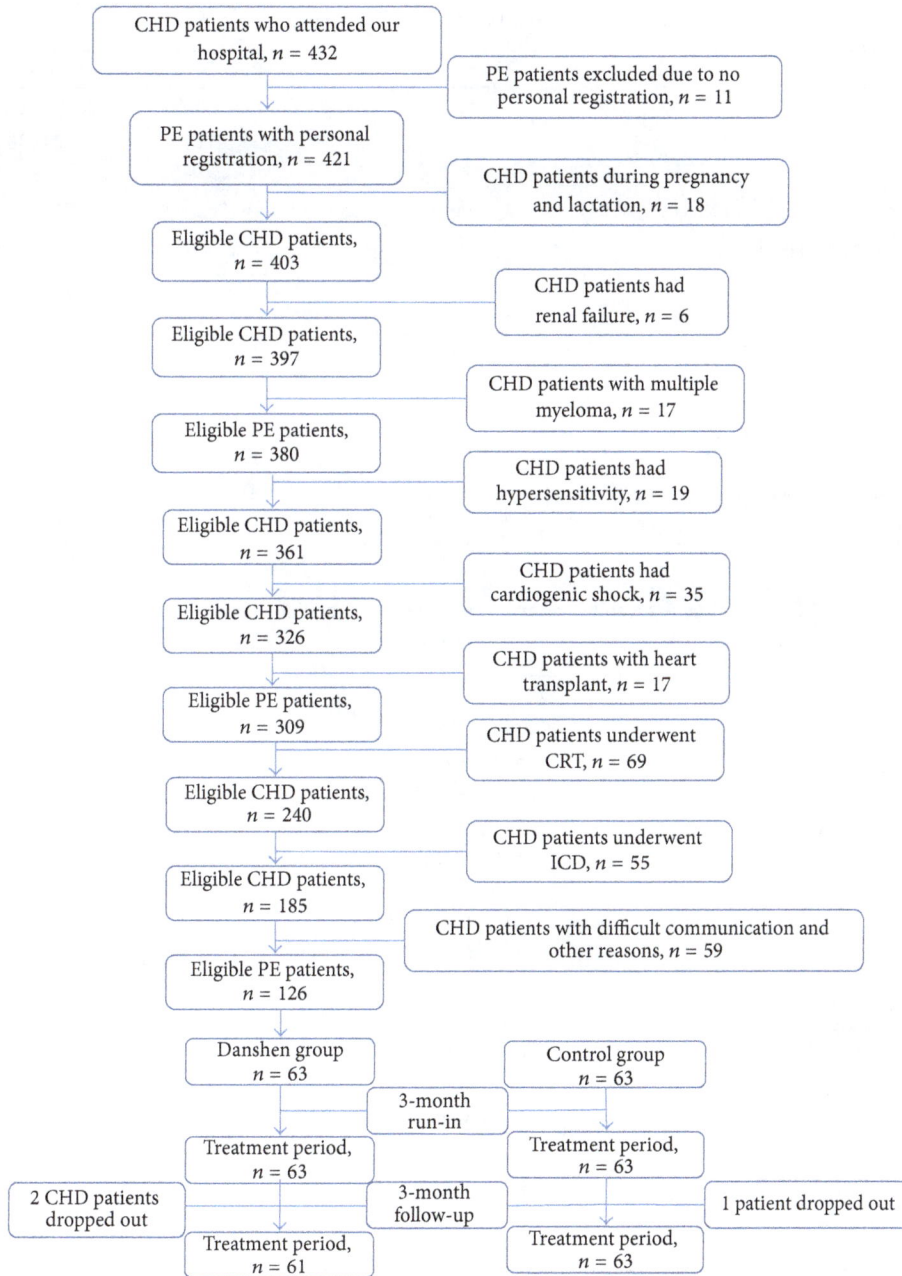

FIGURE 1: The flowchart of this study. CHD, coronary heart disease. The changes for CHD normal therapy, lifestyle, and daily food calories intake were discouraged in three-month run-in and three-month treatment periods. Finally, 61 and 62 CHD patients finished the whole procedure. Danshen pills were the extracts of *Salvia miltiorrhiza* and provided as 27 mg/pill by Tianjin Tasly Group Co., Ltd (Tianjin, China).

for these biochemical parameters in control groups between run-in and treatment periods (Tables 3 and 4) ($P > 0.05$).

4. Discussion

The TCM Danshen has been long regarded as effective in "activating circulation and dispersing blood stasis" [45]. According to the classic theory of TCM, it has been said that "pain will be relieved when blockage is removed." The concept suggests that low blood circulation will do damage

to human tissues and organs. Thus, such theory can be used for the management of CHD.

We assessed the therapeutic efficacy of Danshen, which is associated with the changes of lipid profiles in CHD patients. Multiple markers of biochemical indices of CHD patients were measured in the serum. The results indicated that Danshen presence may cause an improvement of several studied biochemical indices of CHD patients. Levels of TG, TC, LDL-C, Lp(a), GGT, DBil, the AU, and Hcy were statistically significantly reduced ($P < 0.05$, resp.)

Essentials of Complementary and Alternative Medicine

TABLE 1: Baseline characters of CHD patients.

Characteristic	Danshen ($n = 63$)	Control ($n = 63$)	P values
Age (years)	65.9 ± 5.7	67.1 ± 6.4	0.269
Gender, male (%)	26 (41.3)	24 (38.1)	0.716
Hypertension			
Systolic blood pressure ≥ 140 mmHg or diastolic blood pressure ≥ 90 mmHg (%)	48 (76.2)	50 (79.4)	0.668
Hypercholesterolemia (>200 mg/dL) (%)	21 (33.3)	22 (34.9)	0.851
Diabetes mellitus (%)	17 (27)	14 (22.2)	0.535
BMI (kg/m^2)	25.2 ± 5.6	25.8 ± 5.4	0.541
Cigarette smokers (%)	31 (49.2)	29 (46)	0.721
Chronic kidney disease (%)	2 (3.2)	1 (1.6)	1.000
Clinical presentation			
Unstable angina (%)	37 (58.7)	34 (54)	0.590
Non-ST-segment elevation myocardial infarction (%)	11 (17.5)	13 (20.6)	0.650
ST-segment elevation myocardial infarction (%)	12 (19)	14 (22.2)	0.660

TABLE 2: Biochemical indices measure at baseline, median (range), mg/dL.

	Danshen group ($n = 63$)	Placebo group ($n = 63$)	P values
Lipid profile			
LDL cholesterol	118 (95–151)	123 (94–154)	0.875
HDL cholesterol	52 (43–64)	54 (46–67)	0.436
Total cholesterol	197 (178–239)	191 (172–243)	0.527
Triglycerides	117 (85–168)	121 (84–171)	0.329
Apolipoprotein A	93 (83–126)	94 (85–128)	0.811
Apolipoprotein B	71 (62–104)	73 (65–99)	0.743
Apolipoprotein E	6.9 (5.2–8.6)	7.2 (5.3–8.5)	0.632
Lipoprotein (a)	30 (20–45)	33 (24–41)	0.237
Liver function			
Gamma-glutamyl transpeptidase (IU/dL)	2.8 (2.1–5.3)	3.0 (2.5–5.1)	0.165
Total bilirubin	0.5 (0.3–0.6)	0.6 (0.4–0.8)	0.175
Indirect bilirubin	0.4 (0.3–0.6)	0.5 (0.3–0.5)	0.268
Direct bilirubin	0.4 (0.2–0.5)	0.3 (0.2–0.4)	0.377
Renal function			
Uric acid	5.1 (4.5–6.9)	5.5 (4.1–6.4)	0.264
Risk factor of heart disease			
Homocysteine	22 (19–40)	23 (21–42)	0.459

(Tables 3 and 4), while the levels of HDL-C, ApoA, ApoB, ApoE, TBIL, and IBil were significantly elevated (Tables 3 and 4), ($P < 0.05$, resp.). Most of these results are accordant with previous reports.

Danshen was able to improve liver function by increasing the level of total bilirubin [46] and reduce the level of UA in volunteers [47]. Hcy is a byproduct of methionine metabolism and its imbalance will result in hyperhomocysteinemia [48, 49], which is responsible for CHD development [50]. *S. miltiorrhiza* extract also inhibited unwanted adverse effects for HUVECs [51]. All these results suggest that the medicine can improve heart functions and is a potential drug in CHD therapy.

Danshen has been proved to suppress the intake of low-density lipoprotein, increase the expression of intercellular adhesion molecule, and modulate key events in atherosclerosis [52]. The combination of the medicine and Gegen can improve the ratios of TG/HDL-C and LDL-C/HDL-C [53]. The main compositions in Danshen may be beneficial to the improvement of lipid profiles. Cryptotanshinone showed protective effects on atherosclerosis of ApoE-deficient mice and can improve the situation caused by apolipoprotein shortage [54], which also was able to inhibit expression of oxidized adhesion molecules induced by LDL [55]. Tanshinone IIA showed scavenging effects on lipid free radicals in cardiac sarcoplasmic reticulum [56] and inhibited expression of oxidized low-density lipoprotein receptor-1 [57]. Ethanol extract of *S. miltiorrhiza* increased in vivo serum level of HDL to prevent the occurrence of osteoporosis [58]. Lipid peroxidation prevention was also observed in the case of its

TABLE 3: Biochemical indices measure after three-month run-in period, median (range), mg/dL.

	Danshen group ($n = 63$)	Placebo group ($n = 63$)	P values
Lipid profile			
LDL cholesterol	113 (90–147)	120 (91–150)	0.324
HDL cholesterol	55 (44–68)	51 (47–65)	0.512
Total cholesterol	190 (172–234)	189 (176–248)	0.763
Triglycerides	114 (87–173)	118 (82–166)	0.262
Apolipoprotein A	98 (82–126)	99 (85–128)	0.899
Apolipoprotein B	76 (66–103)	78 (62–109)	0.842
Apolipoprotein E	7.0 (5.8–8.5)	7.2 (5.4–8.8)	0.763
Lipoprotein (a)	32 (22–45)	34 (25–48)	0.268
Liver function			
Gamma-glutamyl transpeptidase (IU/dL)	3.3 (2.5–5.4)	3.1 (2.5–5.3)	0.275
Total bilirubin	0.5 (0.4–0.7)	0.6 (0.4–0.8)	0.431
Indirect bilirubin	0.5 (0.3–0.5)	0.4 (0.3–0.5)	0.176
Direct bilirubin	0.4 (0.2–0.6)	0.4 (0.2–0.5)	0.185
Renal function			
Uric acid	5.1 (4.2–6.8)	5.3 (4.2–6.4)	0.267
Risk factor of heart disease			
Homocysteine	23 (20–43)	25 (20–46)	0.341

TABLE 4: Biochemical indices after three-month follow-up, median (range), mg/dL.

	Danshen group ($n = 61$)	Placebo group ($n = 62$)	P values
Lipid profile			
LDL cholesterol	98 (82–133)	123 (94–157)	0.017
HDL cholesterol	62 (49–77)	50 (49–69)	0.039
Total cholesterol	155 (147–195)	192 (179–251)	0.001
Triglycerides	101 (80–158)	121 (84–172)	0.016
Apolipoprotein A	119 (103–143)	96 (81–123)	0.023
Apolipoprotein B	93 (78–114)	75 (65–101)	0.009
Apolipoprotein E	8.7 (6.8–10.7)	7.3 (5.6–8.7)	0.024
Lipoprotein (a)	18 (15–20)	31 (21–43)	0.001
Liver function			
Gamma-glutamyl transpeptidase (IU/dL)	1.6 (1.2–1.8)	3.1 (2.3–5.2)	0.001
Total bilirubin	0.8 (0.6–1.0)	0.6 (0.4–0.7)	0.032
Indirect bilirubin	0.6 (0.5–0.8)	0.4 (0.3–0.5)	0.025
Direct bilirubin	0.2 (0.1–0.3)	0.3 (0.2–0.4)	0.037
Renal function			
Uric acid	4.5 (3.6–5.5)	5.4 (4.2–6.7)	0.040
Risk factor of heart disease			
Homocysteine	14 (11–17)	24 (20–41)	0.001

active compound—rosmarinic acid [59]. All these compositions may be beneficial to the improvement of lipid profiles of CHD patients.

The incidence of CHD differs widely among different studies. The determination of degree of correlation between the risk profiles and the prevalence of factors of CHD patients is often very complicated, especially in the patients with cooccurring diseases such as hypertension [60, 61], diabetes mellitus [62, 63], renal disease [64], and others making such results more variable. Other activities also can make CHD become worse, such as oxidative stress [65, 66] and

the production of proinflammatory cytokines [67]. Thus, the prevention of these accompanying diseases and these processes may improve the clinical outcome of CHD patients. More importantly, the progression of CHD by Danshen seems to be depended on its multiple functions and beneficial effects were demonstrated in several studies. For example, the medicine has the main components with antioxidant activities [10], which can prevent vascular injury [68]. It possesses anti-inflammatory properties [12], inhibits the aggregation of platelet [69], prevents thrombosis [70], reduces blood viscosity, and improves myocardial ischemia [71].

All these results suggest that Danshen is superior to most present medicine with multiple activities, which are beneficial to improve the symptoms of CHD. However, here, we only consider Danshen improving the lipid profiles of CHD patients. Much work needs to be done to better understand its function for ameliorating the severity of CHD.

It should be emphasized that the values of obtained results even with the clinical trial's limitation could have an impact; for example, (1) the sample size seems small only with 126 selected CHD patients, which is caused by the strict criteria given in this study; (2) the whole follow-up period is 6 months, while the period for administration of Danshen is only three months. In such short period, reduction of cardiac death and heart failure cannot be detected; (3) the safety of the medicine is not identified, although it has been widely used clinically in China. Our results should be counted as a promising, although preliminary. Much more evidence is needed to support the clinical use of Danshen for CHD patients.

5. Conclusion

Danshen was able to improve biochemical indices of CHD patients. In a prespecified exploratory analysis, there was evidence of a reduction in the rate of CHD events among patients who had received the medicine therapy. Presently, it is the most popular Chinese herbal drug and is often used either alone or in combination with other drugs, especially for the therapies of cardiovascular diseases. Results of our study reflect the global trend of studies in the field of the role of Danshen in therapy development for CHD patients.

Competing Interests

The authors declare that there are no competing interests regarding the publication of this paper.

Acknowledgments

The authors thank Dr. Wang for her technical assistance during data collection.

References

[1] J. A. Leigh, M. Alvarez, and C. J. Rodriguez, "Ethnic minorities and coronary heart disease: an update and future directions," *Current Atherosclerosis Reports*, vol. 18, no. 2, article 9, 2016.

[2] J. S. Kanu, Y. Gu, S. Zhi et al., "Single nucleotide polymorphism rs3774261 in the AdipoQ gene is associated with the risk of coronary heart disease (CHD) in Northeast Han Chinese population: a case-control study," *Lipids in Health and Disease*, vol. 15, no. 1, p. 6, 2016.

[3] L. Anderson, D. R. Thompson, N. Oldridge et al., "Exercise-based cardiac rehabilitation for coronary heart disease," *Journal of the American College of Cardiology*, vol. 67, no. 1, pp. 1–12, 2016.

[4] X.-Y. Zhang, L. Shu, C.-J. Si et al., "Dietary patterns, alcohol consumption and risk of coronary heart disease in adults: a meta-analysis," *Nutrients*, vol. 7, no. 8, pp. 6582–6605, 2015.

[5] S. Zhao, H. Zhao, L. Wang, S. Du, and Y. Qin, "Education is critical for medication adherence in patients with coronary heart disease," *Acta Cardiologica*, vol. 70, no. 2, pp. 197–204, 2015.

[6] S. K. Agarwal, A. Kapoor, S. Pande et al., "Comparison of release kinetics of different cardiac biomarkers in patients undergoing off pump coronary artery bypass surgery and valve replacement surgery for rheumatic heart disease," *Journal of Cardiothoracic Surgery*, vol. 10, supplement 1, article A208, 2015.

[7] H. Cao, J. Zhai, W. Mu et al., "Use of comparative effectiveness research for similar Chinese patent medicine for angina pectoris of coronary heart disease: a new approach based on patient-important outcomes," *Trials*, vol. 15, article 84, 2014.

[8] J. Luo, W. Song, G. Yang, H. Xu, and K. Chen, "Compound Danshen (*Salvia miltiorrhiza*) dripping pill for coronary heart disease: an overview of systematic reviews," *The American Journal of Chinese Medicine*, vol. 43, no. 1, pp. 25–43, 2015.

[9] T. O. Cheng, "Danshen: a versatile Chinese herbal drug for the treatment of coronary heart disease," *International Journal of Cardiology*, vol. 113, no. 3, pp. 437–438, 2006.

[10] G.-J. Zhou, W. Wang, X.-M. Xie, M.-J. Qin, B.-K. Kuai, and T.-S. Zhou, "Post-harvest induced production of salvianolic acids and significant promotion of antioxidant properties in roots of *Salvia miltiorrhiza* (Danshen)," *Molecules*, vol. 19, no. 6, pp. 7207–7222, 2014.

[11] J.-Y. Han, J.-Y. Fan, Y. Horie et al., "Ameliorating effects of compounds derived from *Salvia miltiorrhiza* root extract on microcirculatory disturbance and target organ injury by ischemia and reperfusion," *Pharmacology and Therapeutics*, vol. 117, no. 2, pp. 280–295, 2008.

[12] C. Stumpf, Q. Fan, C. Hintermann et al., "Anti-inflammatory effects of *Danshen* on human vascular endothelial cells in culture," *The American Journal of Chinese Medicine*, vol. 41, no. 5, pp. 1065–1077, 2013.

[13] C. Wang, R. Zhao, B. Li, L. Y. Gu, and H. Gou, "An in vivo and in vitro study: high-dosage Danshen injection induces peripheral vascular endothelial cells injury," *Human & Experimental Toxicology*, vol. 35, no. 4, pp. 404–417, 2016.

[14] Y. Chen, N. Zhang, J. Ma et al., "A Platelet/CMC coupled with offline UPLC-QTOF-MS/MS for screening antiplatelet activity components from aqueous extract of Danshen," *Journal of Pharmaceutical and Biomedical Analysis*, vol. 117, pp. 178–183, 2016.

[15] C. M. Gamboa, M. M. Safford, E. B. Levitan et al., "Statin underuse and low prevalence of LDL-C control among U.S. adults at high risk of coronary heart disease," *American Journal of the Medical Sciences*, vol. 348, no. 2, pp. 108–114, 2014.

[16] Y. Huang, H. D. Ye, X. Gao et al., "Significant interaction of APOE rs4420638 polymorphism with HDL-C and APOA-I levels in coronary heart disease in Han Chinese men," *Genetics and Molecular Research*, vol. 14, no. 4, pp. 13414–13424, 2015.

[17] P. Gong, S. Li, L. Hu et al., "Total cholesterol mediates the effect of ABO blood group on coronary heart disease," *Zhonghua Xin Xue Guan Bing Za Zhi*, vol. 43, no. 5, pp. 404–407, 2015.

[18] A. Onat, "Influence of gender, C- reactive protein and triglycerides in risk prediction of coronary heart disease," *Anadolu Kardiyoloji Dergisi*, vol. 13, no. 3, pp. 287–288, 2013.

[19] L. Zhu, Z. Lu, and Y. Y. Song, "Advances in the association between apolipoprotein (a) gene polymorphisms and coronary heart disease," *Zhongguo Yi Xue Ke Xue Yuan Xue Bao*, vol. 37, no. 4, pp. 482–488, 2015.

[20] J. Z. Zhang, Y. Y. Zheng, Y. N. Yang et al., "Association between apolipoprotein B gene polymorphisms and the risk of coronary heart disease (CHD): an update meta-analysis," *Journal of the Renin-Angiotensin-Aldosterone System*, vol. 16, no. 4, pp. 827–837, 2015.

[21] G. D. Kolovou, V. Kolovou, D. B. Panagiotakos et al., "Study of common variants of the apolipoprotein E and lipoprotein lipase genes in patients with coronary heart disease and variable body mass index," *Hormones*, vol. 14, no. 3, pp. 376–382, 2015.

[22] E. V. Mazdorova, K. Y. Nikolaev, Y. V. Polonskaya et al., "Valuing the lipid marker of lipoprotein (a) in the diagnosis of patients with coronary heart disease," *Kardiologiia*, vol. 55, no. 8, p. 49, 2015.

[23] Y. Hashimoto, A. Futamura, H. Nakarai, and K. Nakahara, "Relationship between response of γ-glutamyl transpeptidase to alcohol drinking and risk factors for coronary heart disease," *Atherosclerosis*, vol. 158, no. 2, pp. 465–470, 2001.

[24] E. Oda and R. Kawai, "A possible cross-sectional association of serum total bilirubin with coronary heart disease and stroke in a Japanese health screening population," *Heart and Vessels*, vol. 27, no. 1, pp. 29–36, 2012.

[25] C. Ghem, R. E. Sarmento-Leite, A. S. de Quadros, S. Rossetto, and C. A. M. Gottschall, "Serum bilirubin concentration in patients with an established coronary artery disease," *International Heart Journal*, vol. 51, no. 2, pp. 86–91, 2010.

[26] F. Lin, H. Zhang, F. Huang, H. Chen, C. Lin, and P. Zhu, "Influence of changes in serum uric acid levels on renal function in elderly patients with hypertension: a retrospective cohort study with 3.5-year follow-up," *BMC Geriatrics*, vol. 16, no. 1, article 35, 2016.

[27] D. R. Kannangara, G. G. Graham, K. M. Williams, and R. O. Day, "Effect of xanthine oxidase inhibitors on the renal clearance of uric acid and creatinine," *Clinical Rheumatology*, 2016.

[28] B. Ekici, U. Kütük, A. Alhan, and H. F. Töre, "The relationship between serum uric acid levels and angiographic severity of coronary heart disease," *Kardiologia Polska*, vol. 73, no. 7, pp. 533–538, 2015.

[29] L. Han, Q. Wu, C. Wang et al., "Homocysteine, ischemic stroke, and coronary heart disease in hypertensive patients: a population-based, prospective cohort study," *Stroke*, vol. 46, no. 7, pp. 1777–1786, 2015.

[30] E. Sertoglu, H. Kayadibi, and M. Uyanik, "Biochemical view on 'Homocysteine and metabolic syndrome: from clustering to additional utility in prediction of coronary heart disease'," *Journal of Cardiology*, vol. 65, no. 5, p. 439, 2015.

[31] Z. Li, L. Zhu, and B. Huang, "Effects of purified herbal extract of *Salvia miltiorrhiza* on lipid profile in hyperlipidemic patients," *Journal of Geriatric Cardiology*, vol. 6, no. 2, pp. 99–101, 2009.

[32] C. Zhu, H. Cao, X. Zhou et al., "Meta-analysis of the clinical value of danshen injection and huangqi injection in liver cirrhosis," *Evidence-Based Complementary and Alternative Medicine*, vol. 2013, Article ID 842824, 8 pages, 2013.

[33] X. Lu, Y. Jin, L. Ma, and L. Du, "Danshen (*Radix Salviae Miltiorrhizae*) reverses renal injury induced by myocardial infarction," *Journal of Traditional Chinese Medicine*, vol. 35, no. 3, pp. 306–311, 2015.

[34] General Assembly of the World Medical Association, "World Medical Association Declaration of Helsinki: ethical principles for medical research involving human subjects," *The Journal of the American College of Dentists*, vol. 81, no. 3, pp. 14–18, 2014.

[35] American College of Cardiology and American Heart Association Task Force on Practice, "ACC/AHA guidelines for the management of patients with unstable angina and non-ST segment elevation myocardial infarction: executive summary and recommendations," *Catheterization and Cardiovascular Interventions*, vol. 51, no. 4, pp. 505–521, 2000.

[36] S. Senol, M. U. Es, G. Gokmen, O. Ercin, B. A. Tuylu, and K. Kargun, "Genetic polymorphisms in preoperative myocardial infarction," *Asian Cardiovascular and Thoracic Annals*, vol. 23, no. 4, pp. 389–393, 2015.

[37] T. N. Sheth, O. A. Kajander, S. Lavi et al., "Optical coherence tomography-guided percutaneous coronary intervention in ST-segment-elevation myocardial infarction: a prospective propensity-matched cohort of the thrombectomy versus percutaneous coronary intervention alone trial," *Circulation: Cardiovascular Interventions*, vol. 9, no. 4, Article ID e003414, 2016.

[38] M. A. Becker, H. R. Schumacher Jr., R. L. Wortmann et al., "Febuxostat, a novel nonpurine selective inhibitor of xanthine oxidase: a twenty-eight–day, multicenter, phase II, randomized, double-blind, placebo-controlled, dose-response clinical trial examining safety and efficacy in patients with gout," *Arthritis & Rheumatism*, vol. 52, no. 3, pp. 916–923, 2005.

[39] S. H. Park, M. H. Jeong, I. H. Park et al., "Effects of combination therapy of statin and N-acetylcysteine for the prevention of contrast–induced nephropathy in patients with ST-segment elevation myocardial infarction undergoing primary percutaneous coronary intervention," *International Journal of Cardiology*, vol. 212, pp. 100–106, 2016.

[40] A. Auricchio, C. Stellbrink, S. Sack et al., "Long-term clinical effect of hemodynamically optimized cardiac resynchronization therapy in patients with heart failure and ventricular conduction delay," *Journal of the American College of Cardiology*, vol. 39, no. 12, pp. 2026–2033, 2002.

[41] F. Qiu, J. Jiang, Y. Ma et al., "Opposite effects of single-dose and multidose administration of the ethanol extract of danshen on CYP3A in healthy volunteers," *Evidence-Based Complementary and Alternative Medicine*, vol. 2013, Article ID 730734, 8 pages, 2013.

[42] X. Gong, Y. Li, and H. Qu, "Removing tannins from medicinal plant extracts using an alkaline ethanol precipitation process: a case study of Danshen injection," *Molecules*, vol. 19, no. 11, pp. 18705–18720, 2014.

[43] Y. Jia, F. Huang, S. Zhang, and S.-W. Leung, "Is danshen (*Salvia miltiorrhiza*) dripping pill more effective than isosorbide dinitrate in treating angina pectoris? A systematic review of randomized controlled trials," *International Journal of Cardiology*, vol. 157, no. 3, pp. 330–340, 2012.

[44] C. L. Ogden and M. D. Carroll, *Prevalence of Overweight, Obesity, and Extreme Obesity among Adults: United States, Trends 1960-1962 through 2007-2008*, vol. 6, National Center for Health Statistics, Hyattsville, Md, USA, 2010.

[45] T. O. Cheng, "Cardiovascular effects of Danshen," *International Journal of Cardiology*, vol. 121, no. 1, pp. 9–22, 2007.

[46] G.-I. Zhang, X.-D. Wei, B.-J. Fang et al., "The study of preventing hepatic veno-occlusive disease with danshen for injection," *Proceeding of Clinical Medicine*, vol. 8, article 30, 2010.

[47] H. Wu and X. Zhang, "The study on the effect of compound danshen dripping pills on the activity of CYP1A2, NAT2, and XO," *Chinese Journal of Modern Applied Pharmacy*, vol. 1, article 5, 2009.

[48] A. H. Hainsworth, N. E. Yeo, E. M. Weekman, and D. M. Wilcock, "Homocysteine, hyperhomocysteinemia and vascular

contributions to cognitive impairment and dementia (VCID)," *Biochimica et Biophysica Acta*, vol. 1862, no. 5, pp. 1008–1017, 2016.

[49] E. Bukharaeva, A. Shakirzyanova, V. Khuzakhmetova, G. Sitdikova, and R. Giniatullin, "Homocysteine aggravates ROS-induced depression of transmitter release from motor nerve terminals: potential mechanism of peripheral impairment in motor neuron diseases associated with hyperhomocysteinemia," *Frontiers in Cellular Neuroscience*, vol. 9, article 391, 2015.

[50] C. Liu, Y. Yang, D. Peng, L. Chen, and J. Luo, "Hyperhomocysteinemia as a metabolic disorder parameter is independently associated with the severity of coronary heart disease," *Saudi Medical Journal*, vol. 36, no. 7, pp. 839–846, 2015.

[51] K. Chan, S. H. Chui, D. Y. L. Wong, W. Y. Ha, C. L. Chan, and R. N. S. Wong, "Protective effects of Danshensu from the aqueous extract of *Salvia miltiorrhiza* (Danshen) against homocysteine-induced endothelial dysfunction," *Life Sciences*, vol. 75, no. 26, pp. 3157–3171, 2004.

[52] D. P. Sieveking, K.-S. Woo, K. P. Fung, P. Lundman, S. Nakhla, and D. S. Celermajer, "Chinese herbs Danshen and Gegen modulate key early atherogenic events in vitro," *International Journal of Cardiology*, vol. 105, no. 1, pp. 40–45, 2005.

[53] J. Li, X. Cheng, J. Gu et al., "The effects of Gegen-Danshen prescription on the lipid metabolism in hyperlipidemia rats," *Journal of Southwest University for Nationalities: Natural Science Edition*, vol. 36, no. 6, pp. 926–924, 2012.

[54] Z. Liu, S. Xu, X. Huang et al., "Cryptotanshinone, an orally bioactive herbal compound from Danshen, attenuates atherosclerosis in apolipoprotein E-deficient mice: role of lectin-like oxidized LDL receptor-1 (LOX-1)," *British Journal of Pharmacology*, vol. 172, no. 23, pp. 5661–5675, 2015.

[55] W. Zhao, C. Wu, and X. Chen, "Cryptotanshinone inhibits oxidized LDL-induced adhesion molecule expression *via* ROS dependent NF-κB pathways," *Cell Adhesion & Migration*, 2015.

[56] W. Jiang, Y. Zhao, B. Zhao, Q. Wan, and W. Xin, "Studies on the scavenging effect of Tanshinone on lipid free radical of cardiac sarcoplasmic reticulum during peroxidation," *Shengwu Wuli Xuebao*, vol. 10, no. 4, pp. 685–689, 1993.

[57] S. Xu, Z. Liu, Y. Huang et al., "Tanshinone II-A inhibits oxidized LDL-induced LOX-1 expression in macrophages by reducing intracellular superoxide radical generation and NF-κB activation," *Translational Research*, vol. 160, no. 2, pp. 114–124, 2012.

[58] Z.-P. Zhang, T.-T. You, L.-Y. Zou, T. Wu, Y. Wu, and L. Cui, "Effect of Danshen root compound on blood lipid and bone biomechanics in mice with hyperlipemia-induced osteoporosis," *Nan Fang Yi Ke Da Xue Xue Bao*, vol. 28, no. 9, pp. 1550–1553, 2008.

[59] O. Fadel, K. El Kirat, and S. Morandat, "The natural antioxidant rosmarinic acid spontaneously penetrates membranes to inhibit lipid peroxidation in situ," *Biochimica et Biophysica Acta (BBA)—Biomembranes*, vol. 1808, no. 12, pp. 2973–2980, 2011.

[60] E. D. Michos and P. L. Lutsey, "25-hydroxyvitamin D levels and coronary heart disease risk reclassification in hypertension—is it worth the 'hype'?" *Atherosclerosis*, vol. 245, pp. 237–239, 2016.

[61] A. A. Nargesi, B. Heidari, S. Esteghamati et al., "Contribution of vitamin D deficiency to the risk of coronary heart disease in subjects with essential hypertension," *Atherosclerosis*, vol. 244, pp. 165–171, 2016.

[62] J. Liu, Y. Zou, Y. Tang et al., "Circulating cell-free mitochondrial deoxyribonucleic acid is increased in coronary heart disease

patients with diabetes mellitus," *Journal of Diabetes Investigation*, vol. 7, no. 1, pp. 109–114, 2016.

[63] R. N. Das, "Relationship between diabetes mellitus and coronary heart disease," *Current Diabetes Reviews*, vol. 12, no. 999, pp. 1–12, 2016.

[64] H. J. Dong, C. Huang, D. M. Luo et al., "Concomitant coronary and renal revascularization improves left ventricular hypertrophy more than coronary stenting alone in patients with ischemic heart and renal disease," *Journal of Zhejiang University SCIENCE B*, vol. 17, no. 1, pp. 67–75, 2016.

[65] N. Katakami, H. Kaneto, T.-A. Matsuoka et al., "Accumulation of oxidative stress-related gene polymorphisms and the risk of coronary heart disease events in patients with type 2 diabetes—an 8-year prospective study," *Atherosclerosis*, vol. 235, no. 2, pp. 408–414, 2015.

[66] I. V. Gorudko, V. A. Kostevich, A. V. Sokolov et al., "Functional activity of neutrophils in diabetes mellitus and coronary heart disease: role of myeloperoxidase in the development of oxidative stress," *Bulletin of Experimental Biology and Medicine*, vol. 154, no. 1, pp. 23–26, 2012.

[67] V. M. Provotorov, A. V. Budnevskii, G. G. Semenkova, and E. S. Shishkina, "Proinflammatory cytokines in combination of coronary heart disease and chronic obstructive pulmonary disease," *Klinicheskaia Meditsina*, vol. 93, no. 2, pp. 5–9, 2015.

[68] G. L. Oktar, M. Kirisci, A. D. Dursun et al., "Antioxidative effects of adrenomedullin and vascular endothelial growth factor on lung injury induced by skeletal muscle ischemia-reperfusion," *Bratislava Medical Journal*, vol. 114, no. 11, pp. 625–628, 2013.

[69] S. T. Ma, G. L. Dai, X. G. Cheng et al., "Synergistic action of Compound Danshen Dripping Pill (CDDP) on Clopidogrel Bisulfate (CPG) counteracting platelet aggregation," *Zhong Yao Cai*, vol. 37, no. 10, pp. 1820–1825, 2014.

[70] Z. S. Huang, C. L. Zeng, L. J. Zhu, L. Jiang, N. Li, and H. Hu, "Salvianolic acid A inhibits platelet activation and arterial thrombosis via inhibition of phosphoinositide 3-kinase," *Journal of Thrombosis and Haemostasis*, vol. 8, no. 6, pp. 1383–1393, 2010.

[71] T. Y. K. Chan, "Interaction between warfarin and danshen (*Salvia miltiorrhiza*)," *Annals of Pharmacotherapy*, vol. 35, no. 4, pp. 501–504, 2001.

19

Acupuncture for Chronic Urinary Retention due to Spinal Cord Injury

Jia Wang,[1] **Yanbing Zhai,**[1,2] **Jiani Wu,**[1] **Shitong Zhao,**[2] **Jing Zhou,**[2] **and Zhishun Liu**[1]

[1]*Department of Acupuncture, Guang'anmen Hospital, China Academy of Chinese Medical Sciences, No. 5 Beixiange Street, Xicheng District, Beijing 100053, China*
[2]*Beijing University of Chinese Medicine, No. 11 North Third Ring Road, Chaoyang District, Beijing 100029, China*

Correspondence should be addressed to Zhishun Liu; liuzhishun@aliyun.com

Academic Editor: Roja Rahimi

No systematic review has been published on the use of acupuncture for the treatment of chronic urinary retention (CUR) due to spinal cord injury (SCI). The aim of this review was to assess the effectiveness and safety of acupuncture for CUR due to SCI. Three randomized controlled trials (RCTs) including 334 patients with CUR due to SCI were included. Meta-analysis showed that acupuncture plus rehabilitation training was much better than rehabilitation training alone in decreasing postvoid residual (PVR) urine volume (MD −109.44, 95% CI −156.53 to −62.35). Likewise, a combination of acupuncture and aseptic intermittent catheterization was better than aseptic intermittent catheterization alone in improving response rates (RR 1.23, 95% CI 1.10 to 1.38). No severe adverse events were reported. In conclusion, acupuncture as a complementary therapy may have a potential effect in CUR due to SCI in decreasing PVR and improving bladder voiding. Additionally, acupuncture may be safe in treating CUR caused by SCI. However, due to the lack of high quality RCTs, we could not draw any definitive conclusions. More well-designed RCTs are needed to provide strong evidence.

1. Introduction

Urinary retention is described as a bladder that either empties incompletely or does not empty at all [1]. The International Continence Society (ICS) defines chronic urinary retention (CUR) as "a non-painful bladder, which remains palpable or percussable [sic] after the patient has passed urine" [2]. Most studies and the UK National Institute for Health and Clinical Excellence guidelines for lower urinary tract symptoms describe CUR as either a postvoid residual (PVR) urine volume > 300 mL in patients who are able to void or PVR urine volume > 1,000 mL in patients who are unable to void [3–8]. CUR can be caused by obstructive, neurologic, myogenic, or other pathogeneses, such as spinal cord injury (SCI), pelvic nerve injury, peripheral neuropathy, and detrusor overdistention injury [9, 10]. SCI is an important nonobstructive pathogenesis of CUR, which can disrupt the reflex circuitry controlling micturition [11]. To the best of our knowledge, the exact incidence and prevalence of CUR due to SCI are still

unclear. This disease has a serious impact on patients' health and their quality of life. Long-term neglect of CUR may lead to chronic urinary tract infections, upper urinary tract damage, and renal failure [1, 12, 13]. Therefore, timely diagnosis and treatment are vital.

CUR due to SCI can be treated by pelvic floor training [2, 14], sacral neuromodulation (SNM) [15, 16], and intravesical electrostimulation (IVES) [17, 18]. However, IVES provides only short-term efficacy, and the potential complications of SNM include implant infection, pain, and superficial dehiscence [15, 17, 18]. CUR due to SCI can also be relieved using an intermittent or indwelling catheter [4, 19, 20]; although these relief methods have some benefits, catheterization cannot help patients restore their voiding function. Furthermore, long-term catheterization may be associated with complications such as discomfort, urethral injury, and urinary tract infection [19–24].

Acupuncture originates from ancient China and has been used to manage various clinical disorders for thousands of years. Although acupuncture plays an important role in Traditional Chinese Medicine (TCM) and is commonly used for treating CUR due to SCI in Mainland China, no systematic review of this treatment for CUR due to SCI exists; hence, the effectiveness and safety of this treatment remain unclear. The aim of our study was to assess the effectiveness and safety of acupuncture for CUR due to SCI.

2. Methods and Analysis

2.1. Search Strategy. The search strategy was decided according to the guidance of the *Cochrane Handbook*. The key words included "urinary retention", "chronic urinary retention", "CUR", "chronic retention of urine", "spinal cord injury", "traumatic myelopathy", "spinal cord laceration", "post traumatic myelopathy", "spinal cord contusion", "spinal cord trauma", "acupuncture", "manual acupuncture", "electrical acupuncture", "auricular acupuncture", "scalp needle", and "elongated needle". We electronically searched the following databases from their inception: PubMed, EMBASE, Cochrane Central Register of Controlled Trials, ClinicalTrials.gov, China National Knowledge Infrastructure (CNKI), Wan-Fang Database, Chinese Scientific Journal Database (VIP database), and the Chinese Biomedical Literature Database (CBM). In addition, CNKI was searched for unpublished articles, including conference articles and Chinese Doctoral and Master's theses.

2.2. Criteria for Study Inclusion in This Review

2.2.1. Type of Studies. Only randomized controlled trials (RCTs) investigating acupuncture for CUR due to SCI in English or Chinese without restrictions on publication status were included. Nonrandomized studies, quasi-randomized studies, retrospective studies, case reports, case series, literature reviews, animal experiments, clinical empirical summaries, journal indexes, and epidemiological surveys were excluded.

2.2.2. Type of Participants. Patients who had experienced CUR due to SCI, which is defined as a nonpainful bladder that remained palpable or percussible after they had passed urine, were included. Additionally, patients who are able to void with a PVR > 300 mL or unable to void with a PVR > 1,000 mL were included. There were no limitations on sex, age, and race. Patients with CUR caused by other pathogeneses, such as prostate cancer, bladder tumors, and benign prostatic hyperplasia, were excluded [25].

2.2.3. Type of Intervention. All types of TCM acupuncture, including manual acupuncture, electrical acupuncture, auricular acupuncture, elongated needle, and scalp needle, were included. Moxibustion, warm needling, fire needling, acupoint injection, and other non-TCM acupuncture therapies were excluded. RCTs that had control groups with no intervention, sham acupuncture, placebo control, drug therapy, rehabilitation training (such as bladder training), or other conservative treatments such as catheterization were eligible. RCTs involving acupuncture combined with another therapy were also included if that other therapy was the same in both experimental and control groups. Trials comparing different types of acupuncture and acupoints were excluded. Acupuncture plus Chinese medicine compared with Chinese medicine was excluded, and acupuncture plus moxibustion compared with moxibustion was also excluded.

2.2.4. Type of Outcomes. Each trial was required to include at least one of the following outcomes: ① the change of PVR from baseline after treatment and follow-up; ② response rates (proportion of patients improved): effective (regaining the ability to automatically urinate with PVR < 100 mL) and ineffective (regaining partial ability to automatically urinate with PVR ≥ 100 mL or keeping the inability to automatically urinate after treatment); ③ health-related quality of life (HRQL) measured by the Short-Form Health Survey Questionnaire (SF-36) or other internationally accepted scoring scales; ④ adverse events during the scheduled treatment time and follow-up. Any available information about safety was extracted from all clinical studies of acupuncture for CUR due to SCI, including other non-RCTs.

2.3. Study Selection. Two reviewers (Jia Wang and Yanbing Zhai) independently screened titles and abstracts of obtained trials to select articles for full-text assessment and then independently screened full-text papers to confirm eligibility of the trials. We included studies that met the predetermined inclusion criteria listed above. Any disagreements were resolved by consensus discussion between reviewers or with a third party (Zhishun Liu) if necessary. A PRISMA flow diagram was used to describe the process of study selection (Figure 1).

2.4. Data Extraction and Management. Two reviewers (Jia Wang and Yanbing Zhai) independently used a predesigned data extraction form for rigorous data collection, including general information such as authors, year of publication, study size, gender and age of the participants, treatment process, and details of the control, as well as trial characteristics such as randomization, allocation concealment, blinding, incomplete outcome data, selective reporting, and other outcomes.

2.5. Assessment of Risk of Bias in Included Studies. Two authors (Jia Wang and Yanbing Zhai) independently evaluated the methodological quality using the *Cochrane Handbook for Systematic Review of Interventions*, Version 5.1.0 [26], which comprised seven domains: random sequence generation (selection bias), allocation concealment (selection bias), blinding of participants and personnel (performance bias), blinding of outcome assessment (detection bias), incomplete outcome data (attrition bias), selective reporting (reporting bias), and other bias. Each domain was categorized into three levels: low risk, unclear risk, and high risk.

2.6. Measures of Treatment Effect. For dichotomous outcomes, the combination of the risk ratio (RR) and 95% confidence intervals (CI) was applied. For continuous outcomes,

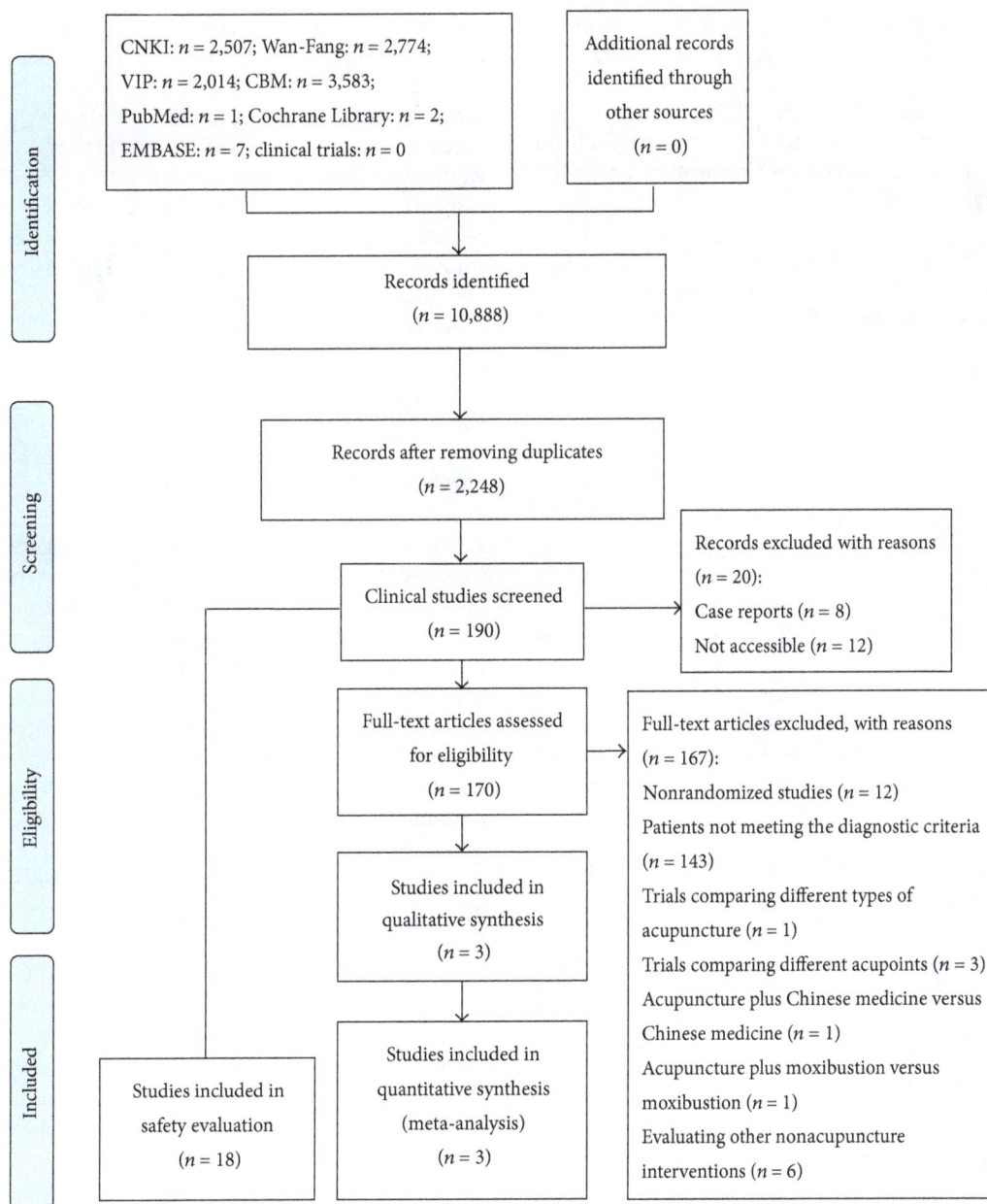

FIGURE 1: Flow diagram for the process of selecting eligible RCTs.

the combination of the mean difference (MD) and 95% CI was used.

2.7. Dealing with Missing Data. We tried to contact the first or corresponding authors by telephone or email to obtain the missing information. In the case of unobtainable missing data, we used the intention-to-treat (ITT) analysis for dichotomous outcomes if possible.

2.8. Assessment of Heterogeneity. The Higgins I^2 test was applied for heterogeneity prior to the meta-analysis to find out if the included studies were heterogeneous. If the I^2 statistics were less than 50%, the heterogeneity was deemed

acceptable. If the I^2 statistics were greater than 50%, this indicated significant heterogeneity among the studies.

2.9. Assessment of Reporting Bias. Funnel plots were used to assess the reporting bias if there were more than 10 studies included in one meta-analysis. The plots were assessed visually or by Egger's test [27].

2.10. Data Synthesis. RevMan V.5.3.1 software from the Cochrane Collaboration was used for the data synthesis [26]. If there was no significant heterogeneity, a combination of RR and 95% CI of each study using the fixed-effect model was applied for dichotomous data, and a combination of

MD and 95% CI of each study using the fixed-effect model was applied for continuous data. If significant heterogeneity was detected, the random-effect model was used. For all the analyses, a P value of less than 0.05 was considered statistically significant. For data that were not appropriate for undergoing quantitative synthesis, we performed a narrative review of the evidence.

2.11. Subgroup Analysis and Sensitivity Analysis. Subgroup analysis was performed according to the use of sham/placebo or positive control when there were more than three trials in each group. A sensitivity analysis was conducted to assess the potential bias of individual trials on the outcome of the meta-analysis for this review if possible.

3. Results

3.1. Study Selection. Through electronic searching, 10,888 records were identified. 2,248 records were eligible for screening after duplicate records were removed. After screening the title and abstract, 190 clinical studies were remained. Then, approximately 170 studies potentially met the inclusion criteria, and these studies were identified for full-text screening. Ultimately, only three RCTs were included for evaluating the effectiveness of acupuncture treatment, while 18 trials were included for safety evaluation [28–30]. All these trials were conducted in China and published in Chinese. The process of study selection was shown in Figure 1.

3.2. Characteristics of Included Trials. The characteristics of included trials were summarized in Table 1.

3.2.1. Patients. A total of 334 participants in three trials were included, with sample sizes ranging from 70 to 132. The age of patients ranged from 11 to 71 years. The disease course ranged from one month to three years. Spinal cord injury was the etiology in all the included trials [28–30].

3.2.2. Acupuncture Interventions. Electroacupuncture was applied in two trials [29, 30], and manual acupuncture was used in one trial [28]. In this trial, manual acupuncture performed was based on disease diagnosis but not based on syndrome differentiation [28]. Patients received acupuncture therapy once a day, and each treatment lasted for 20 [29, 30] or 30 [28] minutes. The treatment duration ranged from two weeks [29, 30] to eight weeks [28]. Zhongji (CV3) [28–30], Qihai (CV6) [28–30], and Guanyuan (CV4) [28–30] were the most frequently used points, with an incidence of 100.0% among these three RCTs. Pangguangshu (BL28) [30], Shenshu (BL23) [29, 30], Qugu (CV2) [29, 30], Yinlingquan (SP9) [29, 30], and Sanyinjiao (SP6) [29, 30] were the next most commonly used acupoints, with an incidence of 66.7% among these three RCTs. Other acupoints mentioned in the included trials were Yaoyangguan (GV3) [28], Mingmen (GV4) [28], Ciliao (BL32) [30], Shangliao (BL31) [30], Zhongliao (BL33) [30], and Xialiao (BL34) [30]. All these acupoints selected were based on disease diagnosis but not due to nerves [28–30]. While acupuncturing, De Qi was obtained of all these acupoints.

3.2.3. Control Interventions. One trial compared acupuncture plus rehabilitation training with rehabilitation training [28]. In this trial, rehabilitation training included bladder sphincter training and urination training. Two trials compared acupuncture plus aseptic intermittent catheterization with aseptic intermittent catheterization [29, 30]. In these three trials, some supportive therapies were applied in both experimental and control groups, including water quantity control [29, 30], neurotrophic drugs [28], dehydrant agents [28], and regulating water, electrolyte, and acid-base balance drugs [28].

3.2.4. Outcome Measures. One trial evaluated postvoid residual (PVR) urine volume [28], while the other two trials evaluated response rates [29, 30]. No trial measured health-related quality of life (HRQL).

3.3. Risk of Bias in the Included RCTs. All three included trials mentioned randomization through the use of random number tables [28–30]. Two trials performed allocation concealment using opaque envelopes [28, 30], and one trial did not perform allocation concealment [28]. Because of the nature of acupuncture, none of the included trials applied the method of blinding acupuncturists and participants. One trial applied the method of blinding outcome assessment [28], but the other two trials did not apply it [29, 30]. One trial reported relevant information regarding drop-outs because of the change in the condition of diseases, but there was no information about the principle used for dealing with the missing data [28]. There was also no information relating to intention-to-treat (ITT) analysis. Therefore, all these trials were evaluated as having high risk of bias. The details of the risks of bias of each trial were presented in Table 2.

3.4. Effects of Interventions. Three trials were divided into two parts to conduct meta-analysis according to different types of comparison groups. Then, trials with similarities were pooled together. Subgroup analysis was not conducted, as there were an insufficient number of studies included in this review.

3.4.1. Acupuncture plus Aseptic Intermittent Catheterization versus Aseptic Intermittent Catheterization

Postvoid Residual (PVR) Urine Volume. In this comparison, no trials applied PVR as the outcome measurement.

Response Rates. Two trials reported response rates, and the RR was 1.23 (95% CI 1.10 to 1.38) using the fixed model [29, 30], which showed that there was a significant difference in the increase in response rates upon comparing acupuncture plus aseptic intermittent catheterization with aseptic intermittent catheterization alone (Figure 2).

Health-Related Quality of Life (HRQL). These two trials did not report the outcome of the improvement of life quality during treatment course and follow-up [29, 30].

TABLE 1: Characteristics of included studies.

Study ID	Sample size (T/C)	Age, y	Etiology	Disease course	Intervention	Control	Treatment duration	Follow-up	Outcomes
Gao et al. 2013 [28]	70 35/35	T: 37.20 ± 7.09 C: 35.20 ± 8.12	SCI	T: 48.34 ± 10.12 d C: 46.03 ± 8.33 d	Acupuncture + RT, 30 min, Qd	RT	8 wk	No	PVR
Qu 2013 [29]	132 66/66	T: 8-66 C: 11-71	SCI	T: 1 mon–3 y C: 2 mon–3 y	EA + AIC 20 min, Qd	AIC	2 wk	No	RR
Wu and Li 2012 [30]	132 68/64	T: 8-66 C: 11-71	SCI	T: 13.6 ± 3.9 mon C: 14.3 ± 4.4 mon	EA + AIC 20 min, Qd	AIC	2 wk	No	RR

T = treatment group; C = control group; SCI = spinal cord injury; RT = rehabilitation training; EA = electrical acupuncture; AIC = aseptic intermittent catheterization; PVR = postvoid residual; RR = response rates.

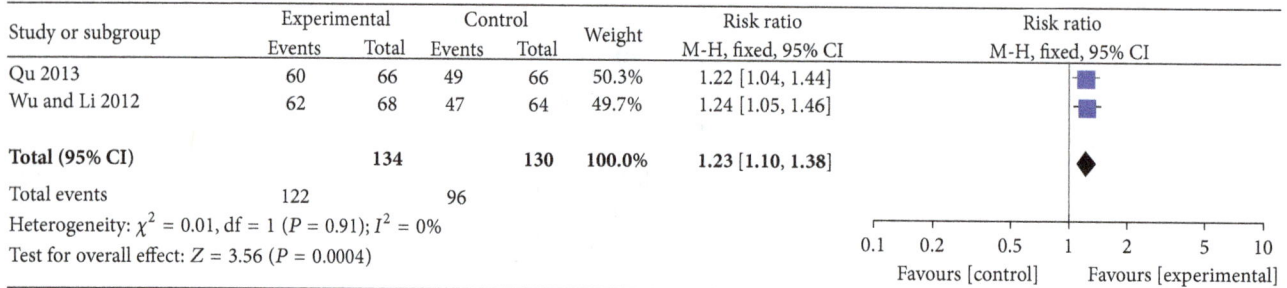

FIGURE 2: Forest plot of the effect of acupuncture plus aseptic intermittent catheterization versus aseptic intermittent catheterization on response rates using the fixed model.

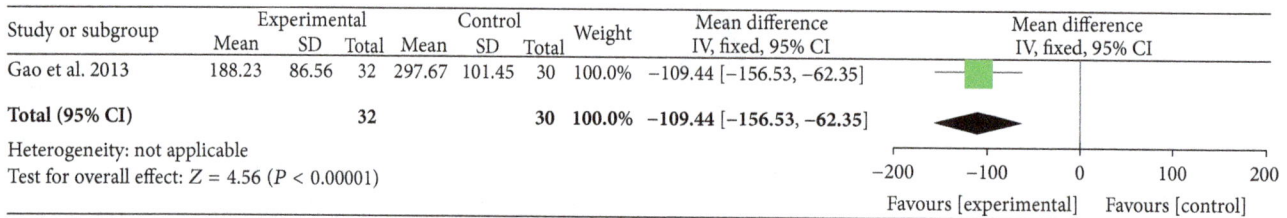

FIGURE 3: Forest plot of the effect of acupuncture plus rehabilitation training versus rehabilitation training on PVR using the fixed model. PVR: postvoid residual.

TABLE 2: Methodological quality of included trials.

Study ID	A	B	C	D	E	F	G
Gao et al. 2013 [28]	−	−	+	−	+	?	?
Qu 2013 [29]	−	+	+	+	−	?	?
Wu and Li 2012 [30]	−	−	+	+	−	?	?

+ = high risk, ? = unclear, and − = low risk. A = random sequence generation (selection bias); B = allocation concealment (selection bias); C = blinding of participants and personnel (performance bias); D = blinding of outcome assessment (detection bias); E = incomplete outcome data (attrition bias); F = selective reporting (reporting bias); G = other bias.

3.4.2. Acupuncture plus Rehabilitation Training versus Rehabilitation Training

PVR. The MD was −109.44 (95% CI −156.53 to −62.35) using the fixed model in one trial [28], which showed that acupuncture plus rehabilitation training was much better than rehabilitation training alone in decreasing PVR from baseline (Figure 3).

Response Rates and HRQL. This trial did not mention any information about the change of response rates and HRQL for CUR patients caused by SCI [28].

3.5. Safety.
There were 18 clinical trials eligible to evaluate the safety of acupuncture for CUR due to SCI. In these trials, 921 patients were treated by acupuncture or by acupuncture combined with other therapies. None of these 18 studies reported any severe adverse events related to acupuncture. And only one trial reported adverse events [31], which was a prospective cohort study of electrical acupuncture for CUR due to SCI in 153 patients. It reported the adverse events of pricking, faint, stuck needle, hematoma around the site of needling, infection, and pelvic floor dysfunction, which disappeared after the treatment withdrawal. However, it did not report the incidence of adverse events.

3.6. Publication Bias.
As the number of included trials was <10, funnel plots were not applied to detect potential publication bias.

4. Discussion

Chronic urinary retention (CUR) is a common urological problem that greatly impacts patients' general health, quality of daily life [32], psychological states [32], and social contact. Prestudies reveal that acupuncture may have promising therapeutic effectiveness in urinary retention [31, 33]. This review had evaluated the effectiveness of acupuncture for CUR due to spinal cord injury (SCI). However, only three RCTs met the inclusion criteria.

4.1. Summary of Effectiveness.
In this review, the main findings of effectiveness were the notion that acupuncture plus rehabilitation training was much better than rehabilitation training alone in decreasing postvoid residual (PVR) urine volume for CUR due to SCI [28] and a combination of acupuncture and aseptic intermittent catheterization was more effective than aseptic intermittent catheterization alone in improving response rates for CUR due to SCI [29, 30].

PVR measurement is an important component in the assessment of voiding dysfunction, including CUR due to SCI [34–36]. Accurate determination of PVR is of significant importance for the diagnosis and treatment of urinary retention [36, 37]. It is also a valuable parameter for evaluating the effectiveness of treatments [36]. The decrease in PVR after treatments can reveal the improvement of voiding function. However, in this review the evidence regarding PVR is limited, as only one RCT with a small sample size performed this measurement [28]. Moreover, this trial did not assess patients during the follow-up period [28], and the information about the drop-outs and other missing data was also inadequate, which may have led to attrition bias. Therefore, the evidence on the effectiveness of acupuncture in decreasing PVR was insufficient. Future studies should pay more attention to this outcome measure and provide stronger evidence.

The improvement of response rates can also reflect the effectiveness of acupuncture for CUR due to SCI. In this review, two trials evaluated response rates [29, 30], which were divided into three grades: cured (restoration of the ability to automatically urinate, disappearance of urinary retention symptoms, and PVR < 80 mL); effective (restoration of the ability to automatically urinate, disappearance of urinary retention symptoms, and 80 mL < PVR < 100 mL), and ineffective (persistence of the inability to automatically urinate, PVR > 100 mL). In clinical practice, PVR < 30 mL can be regarded as insignificant [38]. Meanwhile, PVR < 100 mL for CUR patients due to SCI may indicate the complete or partial restoration of lower urinary tract function and the reduction of upper urinary tract impairment [39]. In this review, we merged the cured and effective components into a single effective component.

In these two trials, the information related to the exact process of randomization and allocation concealment was too scarce [29, 30], which may have led to high risks of selection bias. Additionally, these two trials did not blind the outcome assessment [29, 30], which may have caused detection bias. In addition, all these trials were conducted in China and published in Chinese [29, 30], which may have led to publication bias. The exact process of this measurement and the exact data of patients' symptoms and PVR were also not provided, which may have led to some other potential bias. Therefore, the evidence of acupuncture for CUR due to SCI in improving response rates was still inadequate.

In addition, CUR due to SCI can greatly impact patients' health-related quality of life (HRQL) [32] and the improvement of HRQL can also be an important outcome for the effectiveness. Moreover, SF-36 and other internationally accepted scoring scales can help evaluate the patients' general health, which can be applied to measure the HRQL. However, none of the included trials mentioned any information about HRQL. Thus, the evidence on the effectiveness of acupuncture in improving HRQL was still unobtainable in this review. Therefore, we suggested that future studies should attach more importance to the outcome of HRQL.

Based on this evidence, acupuncture may have a potential therapeutic effect in decreasing PVR and improving response rates for CUR due to SCI. However, the evidence was still too weak to draw any firm conclusions.

4.2. *Summary of Safety.* Acupuncture therapy may also be related to some adverse events such as pricking, redness, ecchymosis [40], hematoma [31], fainting, and bleeding in the local skin [41]. Though these adverse events are minor, the safety management of acupuncture should also be taken into account. In this systematic review, 18 clinical trials were eligible to evaluate the safety of acupuncture for CUR due to SCI.

Adverse events related to acupuncture occurred in only one trial, including pricking, fainting, stuck needles, hematoma around the site of needling, infection, and pelvic floor dysfunction, which were all minor. The other 17 clinical trials did not report any adverse events. No severe adverse events were reported, which indicated that acupuncture was a safe treatment for CUR due to SCI. However, as no trials mentioned any relevant information concerning the follow-up, the long-term safety of acupuncture still remains uncertain. Therefore, we suggest that the long-term safety of acupuncture should also be taken into account in future research.

4.3. *Limitations of This Review.* There were some limitations in our systematic review. First, though we attempted to search CNKI for conference articles and Doctoral and Master's theses, it was difficult to obtain all the unpublished articles. Moreover, because of the language barrier, we only searched databases in Chinese and English; Korean, Japanese, and other foreign databases were not covered. Thus, some relevant clinical trials may have been missed. Second, the three included trials were all conducted in China and most of them omitted the exact process of randomization and allocation concealment, which would lead to selection bias. None of the trials blinded the participants and acupuncturists to the treatment, which may have elicited performance bias; two trials did not blind the outcome assessment, which would lead to detection bias; one trial had incomplete outcome data, which would yield attrition bias. These high risks of bias may have influenced our final conclusions. Third, although we tried our best to contact the corresponding or first authors of each included RCT by phone or email, some missing information still remained unobtainable. Finally, the long-term effectiveness of acupuncture could not be determined as none of the included trials assessed the patients at follow-up.

4.4. *Implications for Practice and Research.* In this review, all the included trials were of small sample size and had high risk of bias. Though the data showed effectiveness of acupuncture in CUR due to SCI, the evidence was still insufficient. More attention should be paid to the outcome measures of PVR and HRQL. What is more, whether acupuncture had effect on CUR caused by other pathogeneses remained unknown. Future studies should attach more importance to other types of CUR. Moreover, the long-term effectiveness of acupuncture for CUR due to SCI remained unclear. Therefore, multicenter RCTs with large-scale and long-term follow-up should be conducted to provide more evidence.

5. Conclusions

Based on this systematic review, acupuncture may have some positive effectiveness in decreasing PVR and in improving response rates for chronic urinary retention (CUR) due to spinal cord injury (SCI). Additionally, acupuncture may be safe for treating CUR due to SCI. However, the evidence is still limited due to the lack of high quality trials. RCTs with large samples and high methodological quality are still needed in further clinical research. A convincing demonstration of the positive effectiveness and safety of acupuncture will have valuable implications for future clinical practice.

Competing Interests

The authors declare that there are no competing interests regarding the publication of this paper.

Authors' Contributions

This review was written by Jia Wang and revised by Jiani Wu, Shitong Zhao, and Jing Zhou. The study selection, study assessment, and data extraction were performed by Jia Wang and Yanbing Zhai. Jia Wang performed data analysis and wrote the completed review. Zhishun Liu arbitrated any disagreements and ensured that no errors occurred during the study. All authors contributed to the conception of the study and approved the publication of this review.

References

[1] C. L. A. Negro and G. H. Muir, "Chronic urinary retention in men: how we define it, and how does it affect treatment outcome," *BJU International*, vol. 110, no. 11, pp. 1590–1594, 2012.

[2] P. Abrams, L. Cardozo, M. Fall et al., "The standardisation of terminology of lower urinary tract function: report from the standardisation sub-committee of the international continence society," *Neurourology and Urodynamics*, vol. 21, no. 2, pp. 167–178, 2002.

[3] P. H. Abrams, M. Dunn, and N. George, "Urodynamic findings in chronic retention of urine and their relevance to results of surgery," *British Medical Journal*, vol. 2, no. 6147, pp. 1258–1260, 1978.

[4] I. F. Ghalayini, M. A. Al-Ghazo, and R. S. Pickard, "A prospective randomized trial comparing transurethral prostatic resection and clean intermittent self-catheterization in men with chronic urinary retention," *BJU International*, vol. 96, no. 1, pp. 93–97, 2005.

[5] C. D. Jaeger, C. R. Mitchell, L. A. Mynderse, and A. E. Krambeck, "Holmium laser enucleation (HoLEP) and photoselective vaporisation of the prostate (PVP) for patients with benign prostatic hyperplasia (BPH) and chronic urinary retention," *BJU International*, vol. 115, no. 2, pp. 295–299, 2015.

[6] D. E. Neal, R. A. Styles, T. Ng, P. H. Powell, J. Thong, and P. D. Ramsden, "Relationship between voiding pressures, symptoms and urodynamic findings in 253 men undergoing prostatectomy," *British Journal of Urology*, vol. 60, no. 6, pp. 554–559, 1987.

[7] D. E. Neal, R. A. Styles, P. H. Powell, and P. D. Ramsden, "Relationship between detrusor function and residual urine in men undergoing prostatectomy," *British Journal of Urology*, vol. 60, no. 6, pp. 560–566, 1987.

[8] N. J. R. George, P. H. O'Reilly, R. J. Barnard, and N. J. Blacklock, "High pressure chronic retention," *British Medical Journal*, vol. 286, no. 6380, pp. 1780–1783, 1983.

[9] C. V. Comiter, "Sacral nerve stimulation to treat nonobstructive urinary retention in women," *Current Urology Reports*, vol. 9, no. 5, pp. 405–411, 2008.

[10] D. Hernández Hernández, R. B. E. Tesouro, and D. Castro-Diaz, "Urinary retention," *Urologia*, vol. 80, no. 4, pp. 257–264, 2013.

[11] W. C. De Groat and N. Yoshimura, "Plasticity in reflex pathways to the lower urinary tract following spinal cord injury," *Experimental Neurology*, vol. 235, no. 1, pp. 123–132, 2012.

[12] G. Lombardi, S. Musco, M. Celso, F. D. Corso, and G. D. Popolo, "Sacral neuromodulation for neurogenic non-obstructive urinary retention in incomplete spinal cord patients: a ten-year follow-up single-centre experience," *Spinal Cord*, vol. 52, no. 3, pp. 241–245, 2014.

[13] W. M. White, C. Dobmeyer-Dittrich, F. A. Klein, and L. S. Wallace, "Sacral nerve stimulation for treatment of refractory urinary retention: long-term efficacy and durability," *Urology*, vol. 71, no. 1, pp. 71–74, 2008.

[14] F. Bernier and G. W. Davila, "The treatment of nonobstructive urinary retention with high-frequency transvaginal electrical stimulation," *Urologic Nursing*, vol. 20, no. 4, pp. 261–264, 2000.

[15] H. S. Shaker and M. Hassouna, "Sacral root neuromodulation in idiopathic nonobstructive chronic urinary retention," *The Journal of Urology*, vol. 159, no. 5, pp. 1476–1478, 1998.

[16] S. Elneil, B. Abtahi, M. Helal, A. Digesu, and G. Gonzales, "Optimizing the duration of assessment of stage-1 sacral neuromodulation in nonobstructive chronic urinary retention," *Neuromodulation*, vol. 17, no. 1, pp. 66–71, 2014.

[17] G. Lombardi, S. Musco, M. Celso et al., "Intravesical electrostimulation versus sacral neuromodulation for incomplete spinal cord patients suffering from neurogenic non-obstructive urinary retention," *Spinal Cord*, vol. 51, no. 7, pp. 571–578, 2013.

[18] G. Lombardi, M. Celso, M. Mencarini, F. Nelli, and G. Del Popolo, "Clinical efficacy of intravesical electrostimulation on incomplete spinal cord patients suffering from chronic neurogenic non-obstructive retention: a 15-year single centre retrospective study," *Spinal Cord*, vol. 51, no. 3, pp. 232–237, 2013.

[19] Y. Homma, I. Araki, Y. Igawa et al., "Clinical guideline for male lower urinary tract symptoms," *International Journal of Urology*, vol. 16, no. 10, pp. 775–790, 2009.

[20] J. W. Warren, "Catheter-associated urinary tract infections," *International Journal of Antimicrobial Agents*, vol. 17, no. 4, pp. 299–303, 2001.

[21] J. W. Warren, "Catheter-associated urinary tract infections," *Infectious Disease Clinics of North America*, vol. 11, no. 3, pp. 609–622, 1997.

[22] B. S. Buckley and M. C. M. Lapitan, "Drugs for treatment of urinary retention after surgery in adults," *Cochrane Database of Systematic Reviews*, vol. 4, Article ID cd008023, 2010.

[23] B. S. Niël-Weise and P. J. van den Broek, "Urinary catheter policies for long-term bladder drainage," *Cochrane Database of Systematic Reviews*, 2005.

[24] B. S. Niël-Weise, P. J. van den Broek, E. M. K. da Silva, and L. A. Silva, "Urinary catheter policies for long-term bladder drainage," *Cochrane Database of Systematic Reviews*, vol. 8, Article ID CD004201, 2012.

[25] B. A. Selius and R. Subedi, "Urinary retention in adults: diagnosis and initial management," *American Family Physician*, vol. 77, no. 5, pp. 643–650, 2008.

[26] J. P. T. Higgins and S. Green, *Cochrane Handbook for Systematic Reviews of Interventions*, Version 5.1.0, The Cochrane Collaboration, 2011.

[27] M. Egger, G. D. Smith, M. Schneider, and C. Minder, "Bias in meta-analysis detected by a simple, graphical test," *British Medical Journal*, vol. 315, no. 7109, pp. 629–634, 1997.

[28] Y. L. Gao, X. Cheng, and M. Xia, "Observation of acupuncture on Governor meridian and Ren meridian for urinary retention caused by incomplete spinal cord injury," *Traditional Chinese Medicine Journal*, vol. 12, no. 4, pp. 46–47, 2013 (Chinese).

[29] Q. M. Qu, "Governor meridian acupuncture and intermittent catheterization for treating traumatic spinal cord injury," *China Health Care Nutrition*, no. 12, p. 517, 2013 (Chinese).

[30] B. T. Wu and J. J. Li, "Acupuncture plus intermittent catheterization for 68 cases with urinary retention caused by spinal cord injury," *Traditional Chinese Medicine Research*, vol. 25, no. 11, pp. 68–70, 2012 (Chinese).

[31] K. H. Zhou and Z. S. Liu, *Observation of Electroacupuncture for Urinary Retention Caused by Cauda Equina Injury*, Beijing University of Chinese Medicine, 2010.

[32] R. D. Malik, J. A. Cohn, and G. T. Bales, "Urinary retention in elderly women: diagnosis & management," *Current Urology Reports*, vol. 15, no. 11, p. 454, 2014.

[33] Z. Liu, K. Zhou, Y. Wang, and Y. Pan, "Electroacupuncture improves voiding function in patients with neurogenic urinary retention secondary to cauda equina injury: results from a prospective observational study," *Acupuncture in Medicine*, vol. 29, no. 3, pp. 188–192, 2011.

[34] Y. H. Park, J. H. Ku, and S.-J. Oh, "Accuracy of post-void residual urine volume measurement using a portable ultrasound bladder scanner with real-time pre-scan imaging," *Neurourology and Urodynamics*, vol. 30, no. 3, pp. 335–338, 2011.

[35] S. A. Kaplan, A. J. Wein, D. R. Staskin, C. G. Roehrborn, and W. D. Steers, "Urinary retention and post-void residual urine in men: separating truth from tradition," *The Journal of Urology*, vol. 180, no. 1, pp. 47–54, 2008.

[36] S.-J. Chang and S. S.-D. Yang, "Variability, related factors and normal reference value of post-void residual urine in healthy kindergarteners," *The Journal of Urology*, vol. 182, no. 4, pp. 1933–1938, 2009.

[37] N. Simforoosh, F. Dadkhah, S. Y. Hosseini, M. A. Asgari, A. Nasseri, and M. R. Safarinejad, "Accuracy of residual urine measurement in men: comparison between real-time ultrasonography and catheterization," *The Journal of Urology*, vol. 158, no. 1, pp. 59–61, 1997.

[38] A. D. Asimakopoulos, C. De Nunzio, E. Kocjancic, A. Tubaro, P. F. Rosier, and E. Finazzi-Agrò, "Measurement of post-void residual urine," *Neurourology and Urodynamics*, vol. 35, no. 1, pp. 55–57, 2016.

[39] L. M. Liao, J. Wu, Y. H. Ju et al., "Guild of urinary system management and clinical rehabilitation for spinal cord injury patients," *Chinese Journal of Rehabilitation Theory and Practice*, vol. 19, pp. 310–317, 2013 (Chinese).

[40] C.-H. Hsu, K.-C. Hwang, C.-L. Chao, J.-G. Lin, S.-T. Kao, and P. Chou, "Effects of electroacupuncture in reducing weight and waist circumference in obese women: a randomized crossover trial," *International Journal of Obesity*, vol. 29, no. 11, pp. 1379–1384, 2005.

[41] J. Zhou, W. N. Peng, M. Xu, W. Li, and Z. S. Liu, "The effectiveness and safety of acupuncture for patients with Alzheimer disease," *Medicine*, vol. 94, no. 22, p. e933, 2015.

20

Acupuncture Decreases NF-κB p65, miR-155, and miR-21 and Increases miR-146a Expression in Chronic Atrophic Gastritis Rats

Jialing Zhang,[1] Kangbai Huang,[2] Guoxin Zhong,[2] Yong Huang,[1] Suhe Li,[2] Shanshan Qu,[1] and Jiping Zhang[1]

[1]*School of Traditional Chinese Medicine, Southern Medical University, Guangzhou, Guangdong 510515, China*
[2]*Clinical Medical College of Acupuncture, Moxibustion and Rehabilitation, Guangzhou University of Chinese Medicine, Guangzhou, Guangdong 510006, China*

Correspondence should be addressed to Yong Huang; nanfanglihuang@163.com and Suhe Li; hlsh@gzhtcm.edu.cn

Academic Editor: Ching-Liang Hsieh

Acupuncture has been used to treat chronic atrophic gastritis (CAG) in traditional Chinese medicine (TCM) for centuries. In this study, we evaluated the effect of acupuncture at Zusanli (ST36), Zhongwan (CV12), and Pishu (BL20) acupoints on weight changes of rats, histological changes of gastric glands, and expressions changes of nuclear factor-kappa B (NF-κB) p65, microRNA- (miR-) 155, miR-21, and miR-146a in CAG rats induced by N-methyl-N′-nitro-N-nitrosoguanidine (MNNG) combined with irregular diet. Consequently, we found that acupuncture treatment elevated body weight of rats significantly when compared to the model group. By observing histological changes, we found that the acupuncture group showed better improvement of gastric mucosa injury than the model group. Our results also demonstrated upregulation of NF-κB p65, miR-155, and miR-21 in gastric tissue of CAG rats and a positive correlation between miR-155 and miR-21. Relatively, expression of miR-146a was downregulated and negative correlation relationships between miR-146a and miR-155/miR-21 in CAG rats were observed. Additionally, expressions of NF-κB p65, miR-155, and miR-21 were downregulated and miR-146a was upregulated after acupuncture treatment. Taken together, our data imply that acupuncture can downregulate NF-κB p65, miR-155, and miR-21 and upregulate miR-146a expression in CAG rats. NF-κB p65, miR-155, miR-21, and miR-146a may play important roles in therapeutic effect of acupuncture in treating CAG.

1. Introduction

Chronic atrophic gastritis (CAG), characterized by loss of normal gastric glandular structures and accompanied by intestinal metaplasia, is well known as a significant premalignant lesion of gastric cancer [1–3]. Recent researches have provided evidence of a sustained inflammatory reaction in gastritis with activation of immune response and involvement of inflammatory pathway [4–6]. With deepening researches on pathogenesis, treatments for CAG have attracted growing attention. However, except pharmacological agents such as *Helicobacter pylori* eradication, acid suppression, and nonsteroidal anti-inflammatory drug treatment, there is no more available effective treatment for CAG currently [3, 7, 8].

Acupuncture, originated in ancient China, is one of the most commonly used complementary medicine modalities in the world [9, 10]. A lot of researches have demonstrated the efficacy of acupuncture in treating gastric diseases [7, 11–13], especially CAG. Additionally, Zusanli (ST36), Zhongwan (CV12), and Pishu (BL20) acupoints were commonly used to treat CAG in China [7, 14, 15], which were included in clinical practice guideline of traditional Chinese medicine (TCM) for chronic gastritis [16]. Recently, it has been proposed that acupuncture could alleviate inflammatory responses through different inflammatory pathways in treating gastrointestinal lesion [17–19]. However, modulation effect of acupuncture in treating CAG remained inconclusive.

MicroRNAs (miRNAs) are a class of small noncoding RNAs [20], which have been discovered as crucial regulators in gastric carcinogenesis through posttranscriptional regulation [21]. Recently, increasing researches have suggested involvement of miRNAs in different processes of gastric carcinogenesis [21, 22], especially miR-155, miR-21, and miR-146a [22–24]. In addition, accumulating evidences have demonstrated the relationship between gastritis and the abovementioned miRNAs [22, 24–26]. Petrocca et al. showed that chronic gastritis was associated with the alteration of miR-155 [25], which was known to play a major role in regulation of immune response [27] and promote tumor progression [28]. Link et al. observed a gradual increase trend of miR-155 and miR-21 expression in preneoplastic gastric mucosa [22], including CAG stage, indicating that miR-155 and miR-21 were essential to persistent inflammation of gastric mucosa. Furthermore, Liu et al. demonstrated that overexpression of miR-146a in chronic gastritis could significantly decrease activity of nuclear factor-kappa B (NF-κB) pathway [24], a well-known signaling pathway of inflammation response, suggesting that miR-146a might play a crucial role in a negative feedback loop to modulate gastric mucosa inflammation. In conclusion, previous researches have indicated that miR-155, miR-21, and miR-146a may function as inflammation regulators in CAG.

In this study, we evaluated the therapeutic effect of acupuncture on body weight changes and gastric histological structures and investigated expressions of NF-κB p65, miR-155, miR-21, and miR-146a in CAG, thus to explore the therapeutic effect of acupuncture in treating CAG.

2. Materials and Methods

2.1. Animals. A total of 60 Sprague-Dawley (SD) rats, half male and half female, 8 weeks old, 180~220 g in weight, provided by the Medical Experimental Animal Center of Guangdong Province (permit number: SCXK (Yue) 2008-0002) were used. Rearing conditions were a laminar flow, specific pathogen-free (SPF) atmosphere, room temperature $(20 \pm 1)°C$, relative humidity 50~60%, automatic ventilation 8~15 times per hour, and 12 h light/dark cycle. The study was carried out adhering to the guidelines provided by the National Institutes of Health for the Care and Use of Laboratory Animals and all efforts were made to minimize suffering of animals.

2.2. CAG Model Preparation [15, 29]. After 1 week of adaptive feeding, the study was begun when the rats behaved normally. A total of 60 rats were randomly divided into 2 groups for control ($n = 20$) and N-methyl-N′-nitro-N-nitrosoguanidine (MNNG) treatment ($n = 40$) by using completely randomized method based on SPSS software (Version 20.0, SPSS Inc., USA). Rats in the MNNG treatment group were induced by MNNG (100 μg/L; Tokyo Kasei Kogyo Co., Ltd.) combined with irregular diet for 12 weeks. MNNG was dissolved in distilled water at a concentration of 1 g/L and kept in a cool (4°C) and dark place. Just before use, the stock solution was diluted to 100 μg/L with distilled water. Rats in the model group were given MNNG solution from a bottle which was covered with

aluminum foil to prevent photolysis of MNNG and used as only water source. The solution was replenished every day. In the meantime, rats in the MNNG treatment group were provided with irregular diet (one day of sufficient feeding and one day of fasting, alternating between the two). Rats in the control group were fed normally and given sterile water *ad libitum*. At week 12, from each group 2 rats were sacrificed to verify whether CAG models were successfully prepared by observing histological changes of gastric structures. After successful modeling (Figure S1 (in Supplementary Material available online at http://dx.doi.org/10.1155/2016/9404629) showed pathologic changes at various time points), rats in the MNNG treatment group were randomly divided into the model group ($n = 18$) and the acupuncture group ($n = 20$). Starting from week 12, all rats in each group were fed normally and given sterile water *ad libitum*. Rats were weighed weekly and their body weight changes were recorded.

2.3. Groups and Treatment. Acupuncture group: starting from week 12, rats in the acupuncture group were given acupuncture treatment daily for 60 consecutive days. Zusanli (ST36, 5 mm lateral to the anterior tubercle of tibia [30], bilateral), Zhongwan (CV12, 9/14 above the pubic crest of the distance measured between the top of the xiphoid process and the pubic crest [30]), and Pishu (BL20, lateral to the lower border of the 11th thoracic vertebra in the back [31], bilateral) acupoints were selected. Rats were lightly immobilized, and the acupuncture needles (Suzhou Medical Appliance Factory; 0.25 mm × 15 mm) were inserted to a depth of 3 mm at the acupoints and retained for 15 min. In the control group, no treatment was performed. In the model group, the same grasping and fixing as the acupuncture group was performed. No rat died in the treatment stage. After acupuncture treatment was finished, all rats in each group were anesthetized and their stomachs were quickly removed. Figure 1 is a flow diagram of the study.

2.4. Histopathological Observation. Gastric tissue samples from each group were collected and fixed in 10% formalin (Invitrogen). Then the samples were embedded in paraffin after tissue was processed. This was followed by sectioning (5 μm thickness) and staining with hematoxylin and eosin (H&E) dye. The sections were observed and analyzed using light microscopy and photographed. Histological score was assessed by the diagnostic criteria of gastritis in Houston in 1996 [32, 33]. Inflammatory score was calculated in 10 microscopic fields of each section and ranked in a 4-score system [34] (0 = normal; 1 = mild, few inflammatory cells' infiltration in pit or basal region of gastric glands; 2 = moderate amount of inflammatory cells infiltration, which localized within two-thirds of gastric glands; 3 = marked, large number of inflammatory cells' infiltration into whole gastric glands). Similarly, atrophy score of gastric glands was calculated in 10 microscopic fields of each section and ranked in a 4-score system (0 = normal; 1 = mild, atrophy less than one-third of gastric glands; 2 = moderate, atrophy localized within two-thirds of gastric glands; 3 = marked, atrophy more than two-thirds of gastric glands). Histological score was composed of inflammatory score and atrophy score.

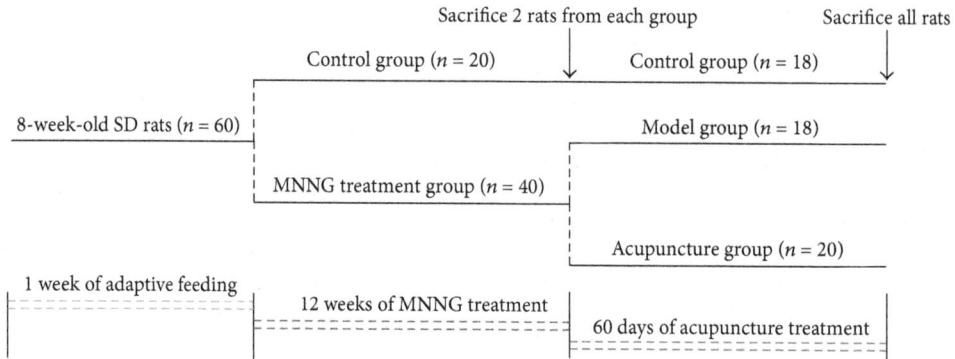

FIGURE 1: Flow diagram of the study.

Besides, morphology and structure of chief cells were also observed by transmission electromicroscope.

2.5. Immunohistochemistry.

Expression of NF-κB p65 in gastric tissue was detected with streptavidin-biotin-peroxidase complex (SABC) immunostain kit (Abcam Co., USA) according to the manufacturer's instructions. Paraffin embedded tissue sections were prepared at 2 μm thickness. After deparaffinization, antigen retrieval was undertaken by high pressure in a buffer composed of sodium citrate (0.01 mol/L). Endogenous peroxidase was cleared with 3% hydrogen peroxide. After blocking with 10% normal goat serum, the sections were incubated with monoclonal antibodies against NF-κB p65 of rabbit anti-rat (1 : 150 dilution, Abcam Co., USA) overnight at 4°C. Afterward, a streptavidin-peroxidase assay kit (Rui Shu Biological Technology Co., Ltd.) was used to develop antibody signal. DAB (Rui Shu Biological Technology Co., Ltd.) was used for staining and hematoxylin for counterstaining. PBS was used as the first antibody for negative control. Images were acquired with microscope and analyzed by Image-Pro Plus 6.0 image system. Under the microscope magnifying at 400 times, 10 random sights of each section were selected to conduct the semiquantitative analysis of the average optical density (OD).

2.6. Real-Time PCR.

Total RNA was extracted from frozen tissues using TRIzol reagent (Invitrogen). The RNA concentration was quantified by NanoDrop® ND-1000. Extracted RNA was reverse transcribed into complementary DNA using MMLV reverse transcriptase (Epicentre) and RT primers (Invitrogen). RT-PCR was carried out using TaqMan probes (Applied Biosystems) according to the manufacturer's instructions, with Gene Amp PCR System 9700 (Applied Biosystems). All reactions were run in triplicate, and average threshold cycle number (Ct) data of each miRNA was recorded. miRNAs expression in cells was normalized to U6 small noncoding RNA.

The ΔCt method and $2^{-\Delta\Delta Ct}$ method were used for analysis. The ΔCt value was the difference between the Ct value of the specific miRNA and the Ct value of U6, $\Delta Ct = Ct$ (miRNA) − Ct (U6). $\Delta\Delta Ct = \Delta Ct$ (sample) −ΔCt (reference). $2^{-\Delta Ct}$ represented miRNAs expression of each sample.

$2^{-\Delta\Delta Ct}$ represented the expression relative quotient (RQ) of target RNA to control RNA.

2.7. Statistical Analysis.

The results were expressed as mean ± SD. One-way analysis of variance (ANOVA) followed by Bonferroni post hoc tests was used to compare contents of miRNAs in different groups; repeated measures analysis of variance was used to compare body weights among groups, using SPSS software (Version 20.0, SPSS Inc., USA). Pearson's test was applied to analyze correlations of RQ values of miRNAs. $P < 0.05$ was considered to be statistically significant.

3. Results

3.1. Body Weight Changes.

Table 1 showed body weight changes in different groups. Body weights in the model group and the acupuncture group were significantly lower than the control group at week 8, week 12, and 60 days after treatment ($P < 0.001$). However, after 60 days of acupuncture treatment, body weights in the acupuncture group were significantly higher than that in the model group ($P < 0.001$).

3.2. Histopathological Evaluation.

Histological observation of gastric lesion induced by MNNG combined with irregular diet in the model group showed cystic dilation, irregular arrangement, reduction, and inflammatory cells infiltration in gastric glands. On the other hand, the acupuncture group showed relatively better protection of gastric mucosa as seen by regular arrangement and increased number of gastric glands and significant reduction in inflammatory cells infiltration. Relatively, gastric mucosa tissue in the control group showed intact appearance of gastric glands when compared with the model group, as shown in Figure 2.

It could be observed that inflammatory score, atrophy score, and histological score in the model group were significantly elevated when compared to the control group ($P < 0.001$). These data indicated that the experimental CAG in rats was successfully established. After acupuncture treatment, scores in the acupuncture group were significantly decreased when compared to the model group ($P < 0.001$). It could be indicated that acupuncture treatment had significant

TABLE 1: Body weight in different groups at various time points ($\overline{X} \pm S$).

Group	N	Before MNNG treatment	Week 8	Week 12	60 days later
Control group	18	201.45 ± 8.95	276.62 ± 10.21	340.33 ± 11.54	413.90 ± 10.69
Model group	18	200.98 ± 9.46	263.09 ± 9.09[*]	301.81 ± 10.88[*]	339.15 ± 13.79[*]
Acupuncture group	20	201.50 ± 9.05	261.75 ± 8.61[*]	300.83 ± 10.47[*]	374.21 ± 12.88[*△]

Note: at week 8/week 12/60 days later, compared with the control group, [*]$P < 0.001$. 60 days later, compared with the model group, [△]$P < 0.001$. Repeated measures analysis of variance was used.

TABLE 2: Histological scores of gastric glands in different groups ($\overline{X} \pm S$).

Group	N	Inflammatory score	Atrophy score	Histological score
Control group	9	1.04 ± 0.23	0.21 ± 0.11	1.26 ± 0.27
Model group	9	2.56 ± 0.42[*]	2.11 ± 0.19[*]	4.70 ± 0.60[*]
Acupuncture group	9	1.30 ± 0.22[△]	0.70 ± 0.22[*△]	2.00 ± 0.25[*△]

Note: compared with the control group, [*]$P < 0.001$. Compared with the model group, [△]$P < 0.001$. ANOVA (2-tailed) was used.

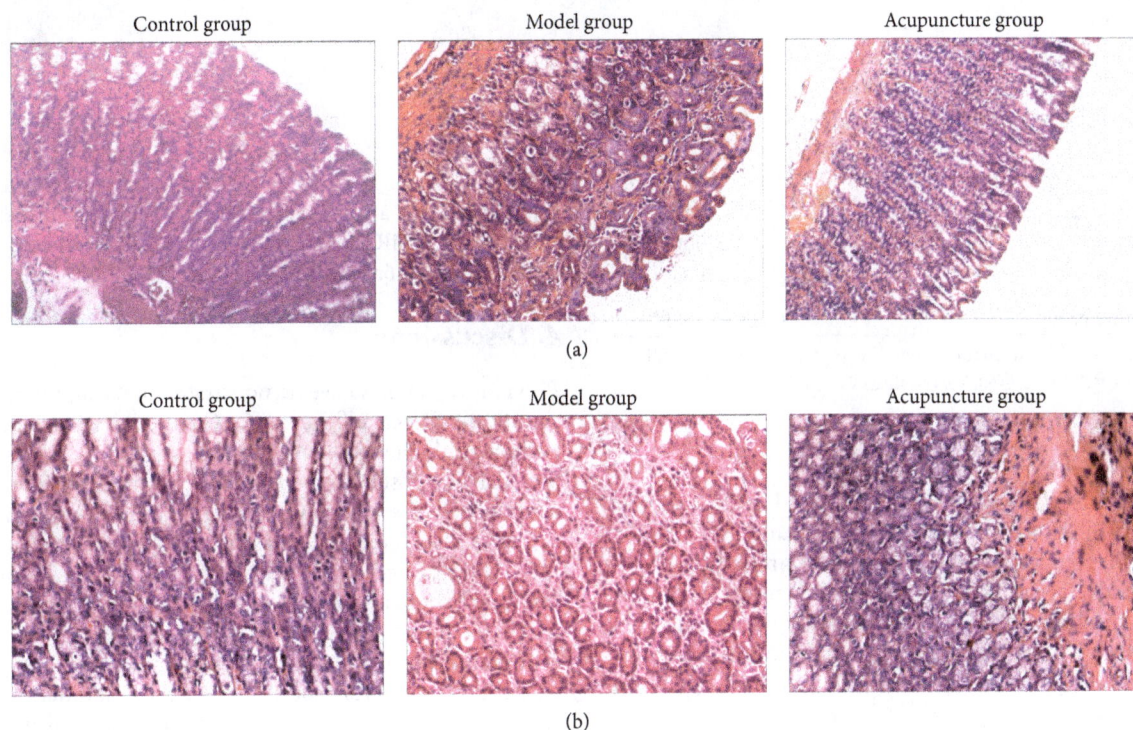

FIGURE 2: Histological evaluation of gastric glands in rats. (a) H&E (×100) staining of gastric glands. Rats in the control group showed complete glandular structure (left diagram). Rats in the model group showed irregular arrangement and reduction of gastric glands with atrophic gastritis (middle). Rats in the acupuncture group showed regular arrangement and increase of gastric glands after acupuncture treatment (right diagram). (b) H&E (×200) staining of gastric glands. Rats in the model group showed cystic dilation and neutrophils and lymphocytes infiltrated into gastric glands with atrophic gastritis (middle). Rats in the acupuncture group showed an increased number of gastric glands and inflammatory cells were reduced (right diagram).

effects on improving structure of gastric glands, as shown in Table 2.

We also evaluated the morphology and structure of chief cells by transmission electromicroscope (Figure 3). In the model group dilation of endoplasmic reticulum and reduction of Golgi complex and zymogen granules in gastric chief cells in rats with CAG could be observed. On the contrary, after acupuncture treatment, increase of endoplasmic reticulum, Golgi complex, and zymogen granules in gastric chief cells was observed in rats of the model group.

(a)   (b)   (c)

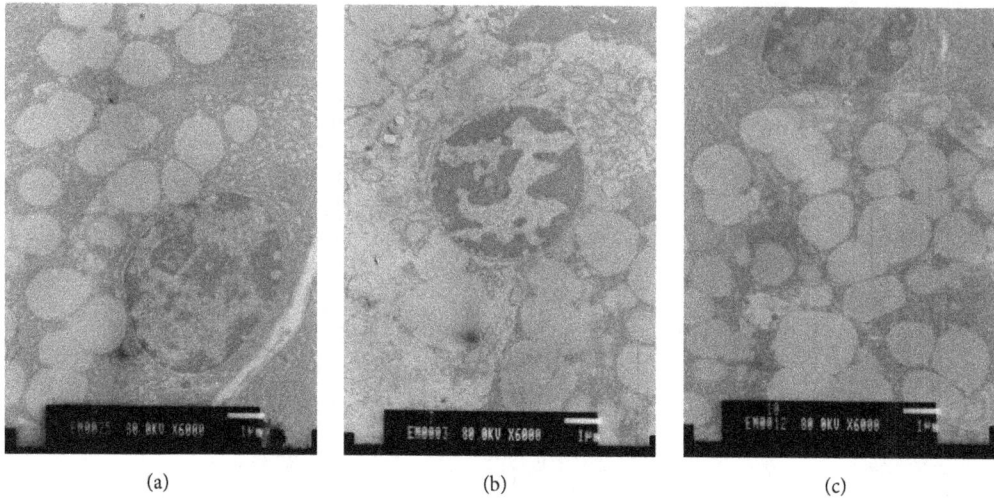

FIGURE 3: Histological evaluation of chief cells by TEM (×6000). (a) Control group. (b) Model group. TEM observation showed dilation of endoplasmic reticulum and reduction of Golgi complex and zymogen granules in chief cells in rats with atrophic gastritis. (c) Acupuncture group. TEM observation showed increase of endoplasmic reticulum, Golgi complex, and zymogen granules in chief cells in rats that received acupuncture treatment.

TABLE 3: Average optical density of NF-κB p65 in different groups ($\overline{X} \pm S$).

Group	N	NF-κB p65 (OD·μm^{-2})
Control group	9	0.180 ± 0.100
Model group	9	$0.290 \pm 0.097^*$
Acupuncture group	9	$0.217 \pm 0.044^\triangle$

Note: compared with the control group, $^*P < 0.01$. Compared with the model group, $^\triangle P < 0.01$. ANOVA (2-tailed) was used.

3.3. Expression of NF-κB p65. Figure 4 and Table 3 showed expression of NF-κB p65 detected by immunohistochemical staining. Expression of NF-κB p65 was significantly higher in the model group than in the control group. Moreover, expression of NF-κB p65 was significantly decreased in the acupuncture group compared to that in the model group, and there was no significant difference between the acupuncture group and the control group.

3.4. $2^{-\Delta Ct}$ Values of miR-155, miR-21, and miR-146a. Table 4 (and Figure S2) showed $2^{-\Delta Ct}$ values of miRNAs obtained from different groups. Expression levels of miR-155 and miR-21 were upregulated significantly in the model group compared to those in the control group and downregulated significantly in the acupuncture group compared to those in the model group, and there was no significance between the acupuncture and control group. Relatively, expression level of miR-146a was downregulated significantly in the model group compared to that in the control group and upregulated significantly in the acupuncture group compared to that in the model group, and there was no significance between the acupuncture and control group.

3.5. Correlations among miR-155, miR-21, and miR-146a. Fold change (RQ = $2^{-\Delta\Delta Ct}$) values of miR-155, miR-21, and miR-146a were shown in Table 5. Pearson's test results indicated that there were a positive correlation relationship between miR-155 and miR-21 and negative correlation relationships between miR-146a and miR-155/miR-21, respectively.

4. Discussions

Previous researches have demonstrated that acupuncture has significant clinical efficacy in CAG patients, with improving pathological changes and clinical symptoms [7, 14, 35]. Similarly, by observing body weight changes, we found that acupuncture therapy could help in gaining weight in CAG rats. We also found that gastric mucosa injuries of CAG rats that received acupuncture therapy were significantly improved compared to those in the model group. Furthermore, we found upregulation of NF-κB p65 in the model group and downregulation in the acupuncture group indicated that acupuncture could alleviate the inflammation reaction in gastric mucosa. These provide experimental evidences for effectiveness of acupuncture in treatment of CAG.

Previous studies have suggested the involvement of miR-NAs in CAG; we further proved that expressions of miR-155 and miR-21 were upregulated and miR-146a was downregulated in gastric tissues of CAG rats. Previous studies have found that acupuncture elicited remarkable miRNAs profiling changes in rats [36, 37]; our finding further demonstrated that acupuncture could regulate miRNAs expressions in CAG rats. To be specific, expressions of miR-155 and miR-21 were downregulated and miR-146a was upregulated after acupuncture treatment. Additionally, our results indicated that there was a positive correlation relationship between miR-155 and miR-21, indicating synergistic effects of these two miRNAs, as what has been reported before [38]. And there were

TABLE 4: 2^{-Ct} values of miR-155, miR-21, and miR-146a.

Group	N	miR-155	miR-21	miR-146a
Control group	9	0.034 ± 0.008	10.103 ± 2.961	5.962 ± 1.063
Model group	9	0.056 ± 0.011*	25.905 ± 3.702*	1.065 ± 0.336*
Acupuncture group	10	0.042 ± 0.008$^{\triangle}$	14.049 ± 3.601$^{\triangle\triangle}$	5.302 ± 0.978$^{\triangle\triangle}$

Note: compared with the control group, $^{*}P < 0.001$. Compared with the model group, $^{\triangle}P < 0.05$ and $^{\triangle\triangle}P < 0.001$. ANOVA (2-tailed) was used.

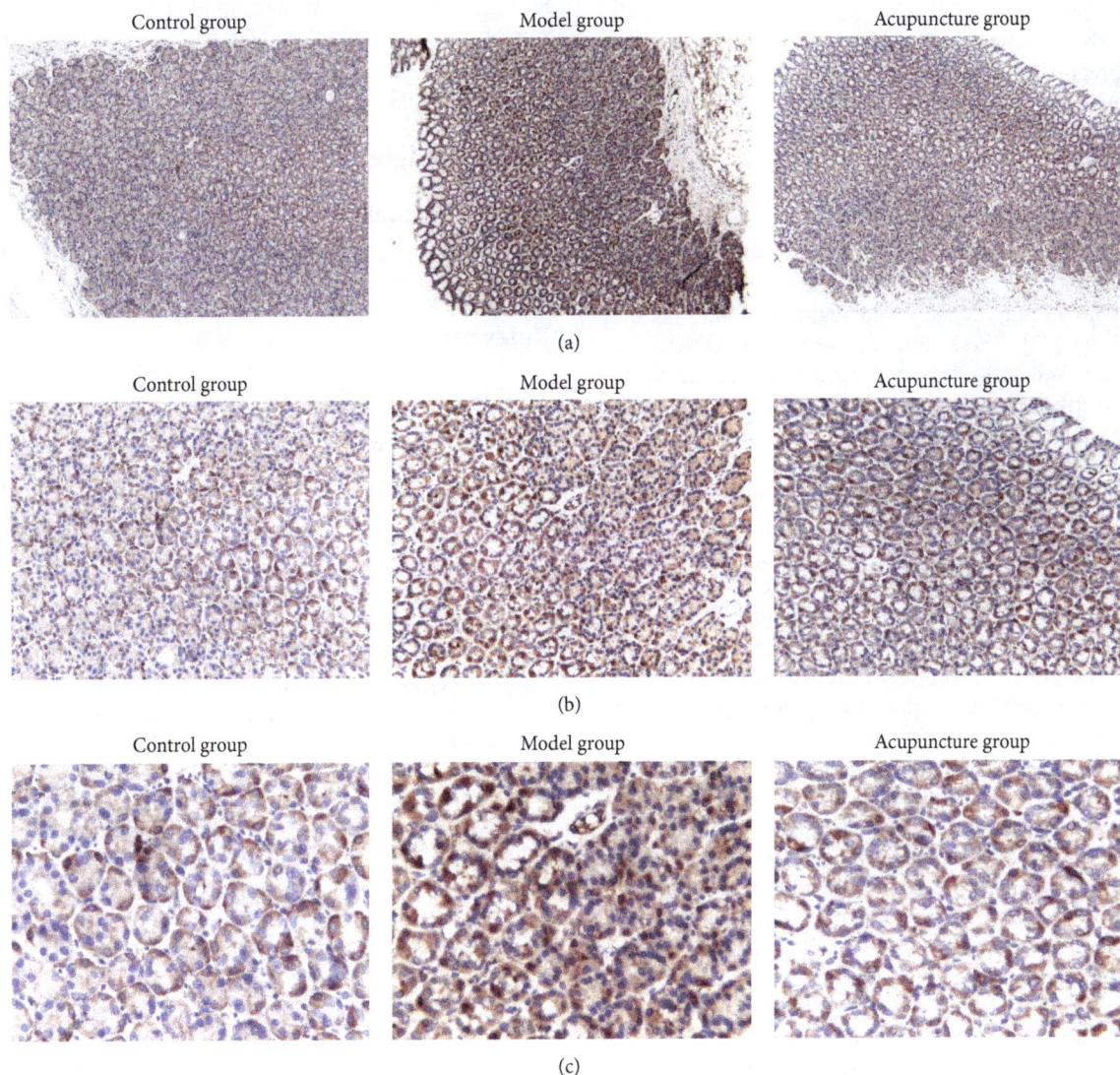

FIGURE 4: Immunohistochemistry stains of NF-κB p65 in gastric glands. (a) ×100. (b) ×200. (c) ×400.

TABLE 5: Fold changes of the expression of miR-155, miR-21, and miR-146a.

miRNAs	r	P value
miR-155 and miR-21	0.722	<0.001
miR-155 and miR-146a	−0.616	<0.05
miR-21 and miR-146a	−0.768	<0.001

Note: Pearson's test (2-tailed) was used.

negative correlation relationships between miR-146a and miR-155/miR-21, respectively, indicating antagonism effects of them on CAG. The abovementioned findings suggested that miR-155, miR-21, and miR-146a were involved in the pathogenesis of CAG and might play an important role in modulation effect of acupuncture in treatment of CAG.

It is well established that miRNAs may serve as functional inflammation regulators in many diseases [39]. Previous researches have shown that miR-155, miR-21, and miR-146a were associated with gastritis [22, 24–26], indicating that miR-155, miR-21, and miR-146a may function as inflammation regulators in CAG. Moreover, miR-155 has been suggested as a crucial effector of immune response in gastric epithelial cell lines and gastric mucosal tissues, which upregulated by activating NF-κB and activator protein-1 pathways [40]. And overexpression of miR-155 could negatively regulate release of proinflammatory cytokines, leading to chronic infection [24]. Similarly, miR-21 was also significantly overexpressed in CAG antrum mucosa [22], which upregulated by activating NF-κB and cyclooxygenase-2/prostaglandin signaling [41, 42]. And knockdown of NF-κB by a specific inhibitor could markedly suppress expression of miR-21 [42], which could slow down the process of gastric cancer. Another important miRNA associated with gastritis is miR-146a. Previous researches have demonstrated that downregulation of miR-146a expression could trigger inflammation response via NF-κB-dependent immunity signaling by increasing thymic stromal lymphopoietin pathway (TSLP) level [43]. These results have suggested that miR-155, miR-21, and miR-146a are potential targets of NF-κB, which are involved in an important signaling pathway in CAG [44], and efficacy of acupuncture in treatment of CAG may take effect by modifying expressions of miR-155, miR-21, and miR-146a via NF-κB pathway, thus to alleviate inflammation reaction of gastric mucosa. Therefore, our findings implied that acupuncture may act through transcription factors and subsequent epigenetic changes, such as NF-κB-miR-155/miR-21/miR-146a signaling. Additionally, significant improvements of histological changes in CAG rats after altering NF-κB/miR-155/miR-21/miR-146a expression levels are powerful evidence to validate therapeutic roles of NF-κB-miR-155/miR-21/miR-146a signaling in response to acupuncture treatment. What is more, downstream targets of miR-155/miR-21/miR-146a including I-kappa B kinase epsilon, Fas-associated death domain protein [40], and TSLP [43] have been reported. However, there is no definite conclusion on downstream targets of NF-κB-miR-155/miR-21/miR-146a signaling. In conclusion, we proposed that acupuncture may exert its therapeutic effects via NF-κB-miR-155/miR-21/miR-146a signaling, including (1) changes of transcription factors (such as NF-κB); (2) changes of miRNAs (miR-155/miR-21/miR-146a); (3) changes of downstream targets (such as TSLP, remaining inconclusive). These changes resulted in remarkable therapeutic effects of acupuncture in CAG rats (as shown in Figure S3).

Possible limitations of the study include the fact that exact function of miR-155/miR-21/miR-146a, interaction between NF-κB, miR-155, miR-21, and miR-146a, and existence of NF-κB-miR-155/miR-21/miR-146a signaling and its definite downstream targets in response to acupuncture therapy remain inconclusive, which require further researches in the future work.

Competing Interests

The authors declare that they have no competing interests.

Authors' Contributions

Jialing Zhang, Kangbai Huang, Yong Huang, and Suhe Li contributed to conception and design. Guoxin Zhong, Shanshan Qu, and Jiping Zhang contributed to acquisition of data or analysis and interpretation of data. Jialing Zhang, Kangbai Huang, Yong Huang, Suhe Li, and Guoxin Zhong contributed to drafting the paper or revising it critically for important intellectual content. Jialing Zhang, Kangbai Huang, and Yong Huang contributed to final approval of the version to be published. Jialing Zhang and Kangbai Huang contributed equally to this paper and should be considered co-first authors.

Acknowledgments

The authors thank Kang Chen Bio-tech for assistance with the experiments. This study was supported by the National Natural Science Foundation of China (no. 81072876).

References

[1] P. Correa, "Chronic gastritis: a clinico-pathological classification," *The American Journal of Gastroenterology*, vol. 83, no. 5, pp. 504–509, 1988.

[2] A. C. de Vries, N. C. T. van Grieken, C. W. N. Looman et al., "Gastric cancer risk in patients with premalignant gastric lesions: a Nationwide Cohort Study in the Netherlands," *Gastroenterology*, vol. 134, no. 4, pp. 945–952, 2008.

[3] Y. H. Park and N. Kim, "Review of atrophic gastritis and intestinal metaplasia as a premalignant lesion of gastric cancer," *Journal of Cancer Prevention*, vol. 20, no. 1, pp. 25–40, 2015.

[4] M. B. Piazuelo, M. C. Camargo, R. M. Mera et al., "Eosinophils and mast cells in chronic gastritis: possible implications in carcinogenesis," *Human Pathology*, vol. 39, no. 9, pp. 1360–1369, 2008.

[5] A. DeFoneska and J. D. Kaunitz, "Gastroduodenal mucosal defense," *Current Opinion in Gastroenterology*, vol. 26, no. 6, pp. 604–610, 2010.

[6] S.-H. Kim, S.-H. Lee, Y.-L. Choi, L.-H. Wang, C. K. Park, and Y. K. Shin, "Extensive alteration in the expression profiles of TGFB pathway signaling components and TP53 is observed along the gastric dysplasia-carcinoma sequence," *Histology and Histopathology*, vol. 23, no. 12, pp. 1439–1452, 2008.

[7] X. Gao, J. Yuan, H. Li, and S. Ren, "Clinical research on acupuncture and moxibustion treatment of chronic atrophic gastritis," *Journal of Traditional Chinese Medicine*, vol. 27, no. 2, pp. 87–91, 2007.

[8] W. J. Den Hollander and E. J. Kuipers, "Current pharmacotherapy options for gastritis," *Expert Opinion on Pharmacotherapy*, vol. 13, no. 18, pp. 2625–2636, 2012.

[9] K. L. Cooper, P. E. Harris, C. Relton, and K. J. Thomas, "Prevalence of visits to five types of complementary and alternative medicine practitioners by the general population: a systematic review," *Complementary Therapies in Clinical Practice*, vol. 19, no. 4, pp. 214–220, 2013.

[10] S. D. Klein, M. Frei-Erb, and U. Wolf, "Usage of complementary medicine across Switzerland: results of the Swiss Health Survey 2007," *Swiss Medical Weekly*, vol. 142, Article ID w13666, 2012.

[11] X. Gao, H. Rao, Y. Wang, D. Meng, and Y. Wei, "Protective action of acupuncture and moxibustion on gastric mucosa in model rats with chronic atrophic gastritis," *Journal of Traditional Chinese Medicine*, vol. 25, no. 1, pp. 66–69, 2005.

[12] C. Zhao, G. Xie, T. Weng, X. Lu, and M. Lu, "Acupuncture treatment of chronic superficial gastritis by the eight methods of intelligent turtle," *Journal of Traditional Chinese Medicine*, vol. 23, no. 4, pp. 278–279, 2003.

[13] J. Yu, H. Peng, Y. Lin, and S. Yi, "Effect of moxibustion treatment on cell apoptosis and expressions of heat shock protein and second mitochondrial activator of caspase in acute gastric mucosal lesion of rats," *Journal of Traditional Chinese Medicine*, vol. 33, no. 2, pp. 258–261, 2013.

[14] Y. Lu, J. T. Wang, and R. X. Chen, "Observation on therapeutic effect of acupuncture combined with drug for treatment of intestinal metaplasia of chronic atrophic gastritis," *Zhongguo Zhen Jiu*, vol. 25, no. 7, pp. 457–459, 2005.

[15] W. Luo, C.-L. Liu, J.-Y. Wang, C. Huang, and H.-J. Yi, "Effect of electroacupuncture combined with cutaneous 'tongluo' stimulation on gastric electrical rhythms and gastromucosal prostaglandin content in rats with chronic atrophic gastritis," *Zhen Ci Yan Jiu*, vol. 39, no. 6, pp. 482–486, 2014.

[16] X.-D. Tang, B. Lu, L.-Y. Zhou et al., "Clinical practice guideline of Chinese medicine for chronic gastritis," *Chinese Journal of Integrative Medicine*, vol. 18, no. 1, pp. 56–71, 2012.

[17] Y. Peng, S.-X. Yi, Y.-S. Feng, D.-M. Shi, Y.-L. Hou, and Y.-P. Lin, "Serumimmunological study of moxibustion on *Helicobacter pylori* gastritis in rats," *Zhongguo Zhen Jiu*, vol. 34, no. 8, pp. 783–790, 2014.

[18] Y. Han, T.-M. Ma, M.-L. Lu, L. Ren, X.-D. Ma, and Z.-H. Bai, "Role of moxibustion in inflammatory responses during treatment of rat ulcerative colitis," *World Journal of Gastroenterology*, vol. 20, no. 32, pp. 11297–11304, 2014.

[19] T.-M. Ma, Y. Han, X.-D. Ma, X.-X. Zeng, and W. Ge, "Influence of moxibustion with different duration on colonic epithelial structure, serum inflammatory cytokines, and intestinal mucosa inflammatory cell signal transduction pathways," *Zhen Ci Yan Jiu*, vol. 39, no. 1, pp. 20–26, 2014.

[20] D. P. Bartel, "MicroRNAs: target recognition and regulatory functions," *Cell*, vol. 136, no. 2, pp. 215–233, 2009.

[21] A. Link, J. Kupcinskas, T. Wex, and P. Malfertheiner, "Macrorole of MicroRNA in gastric cancer," *Digestive Diseases*, vol. 30, no. 3, pp. 255–267, 2012.

[22] A. Link, W. Schirrmeister, C. Langner et al., "Differential expression of microRNAs in preoplastic gastric mucosa," *Scientific Reports*, vol. 5, article 8270, 2015.

[23] M. Oertli, D. B. Engler, E. Kohler, M. Koch, T. F. Meyer, and A. Müller, "MicroRNA-155 is essential for the T cell-mediated control of Helicobacter pylori infection and for the induction of chronic gastritis and colitis," *Journal of Immunology*, vol. 187, no. 7, pp. 3578–3586, 2011.

[24] Z. Liu, B. Xiao, B. Tang et al., "Up-regulated microRNA-146a negatively modulate *Helicobacter pylori*-induced inflammatory response in human gastric epithelial cells," *Microbes and Infection*, vol. 12, no. 11, pp. 854–863, 2010.

[25] F. Petrocca, R. Visone, M. R. Onelli et al., "E2F1-regulated MicroRNAs impair TGFβ-dependent cell-cycle arrest and apoptosis in gastric cancer," *Cancer Cell*, vol. 13, no. 3, pp. 272–286, 2008.

[26] M. Sha, J. Ye, L.-X. Zhang, Z.-Y. Luan, and Y.-B. Chen, "Celastrol induces apoptosis of gastric cancer cells by miR-146a inhibition of NF-κB activity," *Cancer Cell International*, vol. 13, article 50, 2013.

[27] A. Rodriguez, E. Vigorito, S. Clare et al., "Requirement of bic/microRNA-155 for normal immune function," *Science*, vol. 316, no. 5824, pp. 608–611, 2007.

[28] S. Chen, L. Wang, J. Fan et al., "Host miR155 promotes tumor growth through a myeloid-derived suppressor cell-dependent mechanism," *Cancer Research*, vol. 75, no. 3, pp. 519–531, 2015.

[29] A. Nagahara, S. Watanabe, H. Miwa, K. Endo, M. Hirose, and N. Sato, "Reduction of gap junction protein connexin 32 in rat atrophic gastric mucosa as an early event in carcinogenesis," *Journal of Gastroenterology*, vol. 31, no. 4, pp. 491–497, 1996.

[30] P. V. Peplow, "Repeated electroacupuncture in obese Zucker diabetic fatty rats: adiponectin and leptin in serum and adipose tissue," *Journal of Acupuncture and Meridian Studies*, vol. 8, no. 2, pp. 66–70, 2015.

[31] W. P. Zhang, M. Kanehara, Y. Zhang et al., "Acupuncture increases bone strength by improving mass and structure in established osteoporosis after ovariectomy in rats," *Journal of Traditional Chinese Medicine*, vol. 26, no. 2, pp. 138–147, 2006.

[32] M. F. Dixon, R. M. Genta, J. H. Yardley et al., "Classification and grading of gastritis: the updated Sydney System," *The American Journal of Surgical Pathology*, vol. 20, no. 10, pp. 1161–1181, 1996.

[33] J. J. Misiewicz, "The Sydney System: a new classification of gastritis. Introduction," *Journal of Gastroenterology and Hepatology*, vol. 6, no. 3, pp. 207–208, 1991.

[34] S. Chen, J. Zhong, Q. Zhou, X. Lu, L. Wang, and J. Si, "The regenerating gene iα is overexpressed in atrophic gastritis rats with hypergastrinemia," *Gastroenterology Research and Practice*, vol. 2011, Article ID 403956, 7 pages, 2011.

[35] W. Gu and Q.-C. Hu, "Clinical observation on acupuncture for treatment of chronic atrophic gastritis," *Zhongguo Zhen Jiu*, vol. 29, no. 5, pp. 361–364, 2009.

[36] J.-Y. Wang, H. Li, C.-M. Ma, J.-L. Wang, X.-S. Lai, and S.-F. Zhou, "MicroRNA profiling response to acupuncture therapy in spontaneously hypertensive rats," *Evidence-Based Complementary and Alternative Medicine*, vol. 2015, Article ID 204367, 9 pages, 2015.

[37] J.-Y. Wang, H. Li, C.-M. Ma, J.-L. Wang, X.-S. Lai, and S.-F. Zhou, "Acupuncture may exert its therapeutic effect through microRNA-339/Sirt2/NFκB/FOXO1 axis," *BioMed Research International*, vol. 2015, Article ID 249013, 9 pages, 2015.

[38] L. Li, J. Zhang, W. Diao et al., "MicroRNA-155 and microRNA-21 promote the expansion of functional myeloid-derived suppressor cells," *The Journal of Immunology*, vol. 192, no. 3, pp. 1034–1043, 2014.

[39] L. T. Jeker and R. Marone, "Targeting microRNAs for immunomodulation," *Current Opinion in Pharmacology*, vol. 23, pp. 25–31, 2015.

[40] B. Xiao, Z. Liu, B.-S. Li et al., "Induction of microRNA-155 during *Helicobacter pylori* infection and its negative regulatory role in the inflammatory response," *Journal of Infectious Diseases*, vol. 200, no. 6, pp. 916–925, 2009.

[41] P. Zheng, H. Guo, G. Li, S. Han, F. Luo, and Y. Liu, "PSMB4 promotes multiple myeloma cell growth by activating NF-κB-miR-21 signaling," *Biochemical and Biophysical Research Communications*, vol. 458, no. 2, pp. 328–333, 2015.

[42] V. Y. Shin, H. Jin, E. K. O. Ng et al., "NF-κB targets miR-16 and miR-21 in gastric cancer: involvement of prostaglandin E receptors," *Carcinogenesis*, vol. 32, no. 2, pp. 240–245, 2011.

[43] W. Sun, Y. Sheng, J. Chen, D. Xu, and Y. Gu, "Down-regulation of miR-146a expression induces allergic conjunctivitis in mice by increasing TSLP level," *Medical Science Monitor*, vol. 21, pp. 2000–2007, 2015.

[44] H.-Y. Lin, Y. Zhao, J.-N. Yu, W.-W. Jiang, and X.-L. Sun, "Effects of traditional Chinese medicine Wei-Wei-Kang-Granule on the expression of EGFR and NF-KB in chronic atrophic gastritis rats," *African Journal of Traditional, Complementary, and Alternative Medicines*, vol. 9, no. 1, pp. 1–7, 2012.

21

Bioactive Components of Chinese Propolis Water Extract on Antitumor Activity and Quality Control

Hongzhuan Xuan,[1,2] **Yuehua Wang,**[2] **Aifeng Li,**[3] **Chongluo Fu,**[2]
Yuanjun Wang,[2] **and Wenjun Peng**[1]

[1]*Key Laboratory of Pollinating Insect Biology, Ministry of Agriculture, Beijing 100093, China*
[2]*School of Life Science, Liaocheng University, Liaocheng 252059, China*
[3]*College of Chemistry and Chemical Engineering, Liaocheng University, Liaocheng 252059, China*

Correspondence should be addressed to Wenjun Peng; pengwenjun@vip.sina.com

Academic Editor: Michael A. Savka

To understand the material basis of antitumor activity of Chinese propolis water extract (CPWE), we developed a simple and efficient method using macroporous absorptive resin coupled with preparative high performance liquid chromatography and separated and purified eleven chemical components (caffeic acid, ferulic acid, isoferulic acid, 3,4-dimethoxycinnamic acid, pinobanksin, caffeic acid benzyl ester, caffeic acid phenethyl ester, apigenin, pinocembrin, chrysin, and galangin) from CPWE; then we tested the antitumor activities of these eleven components using different human tumor cell lines (MCF-7, MDA-MB-231, HeLa, and A549). Furthermore, cell migration, procaspase 3 level, and reactive oxygen species (ROS) of effective components from CPWE were investigated. Our data showed that antitumor activities of the eleven components from CPWE were different from each other. CPWE and its effective components induced apoptosis by inhibiting tumor cell migration, activating caspase 3, and promoting ROS production. It can be deduced that the antitumor effects of propolis did not depend on a single component, and there must exist "bioactive components," which also provides a new idea for Chinese propolis quality control.

1. Introduction

Propolis is a resinous substance collected by *Apis mellifera* from various tree buds, and it has been used as a folk medicine since ancient time for its widely biological properties, such as antibacterial, antiviral, antioxidant, anti-inflammatory, immunomodulatory, and antitumor. [1–5]. However, in propolis application the biggest problem is the instability of its therapeutic effects and the material basis has not been fully understood, which is caused by the imperfection of propolis quality control and evaluation system. Propolis quality control system is difficult to be established, for there are more than 600 constituents identified from different kinds of propolis in the world, such as polyphenols (flavonoids, phenolic acids, and their esters), terpenoids, steroids, and amino acids [6–8]. And the other major cause is that there is not a unified extract method and solvent

process. Ethanol is the most common solvent during propolis extracting process, and most of the studies and biological activities in propolis are based on propolis ethanolic extract (PEE), which leads to little knowledge known about the biological activities of the propolis water extract, especially "poplar propolis" from China [9, 10].

Recently, we developed a simple and efficient method using macroporous absorptive resin (MAR) coupled with preparative high performance liquid chromatography (PHPLC) for separation of polyphenols from Chinese propolis water extract (CPWE). Six phenolic acids and five flavonoids (caffeic acid, ferulic acid, isoferulic acid, 3,4-dimethoxycinnamic acid, pinobanksin, caffeic acid benzyl ester, caffeic acid phenethyl ester (CAPE), apigenin, pinocembrin, chrysin, and galangin) with high purities were isolated, and the chemical structures were further confirmed by UV and NMR analysis [11].

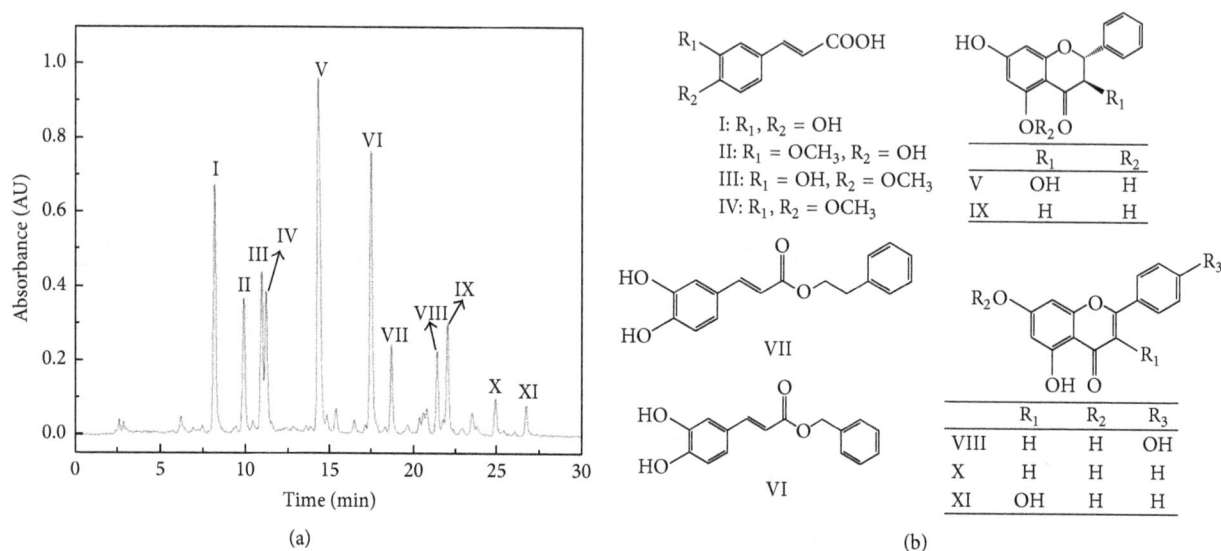

FIGURE 1: HPLC chromatograms of the crude Chinese propolis water extract (CPWE) and the chemical structure of the eleven components. I: caffeic acid, II: ferulic acid, III: isoferulic acid, IV: 3,4-dimethoxycinnamic acid, V: pinobanksin, VI: caffeic acid benzyl ester, VII: caffeic acid phenethyl ester, VIII: apigenin, IX: pinocembrin, X: chrysin, and XI: galangin.

Considering the imperfection of Chinese propolis quality control system and the ambiguity of material basis of antitumor activity of CPWE, in present study we studied the antitumor activities of CPWE and the eleven isolated components from CPWE to determine bioactive components of antitumor activity and provide a new idea for Chinese propolis quality control.

2. Materials and Methods

2.1. Chemicals and Reagents. Dulbecco's modified Eagle's medium (DMEM) was from Gibco (USA). Fetal bovine serum (FBS) was from Hyclone Lab Inc. (USA). Sulforhodamine B (SRB), Hoechst 33258, and $2',7'$-dichlorodihydrofluorescein (DCHF) were from Sigma Co. (USA). Acridine orange was from Amresco (USA). Primary antibodies against β-actin and secondary antibody (horseradish peroxidase) were from Santa Cruz Biotechnology (USA). Primary antibody against procaspase 3 was from Cell Signaling Technology (USA). All other reagents were ultrapure grade.

2.2. Preparation of Propolis Extracts. Chinese propolis was obtained from colonies of honeybees, *A. mellifera* L., in Shandong province of north China and the main plant origin was poplar (*Populus* sp.). Chinese propolis 0.25 kg was frozen, milled, and extracted with boiling water. The water extract was filtered, combined, and concentrated under reduced pressure with a rotary evaporator. Then 95% ethanol was added to the solution to remove polysaccharide until the concentration of ethanol was about 70%. After 12 h, the supernatant was separated and concentrated under reduced pressure. The water-soluble fraction was first "prefractioned" by MAR to obtain four subfractions; and they were all subjected to PHPLC to get different components [11].

2.3. Cell Culture. The human breast cancer cells, MCF-7 (human breast cancer ER (+)) and MDA-MB-231 (human breast cancer ER (−)) cells, lung cancer A549 cells, and human colonic carcinoma HeLa cells were purchased from American Type Culture Collection (ATCC, USA). MCF-7, MDA-MB-231, A549, and HeLa cells were cultured in DMEM medium supplemented with heat-inactivated 10% FBS and 100 U/mL of penicillin and 100 μg/mL streptomycin. Cells were incubated at 37°C in a humidified atmosphere of 5% CO_2 and 95% air.

2.4. Cell Viability Assay. Four different tumor cells were seeded onto 96-well plates and treated with different components separated from CPWE (20, 40, 80, and 160 μM) for 24 and 48 h, respectively. Cell viability was determined by SRB assay. In detail, fix cells by adding 100 μL of cold 10% trichloroacetic acid and incubate for 1 h at 4°C, and then wash the plates with deionized water five times. Add 50 μL of 0.4% SRB solution to each well and shake for 5 min on titer plate shaker. Wash the plate with 1% acetate five times, and subsequently add 100 μL of 10 mM Tris base to dissolve the bound dye. Mix for 5 min on a microtiter plate shaker and read optical densities at the wavelength of 492 nm using Multiskan MK3 microplate reader (Thermo Co., USA). The viability (%) was expressed as (OD of treated group/OD of control group) × 100%. The viability of the control cells was set to 100%.

2.5. Nuclear Fragmentation Assay. The morphological changes of nuclei of MCF-7 cells treated with different components from CPWE were detected by acridine orange staining. At 48 h, cells were washed gently with 1x PBS once and then stained with 5 μg/mL acridine orange at room temperature for 1 min, after that they were washed

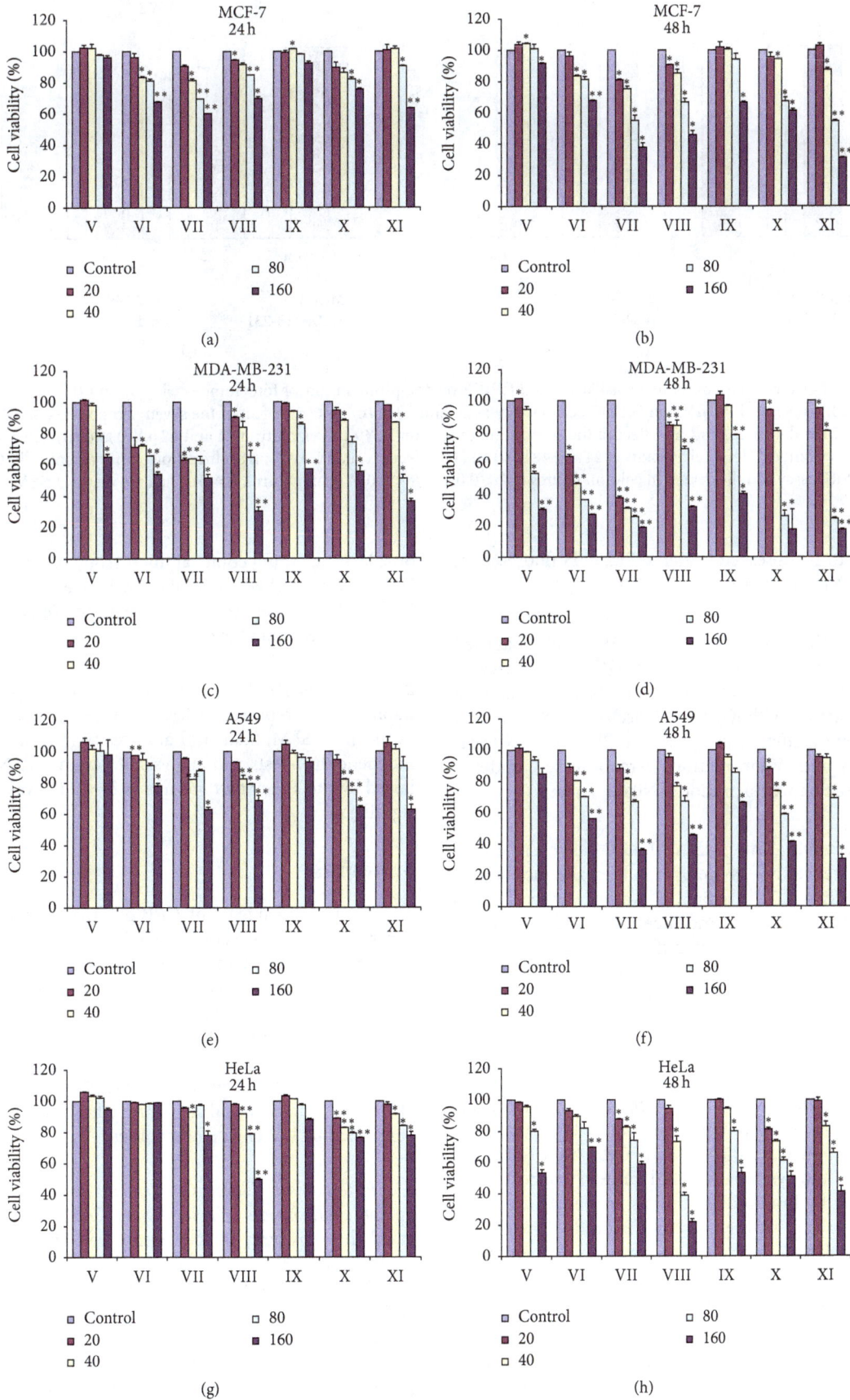

FIGURE 2: Continued.

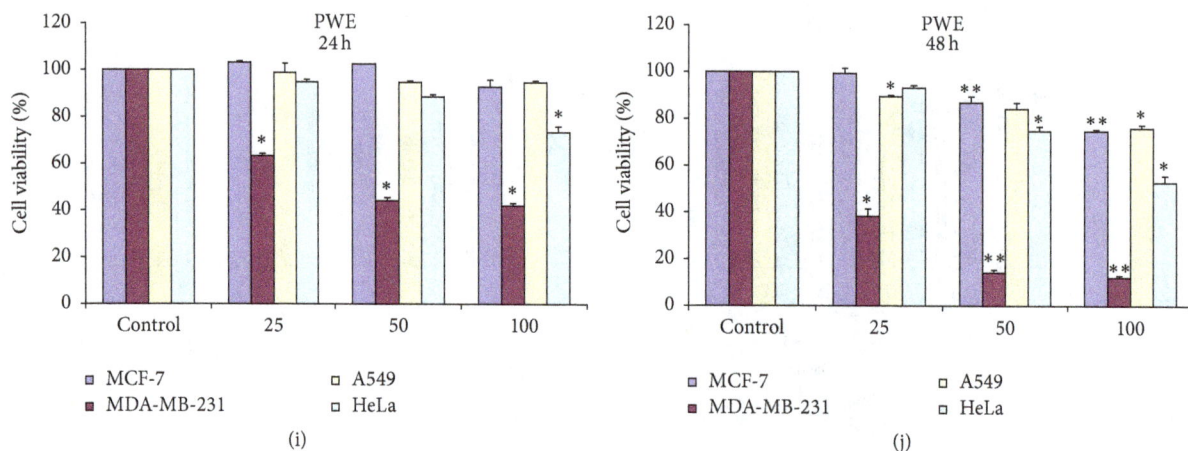

FIGURE 2: Effects of the seven components isolated from CPWE on the proliferation of four tumor cells. (a) and (b), effect of the seven components (20, 40, 80, and 160 μM) on MCF-7 cell viability at 24 and 48 h. (c) and (d), effect of the seven components on MDA-MB-231 cell viability at 24 and 48 h. (e) and (f), effect of the seven components on A549 cell viability at 24 and 48 h. (g) and (h), effect of the seven components on viability of HeLa cell viability at 24 and 48 h. (i) and (j), effect of crude CPWE on proliferation of four tumor cells. Cell viability was tested by SRB assay and illustrated in column figures (*P < 0.05, **P < 0.01 versus control, n = 3). Data are means ± SEM.

gently twice to be observed under a TE2000S fluorescence microscope (Nikon, Japan).

2.6. Hoechst 33258 Staining.

Hoechst 33258 staining was used to observe apoptotic morphology of MCF-7 cells treated with different components from CPWE. At 48 h, cells in all groups were stained with 10 μg/mL Hoechst 33258 for 15 min and then were gently washed with 1x PBS once. Nuclear condensation and fragmentation were observed under a TE2000S fluorescence microscope (Nikon, Japan).

2.7. Wound-Healing Assay.

MDA-MB-231 cells were grown to 80% confluence in a 24-well plate; then the monolayers were scratched with a plastic tip, washed by 1x PBS to remove floating cell debris, and then incubated in medium in the absence or presence of different components from CPWE for 48 h. Cell migration into the wound surface was determined under a TE2000S inverted microscope (Nikon, Japan). Migrated cells across the scratched lines were counted by Image-Pro Plus software (USA).

2.8. Western Blotting Analysis.

Western blotting analysis was used to determine the protein levels in cells treated with different components from CPWE. Cells were collected and lysed in the lysis buffer, and protein concentration was measured by Bradford method as previously described [12]. Protein (30 μg) was separated by running through 12% SDS-PAGE gel and transferred to the PVDF membrane. The transferred proteins were visualized with an enhanced chemiluminescence detection kit.

2.9. Measurement of ROS Production.

ROS production in MCF-7 cells treated with different components from CPWE was determined by use of a fluorescent probe, DCHF as previously described [13]. The fluorescence was observed

on a laser scanning confocal microscopy (Olympus FV1200, Japan). ROS level was quantified by Image-Pro Plus software (USA). Results were shown as relative fluorescence intensity of three independent experiments.

2.10. Statistical Analysis.

All experiments were performed in duplicate and repeated at least 3 times. Data are expressed as means ± SEM. Statistical analyses were performed using independent t-tests and analysis of variance (ANOVA) followed by the Tukey *post hoc test*. A P < 0.05 was considered significant.

3. Results

3.1. Major Components of CPWE.

Finally, eleven components from CPWE were obtained including I: caffeic acid (30 mg), II: ferulic acid (16 mg), III: isoferulic acid (10 mg), IV: 3,4-dimethoxycinnamic acid (12 mg), V: pinobanksin (42 mg), VI: caffeic acid benzyl ester (36 mg), VII: caffeic acid phenethyl ester (12 mg), VIII: apigenin (8 mg), IX: pinocembrin (11 mg), X: chrysin (5 mg), and XI: galangin (4 mg). Their purities were all above 98% as determined by HPLC, and the chemical structures (shown in Figure 1) were confirmed by UV and NMR analysis.

3.2. Effects of the Eleven Components Isolated from CPWE on the Proliferation of Four Tumor Cell Lines.

We investigated the sensitivity of four tumor cell lines to the eleven components (20, 40, 80, and 160 μM) and CPWE (25, 50, and 100 μg/mL) for 24 and 48 h using SRB assay at 24 and 48 h. Caffeic acid, ferulic acid, isoferulic acid, and 3,4-dimethoxycinnamic acid had no significant cytotoxicity to four tumor cells (data were not shown); the other seven components significantly inhibited four tumor cells' proliferation in a dose- and time-dependent manner. The crude CPWE also inhibited cell proliferation of four tumor cells; however,

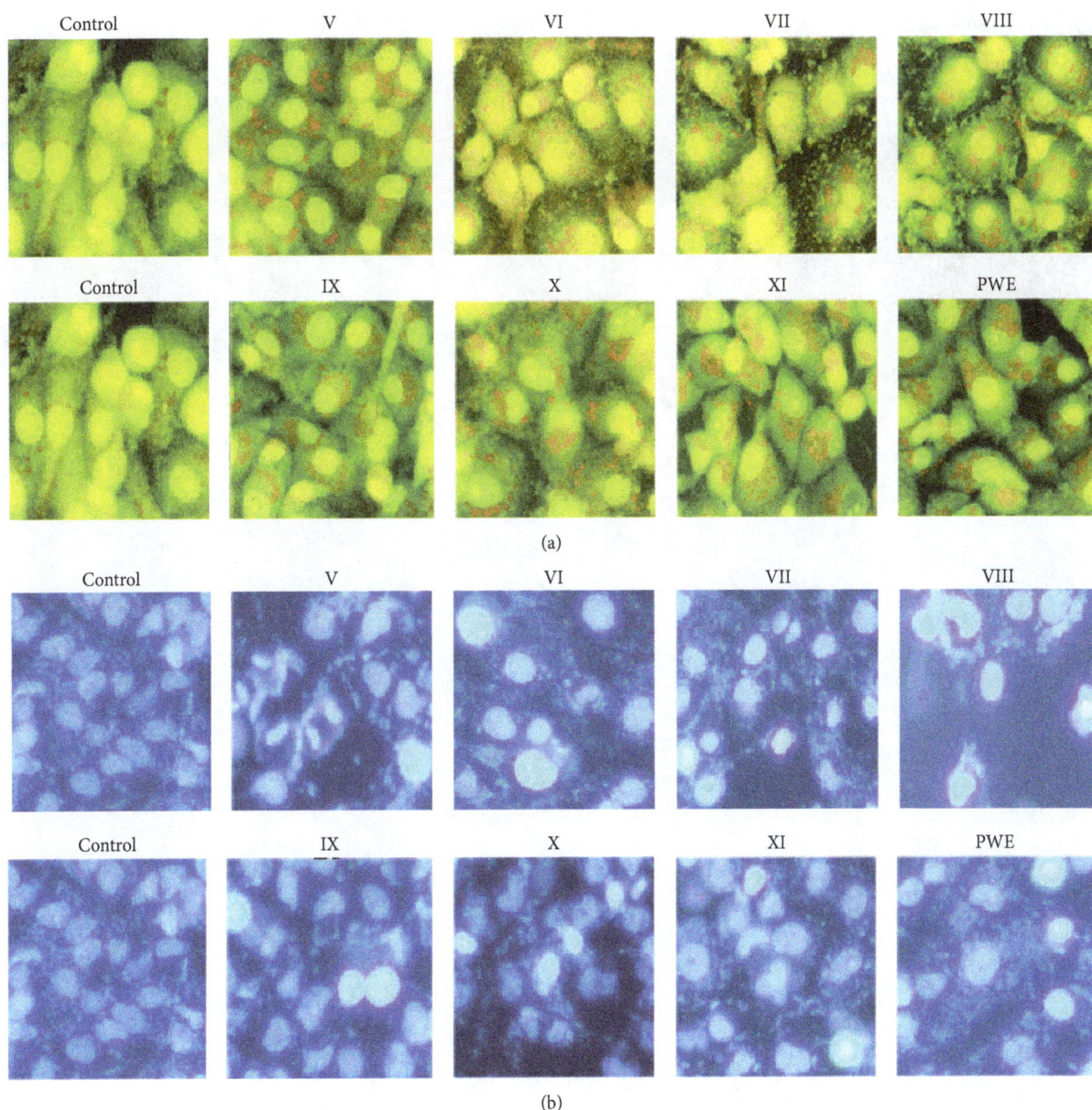

FIGURE 3: Effects of the seven components and crude CPWE on nuclear fragmentations of MCF-7 cells. (a) Morphological changes of nuclei by staining with acridine orange at 48 h (×200). (b) Morphological changes of nuclei by staining with Hoechst 33258 at 48 h (×200).

the inhibitory effect of CPWE was lower than that of ethanol-extracted Chinese propolis, which was tested previously [14]. Furthermore, the sensitivity of four tumor cell lines to the seven components and CPWE from strong to weak was followed by MDA-MB-231, HeLa, A549, and MCF-7 cells ($^*P < 0.05$, $^{**}P < 0.01$; Figure 2).

Notably, the cytotoxicity of pinocembrin to tumor cells was higher than pinobanksin; CAPE was higher than caffeic acid benzyl ester, and the most effective antitumor concentration for seven different components was at concentration higher than 80 μM, so we used 80 μM for the seven components and CPWE 100 μg/mL as the following study dose.

3.3. Effects of the Seven Different Components and CPWE on Apoptosis in MCF-7 Cells. Acridine orange staining and Hoechst 33258 staining results indicated that the seven different components at concentration of 80 μM and CPWE (100 μg/mL) evidently induced nuclear condensation and fragmentation in MCF-7 cells (Figure 3).

3.4. Effects of the Seven Different Components and CPWE on MDA-MB-231 Cells Migration. The migrations of MDA-MB-231 cells were detected by wound-healing assay after being treated with the seven different components at concentration

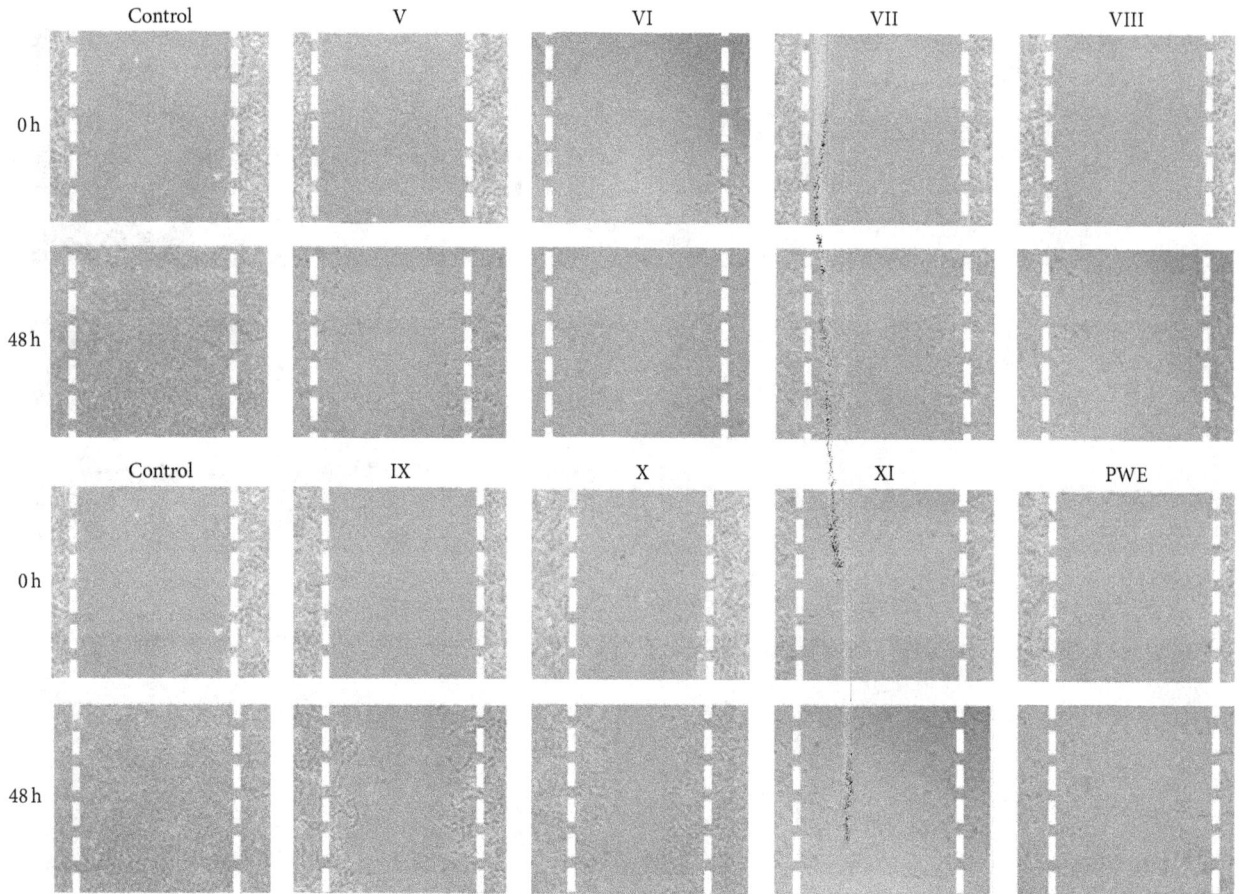

(a)

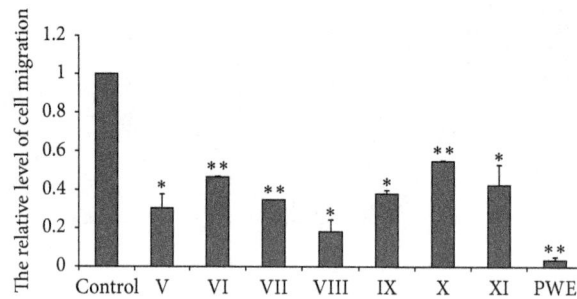

(b)

FIGURE 4: Effects of the seven components and crude CPWE on migration of MDA-MB-231 cells. (a) Cell migration micrographs obtained under a phase contrast microscope at 0 and 48 h (×100). (b) Relative levels of cell migration ($^*P < 0.05$, $^{**}P < 0.01$ versus control, $n = 3$).

of 80 μM and CPWE (100 μg/mL); the results indicated that the seven different components and CPWE significantly inhibited MDA-MB-231 cells migration at 48 h (Figure 4).

3.5. Effects of the Seven Different Components and CPWE on the Level of Procaspase 3 in Two Breast Cancer Cells.
The seven different components at concentration of 80 μM and CPWE (100 μg/mL) significantly activated caspase 3 by western blotting assay in MCF-7 and MDA-MB-231 cells (Figure 5).

3.6. Effects of the Seven Different Components and CPWE on the Production of ROS in MCF-7 Cells.
The seven different components at concentration of 80 μM and CPWE (100 μg/mL) obviously affected ROS production in MCF-7 cells although the ROS levels were different from each other (Figure 6).

4. Discussion

Previous studies from our group reported the biological activities of Chinese propolis [15–17] and the present study

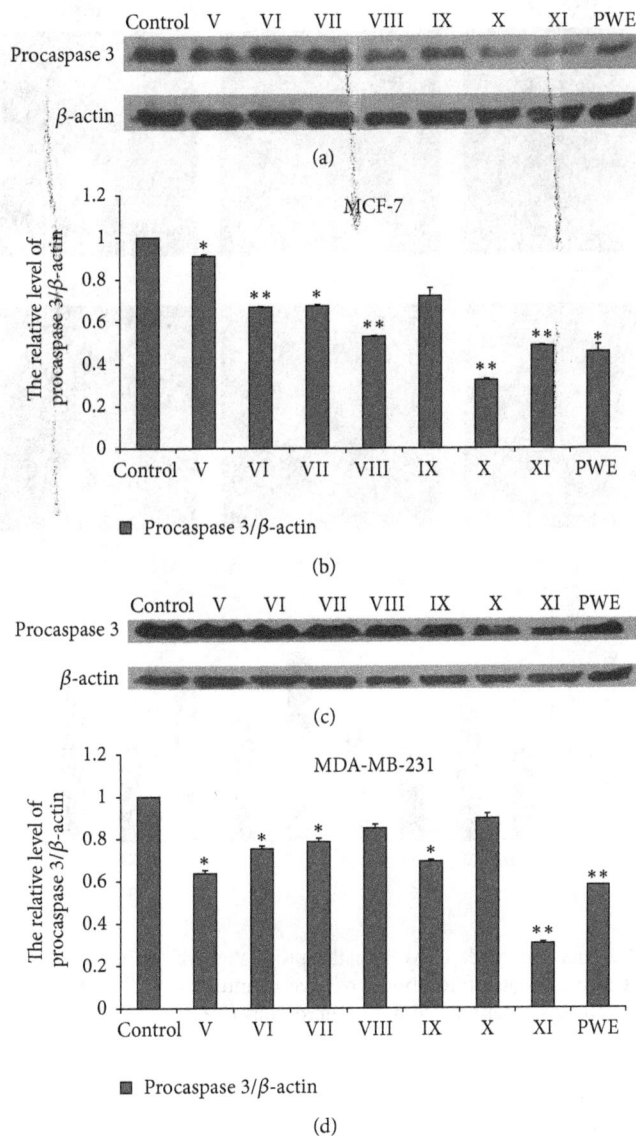

FIGURE 5: Effects of the seven components and crude CPWE on the expression of procaspase 3 in MCF-7 and MDA-MB-231 cells. (a) and (c), expression of procaspase 3 in MCF-7 and MDA-MB-231 cells at 24 h, respectively; (b) and (d) quantification of relative expression quantity in MCF-7 and MDA-MB-231 cells at 24 h, respectively ($^*P < 0.05$, $^{**}P < 0.01$ versus control, $n = 3$).

was the first one to investigate the effective components on antitumor activity in CPWE. Four phenolic acids (caffeic acid, ferulic acid, isoferulic acid, and 3,4-dimethoxycinnamic acid) had little cytotoxicity on four tumor cell lines; the other seven constituents (pinobanksin, caffeic acid benzyl ester, caffeic acid phenethyl ester, apigenin, pinocembrin, chrysin, and galangin) obviously decreased four tumor cells' proliferation, although the inhibitory effects of the seven components were different from each other, which indicated that the antitumor effects of CPWE did not depend on a single component, and at least the seven effective components might be "bioactive components" of antitumor activity. Admittedly, there must be other effective components needed to be studied further.

The standardization of Chinese propolis has caused some interest in recent years in China, and HPLC fingerprint of Chinese propolis from different regions, sources, and seasons has been fully studied, and the authentication standard of Chinese propolis and poplar buds had also been established [18, 19], which greatly promoted the research of quality control system of Chinese propolis. It was pointed out that chrysin, catechol, or another component from propolis could be a candidate for the standardization of Chinese propolis [20, 21]. However, there still exist a lot of problems. For example, propolis has similar biological activities although chemical components vary greatly [22]. And more importantly, a number of studies have confirmed that propolis and its plant sources, poplar buds or gums, have similar biological

(a)

(b)

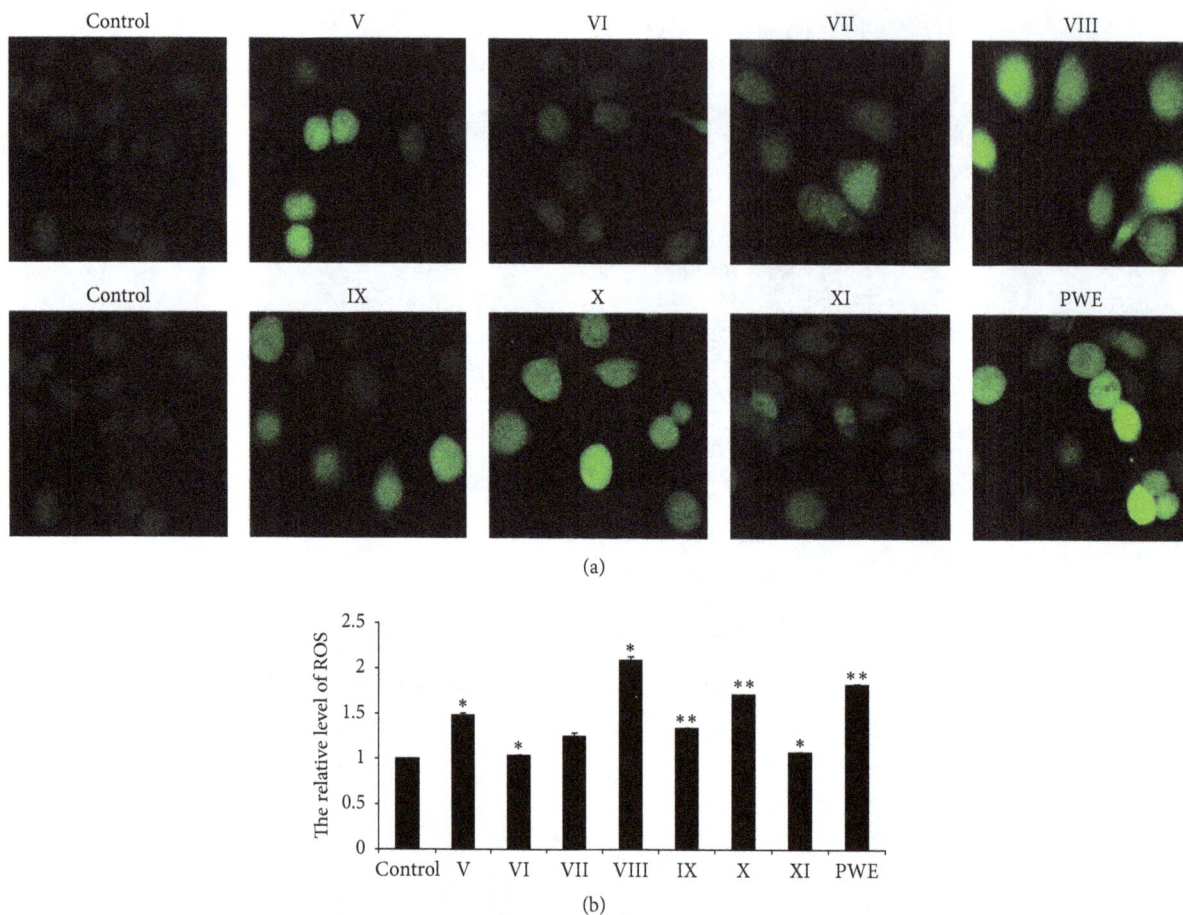

FIGURE 6: Effects of the seven components and crude CPWE on the production of reactive oxygen species (ROS) in MCF-7 cells. (a) Fluorescent micrographs obtained at 48 h. (b) Quantification of relative quantity of ROS in MCF-7 cells. Values represent the relative fluorescent intensity per cell determined by laser scanning confocal microscopy ($^*P < 0.05$, $^{**}P < 0.01$ versus control, $n = 3$).

activities. Wang et al. indicated that ethanol extracts of Chinese propolis (EECP) and buds from poplar had similar anti-inflammatory effects in vivo and in vitro [23]. Another report suggested that the antioxidant mechanisms of EECP and poplar gums were similar, but they also indicated that the antioxidant activities of EECP were stronger than poplar gums. Further analysis indicated that the total content of eight components from EECP (caffeic acid, ferulic acid, p-coumaric acid, apigenin, chrysin, pinocembrin, CAPE, and galangin) was 5.85 g/100 g. However, in poplar gums, caffeic acid, ferulic acid, and p-coumaric acid were not identified, and the total content of the other five components was only 2.59 g/100 g [24]. Based on the facts we deduced that the major cause for EECP with a higher antioxidant than poplar gums was that EECP had more effective components. In present study, we further confirmed that it was not a single component playing the antitumor activity in propolis. Thus, the quality evaluation system of Chinese propolis might be imperfect if it is only based on the quantitative analysis of chemical composition of propolis or some single component, and here we proposed that it was acceptable to perfect

the quality evaluation system of Chinese propolis based on "bioactive components."

The major mechanism of inhibiting tumor cell proliferation of the seven effective components from CPWE was to induce apoptosis by activating caspase 3, the executor of apoptosis, and induce ROS production, which was consistent with our previous studies [14].

In summary, our data highlight the effective components of CPWE on antitumor activity and the probable action mechanisms in inhibiting tumor cell proliferation and provide a novel idea for Chinese propolis quality control.

Competing Interests

The authors declare that they have no competing interests.

Acknowledgments

This work was supported by the grants from the National Natural Science Foundation of China (no. 31201860); Shandong Provincial Natural Science Foundation of China (no.

ZR2012CQ003); Open foundation of Key Laboratory of Pollinating Insect Biology, Ministry of Agriculture, China (no. 2015MFNZS02); and the College Student Innovation Foundation of Liaocheng, University of China (nos. SF2014268, 26312150906).

References

[1] G. C.-F. Chan, K.-W. Cheung, and D. M.-Y. Sze, "The immunomodulatory and anticancer properties of propolis," *Clinical Reviews in Allergy and Immunology*, vol. 44, no. 3, pp. 262–273, 2013.

[2] S. Patel, "Emerging adjuvant therapy for cancer: propolis and its constituents," *Journal of Dietary Supplements*, vol. 13, no. 3, pp. 245–268, 2016.

[3] J. M. Sforcin and V. Bankova, "Propolis: is there a potential for the development of new drugs?" *Journal of Ethnopharmacology*, vol. 133, no. 2, pp. 253–260, 2011.

[4] G. Valenzuela-Barra, C. Castro, C. Figueroa et al., "Anti-inflammatory activity and phenolic profile of propolis from two locations in Región Metropolitana de Santiago, Chile," *Journal of Ethnopharmacology*, vol. 168, pp. 37–44, 2015.

[5] S. Ishiai, W. Tahara, E. Yamamoto, R. Yamamoto, and K. Nagai, "Histone deacetylase inhibitory effect of Brazilian propolis and its association with the antitumor effect in Neuro2a cells," *Food Science & Nutrition*, vol. 2, no. 5, pp. 565–570, 2014.

[6] M. Duman and E. Özpolat, "Effects of water extract of propolis on fresh shibuta (*Barbus grypus*) fillets during chilled storage," *Food Chemistry*, vol. 189, Article ID 16314, pp. 80–85, 2015.

[7] V. Bankova, "Chemical diversity of propolis and the problem of standardization," *Journal of Ethnopharmacology*, vol. 100, no. 1-2, pp. 114–117, 2005.

[8] S. Huang, C.-P. Zhang, K. Wang, G. Q. Li, and F.-L. Hu, "Recent advances in the chemical composition of propolis," *Molecules*, vol. 19, no. 12, pp. 19610–19632, 2014.

[9] F. Hu, H. R. Hepburn, Y. Li, M. Chen, S. E. Radloff, and S. Daya, "Effects of ethanol and water extracts of propolis (bee glue) on acute inflammatory animal models," *Journal of Ethnopharmacology*, vol. 100, no. 3, pp. 276–283, 2005.

[10] T. D. Kwon, M. W. Lee, and K. H. Kim, "The effect of exercise training and water extract from propolis intake on the antioxidant enzymes activity of skeletal muscle and liver in rat," *Journal of Exercise Nutrition and Biochemistry*, vol. 18, no. 1, pp. 9–17, 2014.

[11] A. Li, H. Xuan, A. Sun, R. Liu, and J. Cui, "Preparative separation of polyphenols from water-soluble fraction of Chinese propolis using macroporous absorptive resin coupled with preparative high performance liquid chromatography," *Journal of Chromatography B*, vol. 1012-1013, pp. 42–49, 2016.

[12] A.-Y. Du, B.-X. Zhao, D.-L. Yin, S.-L. Zhang, and J.-Y. Miao, "Discovery of a novel small molecule, 1-ethoxy-3-(3,4-methylenedioxyphenyl)-2-propanol, that induces apoptosis in A549 human lung cancer cells," *Bioorganic and Medicinal Chemistry*, vol. 13, no. 13, pp. 4176–4183, 2005.

[13] N. Suematsu, H. Tsutsui, J. Wen et al., "Oxidative stress mediates tumor necrosis factor-α-induced mitochondrial DNA damage and dysfunction in cardiac myocytes," *Circulation*, vol. 107, no. 10, pp. 1418–1423, 2003.

[14] H. Xuan, Z. Li, H. Yan et al., "Antitumor activity of Chinese propolis in human breast cancer MCF-7 and MDA-MB-231 cells," *Evidence-Based Complementary and Alternative Medicine*, vol. 2014, Article ID 280120, 11 pages, 2014.

[15] Y.-J. Li, H.-Z. Xuan, Q.-Y. Shou, Z.-G. Zhan, X. Lu, and F.-L. Hu, "Therapeutic effects of propolis essential oil on anxiety of restraint-stressed mice," *Human and Experimental Toxicology*, vol. 31, no. 2, pp. 157–165, 2012.

[16] H. Xuan, J. Zhao, J. Miao, Y. Li, Y. Chu, and F. Hu, "Effect of Brazilian propolis on human umbilical vein endothelial cell apoptosis," *Food and Chemical Toxicology*, vol. 49, no. 1, pp. 78–85, 2011.

[17] H. U. Fuliang, H. R. Hepburn, H. Xuan, M. Chen, S. Daya, and S. E. Radloff, "Effects of propolis on blood glucose, blood lipid and free radicals in rats with diabetes mellitus," *Pharmacological Research*, vol. 51, no. 2, pp. 147–152, 2005.

[18] J. Zhou, Y. Li, J. Zhao, X. Xue, L. Wu, and F. Chen, "Geographical traceability of propolis by high-performance liquid-chromatography fingerprints," *Food Chemistry*, vol. 108, no. 2, pp. 749–759, 2008.

[19] Z. Cui-Ping, H. Shuai, W. Wen-Ting et al., "Development of high-performance liquid chromatographic for quality and authenticity control of Chinese propolis," *Journal of Food Science*, vol. 79, no. 7, pp. C1315–C1322, 2014.

[20] S. Huang, C.-P. Zhang, G. Q. Li, Y.-Y. Sun, K. Wang, and F.-L. Hu, "Identification of catechol as a new marker for detecting propolis adulteration," *Molecules*, vol. 19, no. 7, pp. 10208–10217, 2014.

[21] L.-P. Sun, A.-L. Chen, H.-C. Hung et al., "Chrysin: a histone deacetylase 8 inhibitor with anticancer activity and a suitable candidate for the standardization of Chinese propolis," *Journal of Agricultural and Food Chemistry*, vol. 60, no. 47, pp. 11748–11758, 2012.

[22] W. Zhu, Y.-H. Li, M.-L. Chen, and F.-L. Hu, "Protective effects of Chinese and Brazilian propolis treatment against hepatorenal lesion in diabetic rats," *Human and Experimental Toxicology*, vol. 30, no. 9, pp. 1246–1255, 2011.

[23] K. Wang, J. Zhang, S. Ping et al., "Anti-inflammatory effects of ethanol extracts of Chinese propolis and buds from poplar (*Populus×canadensis*)," *Journal of Ethnopharmacology*, vol. 155, no. 1, pp. 300–311, 2014.

[24] J. Zhang, X. Cao, S. Ping et al., "Comparisons of ethanol extracts of Chinese propolis (poplar type) and poplar gums based on the antioxidant activities and molecular mechanism," *Evidence-Based Complementary and Alternative Medicine*, vol. 2015, Article ID 307594, 15 pages, 2015.

22

The Clinical Effect of Acupuncture in the Treatment of Obstructive Sleep Apnea: A Systematic Review and Meta-Analysis of Randomized Controlled Trials

Zheng-tao Lv,[1] Wen-xiu Jiang,[2] Jun-ming Huang,[1] Jin-ming Zhang,[1] and An-min Chen[1]

[1]*Department of Orthopedics, Tongji Hospital, Tongji Medical College, Huazhong University of Science and Technology, Wuhan, Hubei 430030, China*
[2]*Department of Otolaryngology, Tongji Hospital, Tongji Medical College, Huazhong University of Science and Technology, Wuhan, Hubei 430030, China*

Correspondence should be addressed to An-min Chen; anminchen@hust.edu.cn

Academic Editor: Christopher Worsnop

Purpose. This study aims to determine the clinical efficacy of acupuncture therapy in the treatment of obstructive sleep apnea. *Methods.* A systematic literature search was conducted in five databases including PubMed, EMBASE, CENTRAL, Wanfang, and CNKI to identify randomized controlled trials (RCTs) on the effect of acupuncture therapy for obstructive sleep apnea. Meta-analysis was conducted using the RevMan version 5.3 software. *Results.* Six RCTs involving 362 subjects were included in our study. Compared with control groups, manual acupuncture (MA) was more effective in the improvement of apnea/hypopnea index (AHI), apnea index, hypopnea index, and mean SaO_2. Electroacupuncture (EA) was better in improving the AHI and apnea index when compared with control treatment, but no statistically significant differences in hypopnea index and mean SaO_2 were found. In the comparison of MA and nasal continuous positive airway pressure, the results favored MA in the improvement of AHI; there was no statistical difference in the improvement in mean SaO_2. No adverse events associated with acupuncture therapy were documented. *Conclusion.* Compared to control groups, both MA and EA were more effective in improving AHI and mean SaO_2. In addition, MA could further improve apnea index and hypopnea index compared to control.

1. Introduction

Obstructive sleep apnea (OSA) is a major public health issue affecting children and adults which is characterized by reduced airflow during sleep resulting in gas exchange abnormalities and disrupted sleep [1]. The pathogenesis of OSA is complicated but it is probably due to a combination of an anatomically small pharyngeal airway in conjunction with a sleep related decline in upper airway dilator muscle activity [2, 3]. OSA occurs more commonly in men than in women, and predisposing risk factors include obesity, adenotonsillar hypertrophy, retrognathia, hypothyroidism, nasal obstruction, and evening alcohol ingestion [4]. Patients with OSA exhibit reduced quality of life due to daytime symptoms such as excessive sleepiness, irritability, decreased concentration and memory, reduced energy, erectile dysfunction, depressive symptoms, and an association with cardiovascular and metabolic diseases that restrict their social activities [5–12].

The gold standard for documenting severity of OSAS is overnight polysomnography (PSG). Considering the socioeconomic burden of OSA, patients with OSA should be treated immediately after diagnosis. In view of the high prevalence and the relevant impairment of patients with OSA, lots of methods are offered for the improvement of OSA. Nasal continuous positive airway pressure (nCPAP) therapy is accepted as the standard treatment for the management of clinically significant OSA in recent decades [13]. Proper use of nCPAP manages apnea and hypopnea, eliminates hypoxia, restores normal sleep architecture, and significantly improves subjective and objective measures of wakefulness and averts cardiovascular consequences, especially arterial hypertension

[14]. In addition to nCPAP, oral appliances may be considered as a long-term alternative in patients with severe OSAS who do not respond to CPAP or in whom treatment attempts with CPAP fail. Surgery may also be recommended with curative intent for patients with an obvious anatomic obstruction such as large palatine or lingual tonsils or used as a salvage procedure to improve OSA in patients who fail CPAP and/or other treatment measures [15, 16].

The standard treatment, nCPAP, has been proven to reduce upper airway obstructions and improves quality of life. Despite the notable efficacy of nCPAP, many patients suffer from local side effects at the nose or face or discomfort due to the mask [17]. Moreover, CPAP does not allow for a permanent resolution of respiratory disturbances during sleep but only suppresses them while using the devices [17, 18]. Patients often have difficulty in adhering to nCPAP or may switch to complementary and alternative (CAM) therapy [19]. Those with OSA who choose CAM approaches are potentially seeking ways to improve chronic fatigue and fragmented sleep. As a mainstream of CAM therapy, acupuncture has been practiced for thousands of years in China for the treatment of various diseases [20]. Given the lack of now-existing evidence showing the beneficial effect of CAM therapies, they cannot be recommended as a primary treatment of OSA. It seems that there are no alternatives to the conventional treatment of OSAS which provide the same positive outcomes as CPAP, surgical interventions, or oral appliances when used appropriately for selected patients [1]. Thus, the aim of our present work was to evaluate the clinical effect of acupuncture therapy in the treatment of OSA, which could be an affordable treatment for OSA.

2. Materials and Methods

This systematic review and meta-analysis was performed strictly in accordance with the Preferred Reporting Items for Systematic Reviews and Meta-Analyses (PRISMA) guidelines [21].

2.1. Search Strategy. A systematic literature search was conducted using the following electronic databases: Pubmed, EMBASE, CENTRAL, Wanfang, and CNKI. All these electronic databases were searched from their inception dates up to the latest issue (October 2015). The bibliographies of relevant systematic reviews and clinical guidelines were manually searched; no language restriction was imposed. A combination of medical subject headings (MeSH) and free terms was applied to retrieve the potentially eligible studies as possible; MeSH was slightly modified based on the specification of each database.

The search terms of English databases were as follows: ("Sleep Apnea, Obstructive" or osahs OR obstructive sleep apnea OR sleep apnea OR sleep hypopnea OR upper airway resistance sleep apnea syndrome) and ("Acupuncture Therapy" or acupuncture or moxibustion or acupoint or acupressure OR acustimulation); for Chinese databases we used search terms as "zhen" and ("shuimian" and ("huxizanting" or "ditongqi" or "zusexing")). The detailed procedure of

literature search in Pubmed and EMBASE was presented in Appendix.

2.2. Inclusion and Exclusion Criteria. The PICOS (participants, interventions, comparisons, outcomes, and study design) principle was utilized for our inclusion and exclusion criteria.

Participants included in our study had to be diagnosed with OSA according to the results of PSG (AHI > 5). No restrictions on age, sex, and race were imposed. Patients with OSA in the experimental groups mainly received acupuncture therapy including manual acupuncture (MA) and electroacupuncture (EA), without differentiating the needle materials and acupoints selection; subjects allocated in the control groups received no specific treatment or sham acupuncture (SA) or nCPAP treatment. The primary outcome was apnea/hypopnea index (AHI) and the second outcomes included hypopnea index, apnea index, and mean SaO$_2$. To be included in our current review, the study design had to be randomized controlled trial. Animal experiments, review, case report, and studies that were duplicates for retrieving or publishing were excluded.

2.3. Data Extraction. Two independent reviewers (Zhengtao Lv and Wen-xiu Jiang) reviewed each article and each one of them was blinded to the findings of the other. Raw data was independently extracted and collected from the original articles by two reviewers; data extraction was guided by a predetermined standardized collection form which includes first author and year, country, study design, baseline characteristics of participants, diagnostic criteria for OSA, interventions in experimental and control groups, duration of treatment, and main outcome assessments. Any discrepancies between reviewers were resolved through discussion until a consensus was reached. A third author (An-min Chen) was consulted if a consensus could not be reached.

2.4. Risk of Bias Assessment. To assess the methodological quality of selected studies, Cochrane Collaboration's tool [28] was used, which was based on seven items: random sequence generation, allocation concealment, blinding of participants and personnel, blinding of outcome assessment, incomplete outcome data, selective reporting, and other sources of bias. The response for each criterion was reported as low risk of bias, high risk of bias, and unclear risk of bias. Two reviewers evaluated the quality of trials independently.

2.5. Data Synthesis and Analysis. The meta-analysis and statistical analyses were performed using the RevMan 5.3 analyses software of the Cochrane Collaboration. Since the types of all the outcome measurements were continuous variables, mean differences (MD) and the associated 95% confidence interval (CI) were calculated for AHI, hypopnea index, apnea index, and mean SaO$_2$. Heterogeneity among studies was assessed using Chi-squared test and Higgins I^2 test ($I^2 < 50\%$ indicates acceptable heterogeneity); we pooled data across studies using random effect model if obvious heterogeneity existed; otherwise, a fixed effect model would

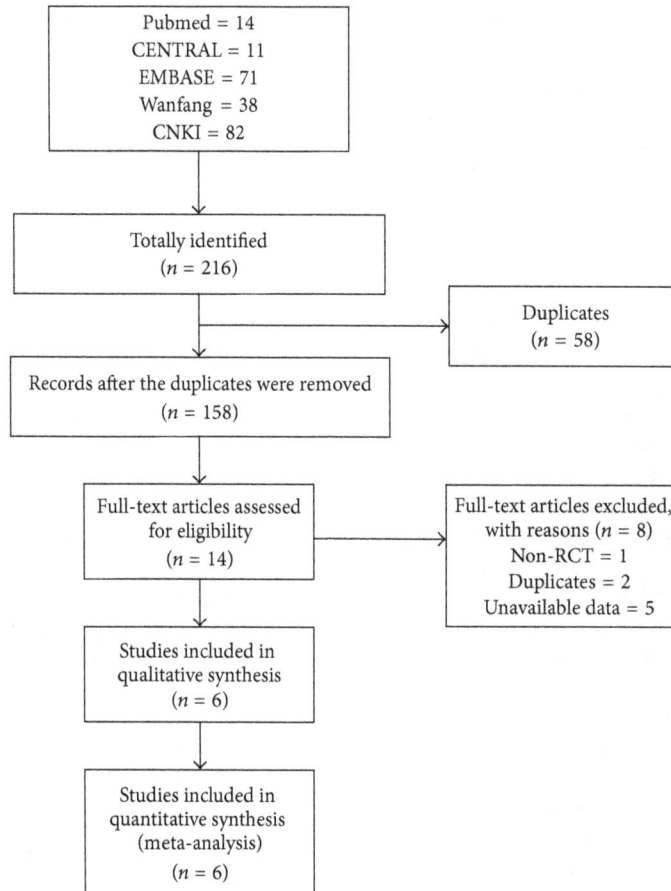

FIGURE 1: Flowchart of the literature search.

be used. In case of obvious heterogeneity, subgroup analysis was conducted based on the specification of acupuncture techniques. Publication bias was detected via a funnel plot if the amount of included studies was greater than 10.

3. Results

3.1. Literature Search. The literature screening process is presented in Figure 1. An initial search yielded 216 potential literature citations, including 14 records from Pubmed, 11 from CENTRAL, 71 from EMBASE, 38 from Wanfang, and 82 from CNKI. 58 records were excluded because they were duplicates. 158 studies were considered potentially eligible by reading their titles and abstracts. According to the predetermined inclusion criteria, 14 articles remained to be evaluated using a full-text screen. Of the remaining 14 studies, one study was excluded because it was not RCT, two studies were excluded because they were duplicates, and five studies were excluded because of unavailable data reported. Finally, six studies [22–27] were deemed eligible to be included in our meta-analysis.

3.2. The Characteristics of Included Trials. The basic demographic information and detailed intervention methods are listed in Tables 1 and 2. Two studies [22, 24] were conducted in Brazil and the other four [23, 25–27] were conducted by

Chinese investigators; each study was performed at a single center. These RCTs were published between 2007 and 2015; a total of 362 patients were enrolled: 197 patients in the acupuncture group and 165 patients in control group. Age of the participants ranged from 35 to 76; baseline similarities were reported in each study. All the studies conducted in China used a two-arm parallel design, two studies [25, 27] were designed to evaluate the clinical effect of EA compared to nonspecific treatment, and the other two studies [23, 26] aimed to compare the efficacy of MA and that of nCPAP. The single-blinded RCT [22] conducted in 2007 used a three-arm parallel design; MA was compared with no treatment and SA. A four-arm parallel RCT [24] was conducted by Freire and colleagues in 2010, the clinical efficacy of MA and EA with different power frequencies was compared with that of control group, and parameters associated with OSA (AHI, apnea index, hypopnea index, and mean SaO_2) were assessed by PSG.

3.3. Risk of Bias Assessment. To assess the risk of bias among included studies, Cochrane Collaboration's tool was employed. All of the six studies reported suggested randomization; however, two studies [25, 26] failed to provide the method of random sequence generation. Only two studies [22, 24] reported the procedure of allocation concealment, and the blinding of participants and personnel was carried

TABLE 1: Characteristics of included studies.

Study	Country	Study design	Population	Age (mean or range)	EC approval
Freire et al., 2007 [22]	Brazil	RCT	MA: 12 SA: 12 Control: 12	MA: 54.0 (51.0–63.0) SA: 53.0 (49.0–63.0) Control: 57.0 (50.0–64.0)	Yes
Chen et al. 2008 [23]	China	RCT	MA: 44 nCPAP: 22	MA: 55.44 ± 11.04 nCPAP: 56.73 ± 10.21	Not reported
Freire et al., 2010 [24]	Brazil	RCT	MA: 10 2 Hz EA: 10 10 Hz EA: 10 Control: 10	MA: 57.7 (44.0–68.0) 2 Hz EA: 52.9 (33.0–69.0) 10 Hz EA: 54.8 (35.0–71.0) Control: 54.3 (35.0–69.0)	Yes
Zhang, 2014 [25]	China	RCT	2 Hz EA: 30 Control: 30	2 Hz EA: 69.45 ± 6.78 Control: 70.01 ± 5.94	Not reported
Zhang et al. 2014 [26]	China	RCT	MA: 45 nCPAP: 45	MA: 48.45 ± 9.76 nCPAP: 51.96 ± 9.87	Not reported
Song et al., 2015 [27]	China	RCT	2 Hz EA + nCPAP: 36 nCPAP: 34	2 Hz EA + nCPAP: 53.17 ± 10.20 nCPAP: 52.71 ± 11.26	Yes

Note. RCT: randomized controlled trial; MA: manual acupuncture; SA: sham acupuncture; EA: electroacupuncture; nCPAP: nasal continuous positive airway pressure; EC: ethical committee.

TABLE 2: Interventions and outcome assessment of included studies.

Study	Diagnostic criteria for OSAHS	Duration of treatment	Experimental treatment	Control treatment	Main outcome
Freire et al., 2007 [22]	PSG $15 < AHI < 30$	10 weeks	MA: (Gv20, Li20, Ren23, P6, Lu7, Li4, St36, St40, Sp6, Kd6) 30 min, deqi	Control: weight reduction advice and sleep hygiene counseling SA: (acupoints were 1 cun from the real point) 30 min, no manipulation	AHI, AI, HI, mean SaO_2
Chen et al., 2008 [23]	PSG $AHI > 5$	20 days	MA: (Cv23, Panglianquan, Si17, L7, K6, Sp4, Cv17, S40, H7, Sp6, extra6) 30 min, deqi	nCPAP: once a day, 20 days in total	AHI, AI, HI, mean SaO_2
Freire et al., 2010 [24]	PSG $15 < AHI < 30$	1 night	MA: (Lu6, Lu7, Li4, Li20, Gv20, Cv23, St36, St40, Sp6, Ki6, Extra12) 30 min, deqi 2 Hz EA: (Cv23, Extra12, Li4, St36) 30 min, 0.6–0.8 mA, 2 Hz 10 Hz EA: (Cv23, Extra12, Li4, St36) 30 min, 0.6–0.8 mA, 10 Hz	No specific treatment reported	AHI, AI, HI, mean SaO_2
Zhang, 2014 [25]	PSG $AHI > 5$	20 days	2 Hz EA: (Cv23, Panglianquan) once a day	No specific treatment reported	AHI, AI, HI
Zhang et al. 2014 [26]	PSG $AHI > 5$	4 weeks	MA: (Li11, S25, Sp9, S40, Liv3) 30 min, deqi; weight reduction advice and smoking cessation	nCPAP: details are not reported; weight reduction advice and smoking cessation	AHI, mean SaO_2
Song et al., 2015 [27]	PSG $AHI > 15$	6 weeks	nCPAP + 2 Hz EA: (Extra8, Extra9, Extra6, H7, St36, Sp6, K6) 2 Hz, 30 min	nCPAP: 3 times a week, 6 weeks in total	AHI

Note. MA: manual acupuncture; SA: sham acupuncture; EA: electroacupuncture; nCPAP: nasal continuous positive airway pressure; PSG: polysomnography; AHI: apnea/hypopnea index; HI: hypopnea index; AI: apnea index.

out appropriately in these two trials; the investigators conducted RCT according to a strict study protocol approved by the ethical committee of the Universidade Federal de Sao Paulo. None of the four remaining studies [23, 25–27] provided detailed information about the allocation concealment and blinding of participants and personnel. The blinding of outcome measure was judged to low risk of bias because all the outcomes were measured depending on the records of PSG; the accuracy and objectivity were unlikely to be influenced by lack of blinding. Regarding the selective reporting, all the trials were judged to low risk of bias, since we only included studies that reported AHI, apnea

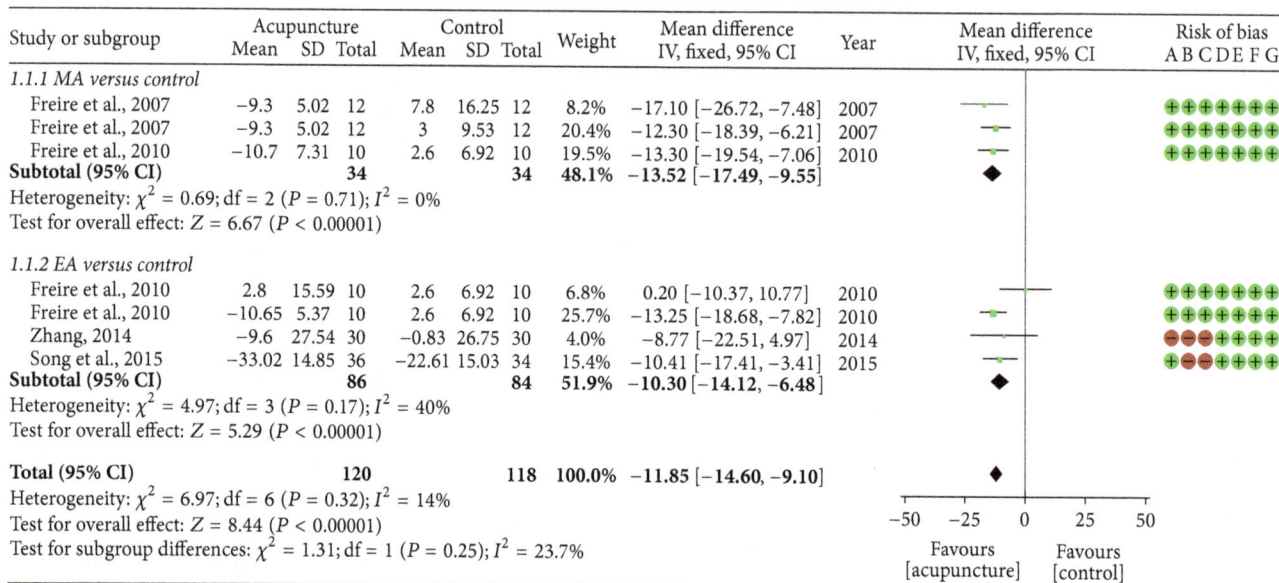

Study or subgroup	Acupuncture Mean	SD	Total	Control Mean	SD	Total	Weight	Mean difference IV, fixed, 95% CI	Year	Mean difference IV, fixed, 95% CI	Risk of bias A B C D E F G
1.1.1 MA versus control											
Freire et al., 2007	−9.3	5.02	12	7.8	16.25	12	8.2%	−17.10 [−26.72, −7.48]	2007		++++++
Freire et al., 2007	−9.3	5.02	12	3	9.53	12	20.4%	−12.30 [−18.39, −6.21]	2007		++++++
Freire et al., 2010	−10.7	7.31	10	2.6	6.92	10	19.5%	−13.30 [−19.54, −7.06]	2010		++++++
Subtotal (95% CI)			34			34	48.1%	−13.52 [−17.49, −9.55]			

Heterogeneity: $\chi^2 = 0.69$; df = 2 ($P = 0.71$); $I^2 = 0\%$
Test for overall effect: $Z = 6.67$ ($P < 0.00001$)

1.1.2 EA versus control											
Freire et al., 2010	2.8	15.59	10	2.6	6.92	10	6.8%	0.20 [−10.37, 10.77]	2010		++++++
Freire et al., 2010	−10.65	5.37	10	2.6	6.92	10	25.7%	−13.25 [−18.68, −7.82]	2010		++++++
Zhang, 2014	−9.6	27.54	30	−0.83	26.75	30	4.0%	−8.77 [−22.51, 4.97]	2014		⊖⊖⊖++++
Song et al., 2015	−33.02	14.85	36	−22.61	15.03	34	15.4%	−10.41 [−17.41, −3.41]	2015		⊖⊖⊖++++
Subtotal (95% CI)			86			84	51.9%	−10.30 [−14.12, −6.48]			

Heterogeneity: $\chi^2 = 4.97$; df = 3 ($P = 0.17$); $I^2 = 40\%$
Test for overall effect: $Z = 5.29$ ($P < 0.00001$)

Total (95% CI)			120			118	100.0%	−11.85 [−14.60, −9.10]	

Heterogeneity: $\chi^2 = 6.97$; df = 6 ($P = 0.32$); $I^2 = 14\%$
Test for overall effect: $Z = 8.44$ ($P < 0.00001$)
Test for subgroup differences: $\chi^2 = 1.31$; df = 1 ($P = 0.25$); $I^2 = 23.7\%$

−50 −25 0 25 50
Favours [acupuncture] Favours [control]

Risk of bias:
(A): random sequence generation (selection bias).
(B): allocation concealment (selection bias).
(C): blinding of participants and personnel (performance bias).
(D): blinding of outcome assessment (detection bias).
(E): incomplete outcome data (attrition bias).
(F): selective reporting (reporting bias).
(G): other biases.

FIGURE 2: Forest plot of acupuncture therapy versus control group: AHI; the authors' judgment about each risk of bias item for each included study.

index, hypopnea index, and mean SaO_2 as outcome. No study reported adverse events associated with acupuncture sessions. Good compliance seemed to be achieved in all studies; each study reported characterized similarity of baseline. Finally, two studies [22, 24] were judged to low risk of bias; the four remaining studies [23, 25–27] were judged to high risk of bias. The risk of bias assessment of each study was listed in corresponding forest plot (Figures 2, 3, 4, 5, 6, and 7).

3.4. Meta-Analysis Results

3.4.1. Acupuncture versus Control

AHI. Four studies [22, 24, 25, 27] measured AHI as outcome; a fixed effect model was employed because there was no obvious heterogeneity among included studies. Compared with control group, both MA (−13.52 [−17.49, −9.55]) and EA (−10.30 [−14.12, −6.48]) could further improve AHI (Figure 2).

Apnea Index. Three studies [22, 24, 25] measure apnea index as outcome measurement; fixed effect model was used, since there was no obvious heterogeneity among the included studies. Compared with control group, both MA (−7.49 [−10.65, −4.34]) and EA (−5.86 [−10.32, −1.40]) could further improve apnea index (Figure 3).

Hypopnea Index. Three studies [22, 24, 25] measured hypopnea index as outcome measurement. Fixed effect model was

used for statistical analysis because there was no obvious heterogeneity among studies. The pooled data showed that MA was more effective in the improvement of hypopnea index compared with control group (−5.52 [−9.17, −1.87]), whereas there was no significant difference between EA (−0.71 [−4.54, 3.13]) and control group (Figure 4).

Mean SaO₂. Two studies [22, 24] measured mean SaO_2 as outcome assessment. Since there was no obvious heterogeneity among studies, fixed effect model was utilized for statistical analysis. The combined data suggested that MA (2.04 [1.09, 3.00]) could further improve mean SaO_2 but EA (1.07 [−0.46, 2.60]) could not (Figure 5).

3.4.2. Acupuncture versus nCPAP

AHI. Two studies [23, 26] employed AHI as outcome; obvious heterogeneity existed among studies (heterogeneity: $\tau^2 = 46.11$; $\chi^2 = 2.66$; df = 1 ($P = 0.10$); $I^2 = 62\%$). Thus, random effect model was utilized for data analysis; the combined data showed that MA was more effective in improving the AHI when compared with nCPAP (−12.49 [−24.08, −0.90]) (Figure 6).

Mean SaO₂. Two studies [23, 26] recorded mean SaO_2 in MA group and nCPAP group; the heterogeneity could be observed so the random effect model was used (heterogeneity: $\tau^2 = 85.99$; $\chi^2 = 34.18$; df = 1 ($P < 0.00001$); $I^2 = 97\%$).

Study or subgroup	Acupuncture Mean	SD	Total	Control Mean	SD	Total	Weight	Mean difference IV, fixed, 95% CI	Year	Mean difference IV, fixed, 95% CI	Risk of bias A B C D E F G
1.2.1 MA versus control											
Freire et al., 2007	−6.6	4.1	12	0	6.38	12	36.1%	−6.60 [−10.89, −2.31]	2007		+ + + + + + +
Freire et al., 2007	−6.6	4.1	12	2.5	8.83	12	21.9%	−9.10 [−14.61, −3.59]	2007		+ + + + + + +
Freire et al., 2010	−4.45	11.19	10	2.7	8.62	10	8.7%	−7.15 [−15.90, 1.60]	2010		+ + + + + + +
Subtotal (95% CI)			34			34	66.6%	**−7.49 [−10.65, −4.34]**			
Heterogeneity: $\chi^2 = 0.50$; df = 2 ($P = 0.78$); $I^2 = 0\%$											
Test for overall effect: $Z = 4.65$ ($P < 0.00001$)											
1.2.2 EA versus control											
Freire et al., 2010	−7.9	9.64	10	2.7	8.62	10	10.3%	−10.60 [−18.62, −2.58]	2010		+ + + + + + +
Freire et al., 2010	−3.7	7.81	10	2.7	8.62	10	12.8%	−6.40 [−13.61, 0.81]	2010		+ + + + + + +
Zhang, 2014	−0.38	16.38	30	0.05	15.39	30	10.3%	−0.43 [−8.47, 7.61]	2014		− − − + + + +
Subtotal (95% CI)			50			50	33.4%	**−5.86 [−10.32, −1.40]**			
Heterogeneity: $\chi^2 = 3.12$; df = 2 ($P = 0.21$); $I^2 = 36\%$											
Test for overall effect: $Z = 2.58$ ($P = 0.010$)											
Total (95% CI)			84			84	100.0%	**−6.95 [−9.53, −4.37]**			
Heterogeneity: $\chi^2 = 3.96$; df = 5 ($P = 0.56$); $I^2 = 0\%$											
Test for overall effect: $Z = 5.29$ ($P < 0.00001$)											
Test for subgroup differences: $\chi^2 = 0.34$; df = 1 ($P = 0.56$); $I^2 = 0\%$											

$$-20 \quad -10 \quad 0 \quad 10 \quad 20$$
Favours [acupuncture]   Favours [control]

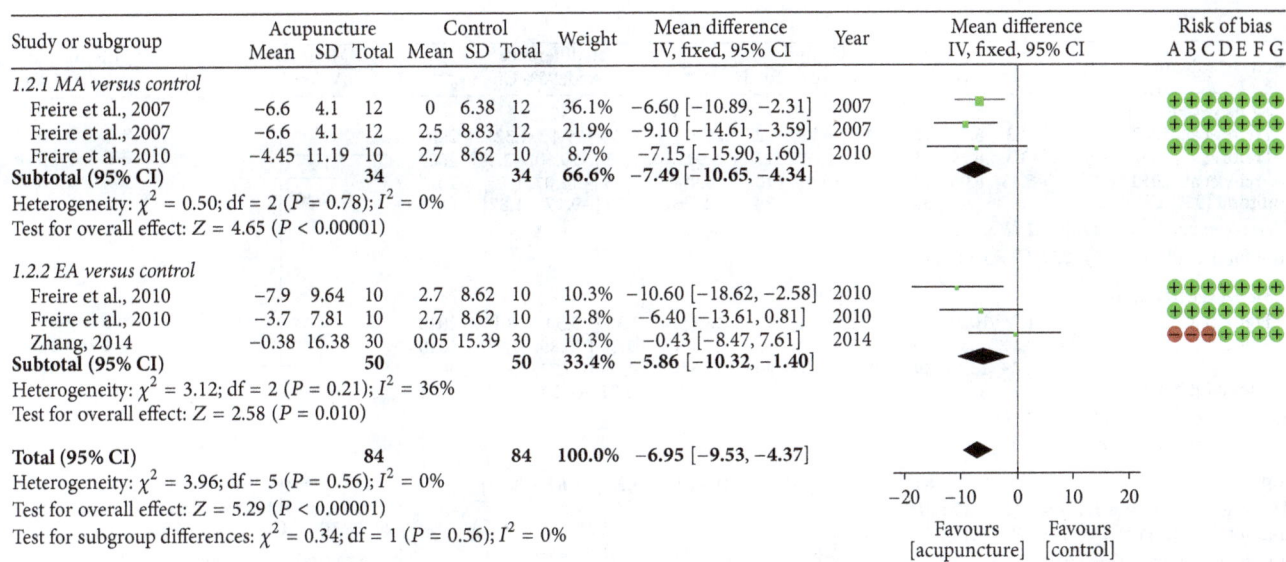

Risk of bias:
(A): random sequence generation (selection bias).
(B): allocation concealment (selection bias).
(C): blinding of participants and personnel (performance bias).
(D): blinding of outcome assessment (detection bias).
(E): incomplete outcome data (attrition bias).
(F): selective reporting (reporting bias).
(G): other biases.

FIGURE 3: Forest plot of acupuncture therapy versus control group: apnea index; the authors' judgment about each risk of bias item for each included study.

Regarding the improvement in mean SaO_2 no significant difference could be detected between MA and nCPAP (5.98 [−7.07, 19.02]) (Figure 7).

3.5. Adverse Events. All the enrolled patients were informed about the possible risks of acupuncture treatment such as infection, fainting, and hematoma. Ideal compliance seemed to be achieved in each study; no adverse events associated with acupuncture therapy were reported.

3.6. Publication Bias. The publication bias in our meta-analysis was not explored since the amount of included studies was insufficient. The potential of publication bias could not be excluded.

4. Discussion

To the best of our knowledge, this is the first meta-analysis aiming to assess the clinical effect of acupuncture therapy in the treatment of OSA; six studies involving 362 subjects were selected in our study. The findings of our work suggest that MA was more effective in the improvement of AHI, apnea index, hypopnea index, and mean SaO_2 when compared with nonspecific treatment; EA could further improve AHI and apnea index; there was no significant difference regarding the improvement of hypopnea index and SaO_2. Regarding the comparison of MA and nCPAP, MA was more effective in improving AHI. No adverse events associated with acupuncture therapy were documented.

The goal of OSA treatment is reduction in sleep disruption and the AHI, with resultant improved overall health and quality of life. Despite the remarkable efficacy of nCPAP, patients often have difficulty in adhering to it or may switch to CAM therapy because of the cumbersome nature of CPAP and the socioeconomic burden. In our current review, acupuncture therapy was compared with nonspecific treatment and nCPAP separately. In the comparison of MA and control group, all included studies showed a consistency regarding the improvement of AHI, apnea index, hypopnea index, and mean SaO_2; heterogeneity among these studies was acceptable. However, compared to control group, EA was only effective in the improvement of AHI and apnea index. In terms of the comparison between MA and nCPAP, MA was more effective in the improvement of AHI; no significant difference was found in the improvement of SaO_2.

Based on the quality assessment of our included studies, only two studies were judged to low risk of bias, whereas the remaining four studies were judged to high risk of bias. The methodological deficiency might limit the paucity of conclusions and lead to overstatement of clinical efficacy of acupuncture therapy. Lack of blinding procedures in RCTs can also exaggerate the conclusions of these trials. In the clinical trial conducted by Ernest and Resch, specific and/or nonspecific effects indicated that a treatment had been successful [29]. Acupuncture has the potential to elicit very powerful placebo effects [30]. Not surprisingly, therefore, almost all patients treated with sham acupuncture may respond positively in some manner [31]. In our study, we

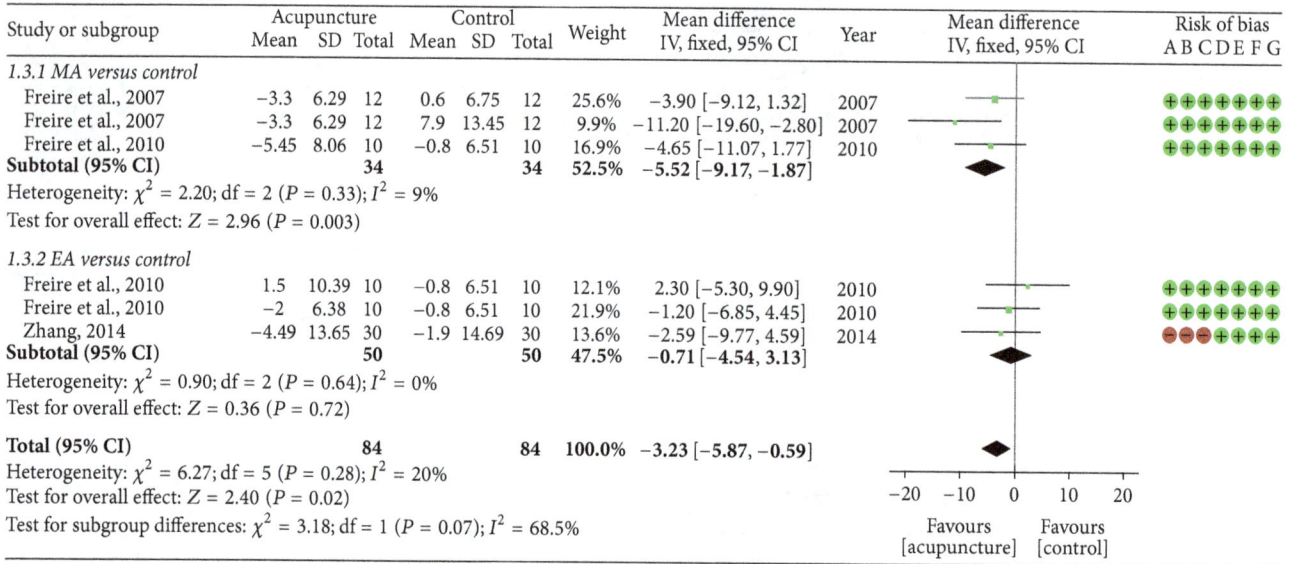

Study or subgroup	Acupuncture Mean	SD	Total	Control Mean	SD	Total	Weight	Mean difference IV, fixed, 95% CI	Year	Mean difference IV, fixed, 95% CI	Risk of bias A B C D E F G
1.3.1 MA versus control											
Freire et al., 2007	−3.3	6.29	12	0.6	6.75	12	25.6%	−3.90 [−9.12, 1.32]	2007		+ + + + + + +
Freire et al., 2007	−3.3	6.29	12	7.9	13.45	12	9.9%	−11.20 [−19.60, −2.80]	2007		+ + + + + + +
Freire et al., 2010	−5.45	8.06	10	−0.8	6.51	10	16.9%	−4.65 [−11.07, 1.77]	2010		+ + + + + + +
Subtotal (95% CI)			34			34	52.5%	−5.52 [−9.17, −1.87]			
Heterogeneity: $\chi^2 = 2.20$; df = 2 ($P = 0.33$); $I^2 = 9\%$											
Test for overall effect: $Z = 2.96$ ($P = 0.003$)											
1.3.2 EA versus control											
Freire et al., 2010	1.5	10.39	10	−0.8	6.51	10	12.1%	2.30 [−5.30, 9.90]	2010		+ + + + + + +
Freire et al., 2010	−2	6.38	10	−0.8	6.51	10	21.9%	−1.20 [−6.85, 4.45]	2010		+ + + + + + +
Zhang, 2014	−4.49	13.65	30	−1.9	14.69	30	13.6%	−2.59 [−9.77, 4.59]	2014		− − − + + + +
Subtotal (95% CI)			50			50	47.5%	−0.71 [−4.54, 3.13]			
Heterogeneity: $\chi^2 = 0.90$; df = 2 ($P = 0.64$); $I^2 = 0\%$											
Test for overall effect: $Z = 0.36$ ($P = 0.72$)											
Total (95% CI)			84			84	100.0%	−3.23 [−5.87, −0.59]			
Heterogeneity: $\chi^2 = 6.27$; df = 5 ($P = 0.28$); $I^2 = 20\%$											
Test for overall effect: $Z = 2.40$ ($P = 0.02$)											
Test for subgroup differences: $\chi^2 = 3.18$; df = 1 ($P = 0.07$); $I^2 = 68.5\%$											

−20 −10 0 10 20
Favours [acupuncture]   Favours [control]

Risk of bias:
(A): random sequence generation (selection bias).
(B): allocation concealment (selection bias).
(C): blinding of participants and personnel (performance bias).
(D): blinding of outcome assessment (detection bias).
(E): incomplete outcome data (attrition bias).
(F): selective reporting (reporting bias).
(G): other biases.

FIGURE 4: Forest plot of acupuncture therapy versus control group: hypopnea index; the authors' judgment about each risk of bias item for each included study.

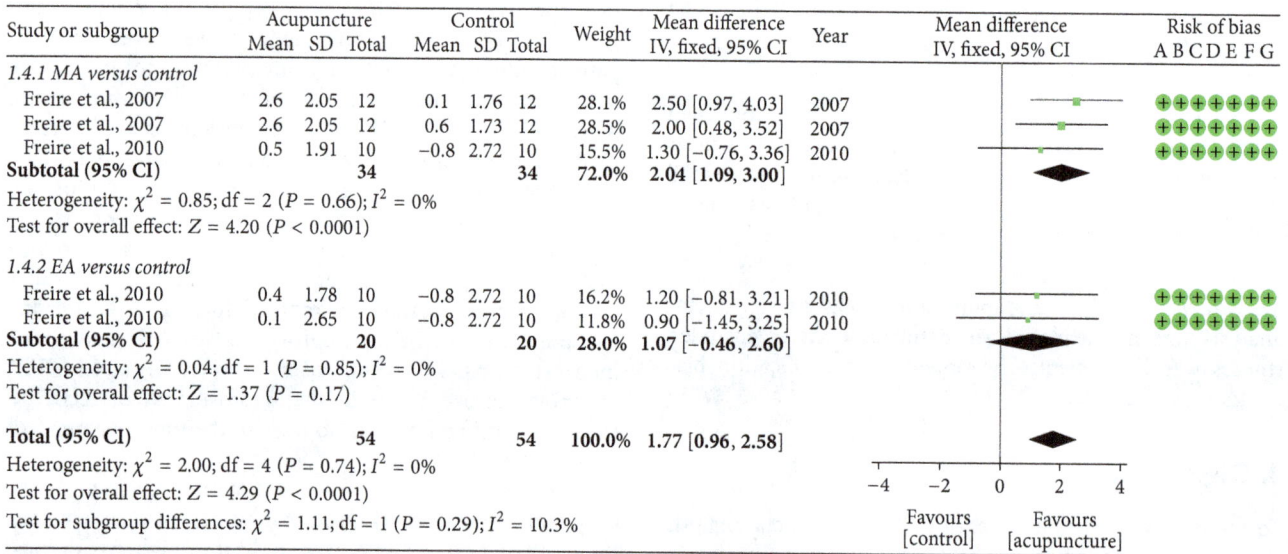

Study or subgroup	Acupuncture Mean	SD	Total	Control Mean	SD	Total	Weight	Mean difference IV, fixed, 95% CI	Year	Mean difference IV, fixed, 95% CI	Risk of bias A B C D E F G
1.4.1 MA versus control											
Freire et al., 2007	2.6	2.05	12	0.1	1.76	12	28.1%	2.50 [0.97, 4.03]	2007		+ + + + + + +
Freire et al., 2007	2.6	2.05	12	0.6	1.73	12	28.5%	2.00 [0.48, 3.52]	2007		+ + + + + + +
Freire et al., 2010	0.5	1.91	10	−0.8	2.72	10	15.5%	1.30 [−0.76, 3.36]	2010		+ + + + + + +
Subtotal (95% CI)			34			34	72.0%	2.04 [1.09, 3.00]			
Heterogeneity: $\chi^2 = 0.85$; df = 2 ($P = 0.66$); $I^2 = 0\%$											
Test for overall effect: $Z = 4.20$ ($P < 0.0001$)											
1.4.2 EA versus control											
Freire et al., 2010	0.4	1.78	10	−0.8	2.72	10	16.2%	1.20 [−0.81, 3.21]	2010		+ + + + + + +
Freire et al., 2010	0.1	2.65	10	−0.8	2.72	10	11.8%	0.90 [−1.45, 3.25]	2010		+ + + + + + +
Subtotal (95% CI)			20			20	28.0%	1.07 [−0.46, 2.60]			
Heterogeneity: $\chi^2 = 0.04$; df = 1 ($P = 0.85$); $I^2 = 0\%$											
Test for overall effect: $Z = 1.37$ ($P = 0.17$)											
Total (95% CI)			54			54	100.0%	1.77 [0.96, 2.58]			
Heterogeneity: $\chi^2 = 2.00$; df = 4 ($P = 0.74$); $I^2 = 0\%$											
Test for overall effect: $Z = 4.29$ ($P < 0.0001$)											
Test for subgroup differences: $\chi^2 = 1.11$; df = 1 ($P = 0.29$); $I^2 = 10.3\%$											

−4 −2 0 2 4
Favours [control]   Favours [acupuncture]

Risk of bias:
(A): random sequence generation (selection bias).
(B): allocation concealment (selection bias).
(C): blinding of participants and personnel (performance bias).
(D): blinding of outcome assessment (detection bias).
(E): incomplete outcome data (attrition bias).
(F): selective reporting (reporting bias).
(G): other biases.

FIGURE 5: Forest plot of acupuncture therapy versus control group: mean SaO_2; the authors' judgment about each risk of bias item for each included study.

Study or subgroup	Acupuncture Mean	SD	Total	Control Mean	SD	Total	Weight	Mean difference IV, random, 95% CI	Year	Mean difference IV, random, 95% CI	Risk of bias A B C D E F G
Bo et al., 2008	−5.31	27.28	44	−0.32	24.89	22	38.3%	−4.99 [−18.15, 8.17]	2008		⊕⊕⊕⊕⊕⊕⊕
Zhang et al., 2014	−13.71	18.71	45	3.44	11.21	45	61.7%	−17.15 [−23.52, −10.78]	2014		⊖⊖⊖⊕⊕⊕⊕
Total (95% CI)			**89**			**67**	**100.0%**	**−12.49 [−24.08, −0.90]**			

Heterogeneity: $\tau^2 = 46.11$; $\chi^2 = 2.66$; df = 1 ($P = 0.10$); $I^2 = 62\%$

Test for overall effect: $Z = 2.11$ ($P = 0.03$)

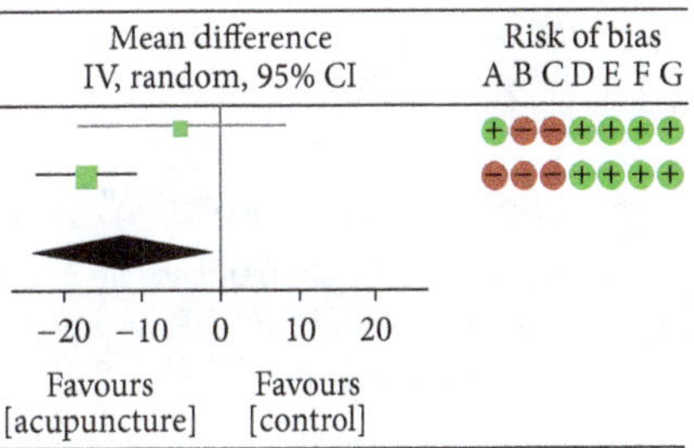

−20 −10 0 10 20

Favours [acupuncture] Favours [control]

Risk of bias:
(A): random sequence generation (selection bias).
(B): allocation concealment (selection bias).
(C): blinding of participants and personnel (performance bias).
(D): blinding of outcome assessment (detection bias).
(E): incomplete outcome data (attrition bias).
(F): selective reporting (reporting bias).
(G): other biases.

FIGURE 6: Forest plot of MA versus nCPAP: AHI; the authors' judgment about each risk of bias item for each included study.

Study or subgroup	Acupuncture Mean	SD	Total	Control Mean	SD	Total	Weight	Mean difference IV, random, 95% CI	Year	Mean difference IV, random, 95% CI	Risk of bias A B C D E F G
Bo et al., 2008	0.65	4	44	1.2	3.31	22	51.0%	−0.55 [−2.37, 1.27]	2008		⊕⊕⊕⊕⊕⊕⊕
Zhang et al., 2014	15.76	9.4	45	3	10.3	45	49.0%	12.76 [8.69, 16.83]	2014		⊖⊖⊖⊕⊕⊕⊕
Total (95% CI)			**89**			**67**	**100.0%**	**5.98 [−7.07, 19.02]**			

Heterogeneity: $\tau^2 = 85,99$; $\chi^2 = 34.18$; df = 1 ($P < 0.00001$); $I^2 = 97\%$

Test for overall effect: $Z = 0.90$ ($P = 0.37$)

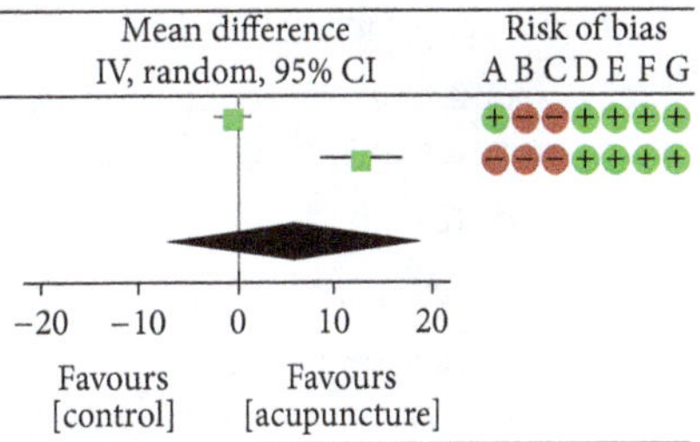

−20 −10 0 10 20

Favours [control] Favours [acupuncture]

Risk of bias:
(A): random sequence generation (selection bias).
(B): allocation concealment (selection bias).
(C): blinding of participants and personnel (performance bias).
(D): blinding of outcome assessment (detection bias).
(E): incomplete outcome data (attrition bias).
(F): selective reporting (reporting bias).
(G): other biases.

FIGURE 7: Forest plot of MA versus nCPAP: mean SaO_2; the authors' judgment about each risk of bias item for each included study.

selected AHI, apnea index, hypopnea index, and mean SaO_2 as outcome assessment because these data could be directly recorded by overnight PSG. Thus, the accuracy and the objectivity of outcome would not be influenced by lack of blinding.

As an alternative modality of MA, EA has been used frequently in clinical and basic search, but the underlying mechanism of EA and MA might differ to some extent, since EA causes the release of beta-endorphin and adrenocorticotrophic hormone into plasma, whereas MA releases only beta-endorphin [20, 32]. Freire et al. found that comparison of the results between the groups after treatment showed that the MA group and the 10 Hz EA group significantly differed from both the 2 Hz EA and control groups in all the polysomnographic parameters, specifically in the primary outcome, AHI. Freire and colleagues attributed this improvement to the involvement of serotonergic pathways in the responses mediated by acupuncture as well as its anti-inflammatory effect [33–35]. In our systematic review, different types of acupuncture including MA, 2 Hz EA, and 10 Hz EA were treated as one type of therapy and the data

were combined without differentiating acupoint selection or acupuncture modalities. Thus, the findings of this review indicate an overall trend of efficacy; definite conclusions could not be drawn.

Proper ethical research needs to take into consideration not only the cost of treatment or wait time for treatment but also a thorough understanding of the nature of acupuncture therapy. Further studies with strict study design and larger sample size are encouraged.

5. Conclusion

In summary, the results of our review suggest that both MA and EA were effective in improving AHI and mean SaO_2; additionally, MA could further improve apnea index and hypopnea index when compared with control treatment. Regarding the comparison of MA and nCPAP, no definite conclusion could be drawn due to the limited evidence. Additional RCTs with rigorous study design and larger sample size are required.

Appendix

Pubmed

(1) "Sleep Apnea, Obstructive" [MeSH]

(2) (OSAHS OR obstructive sleep apnea OR sleep apnea OR sleep hypopnea OR upper airway resistance sleep apnea syndrome)

(3) (1) or (2)

(4) "Acupuncture Therapy" [MeSH]

(5) (acupuncture or moxibustion or acupoint or acupressure OR acustimulation)

(6) (4) or (5)

(7) (3) and (6)

EMBASE

(1) exp acupuncture/

(2) (acupuncture or acupuncture therapy or meridians or moxibustion or ear acupuncture).af.

(3) (1) or (2)

(4) exp sleep disordered breathing/

(5) (Obstructive sleep apnea* or obstructive sleep apnea hypopnea syndrome or sleep apnea*).af.

(6) (4) or (5)

(7) (3) and (6)

Additional Points

This review highlights the clinical effect of manual acupuncture and electroacupuncture in the treatment of patients with obstructive sleep apnea.

Competing Interests

The authors declare that they have no competing interests regarding the publication of this paper.

Acknowledgments

The present study was supported by The National High Technology Research and Development Program of China (863 Program) (no. 2012AA02A612) and the National Natural Science Foundation of China (no. 81472082 and no. 81171696).

References

[1] K. R. Billings and J. Maddalozzo, "Complementary and integrative treatments: managing obstructive sleep apnea," *Otolaryngologic Clinics of North America*, vol. 46, no. 3, pp. 383–388, 2013.

[2] R. J. Schwab, K. B. Gupta, W. B. Gefter, L. J. Metzger, E. A. Hoffman, and A. I. Pack, "Upper airway and soft tissue anatomy in normal subjects and patients with sleep-disordered breathing: significance of the lateral pharyngeal walls," *American Journal of Respiratory and Critical Care Medicine*, vol. 152, no. 5, part 1, pp. 1673–1689, 1995.

[3] J. E. Remmers, W. J. DeGroot, E. K. Sauerland, and A. M. Anch, "Pathogenesis of upper airway occlusion during sleep," *Journal of Applied Physiology: Respiratory Environmental and Exercise Physiology*, vol. 44, no. 6, pp. 931–938, 1978.

[4] American Sleep Disorders Association, "Practice parameters for the treatment of obstructive sleep apnea in adults: the efficacy of surgical modifications of the upper airway. Report of the American Sleep Disorders Association," *Sleep*, vol. 19, no. 2, pp. 152–155, 1996.

[5] R. N. Aurora and N. M. Punjabi, "Obstructive sleep apnoea and type 2 diabetes mellitus: a bidirectional association," *The Lancet Respiratory Medicine*, vol. 1, no. 4, pp. 329–338, 2013.

[6] E. O. Bixler, A. N. Vgontzas, H.-M. Lin et al., "Association of hypertension and sleep-disordered breathing," *Archives of Internal Medicine*, vol. 160, no. 15, pp. 2289–2295, 2000.

[7] A. Głębocka, A. Kossowska, and M. Bednarek, "Obstructive sleep apnea and the quality of life," *Journal of Physiology and Pharmacology*, vol. 57, no. 4, pp. 111–117, 2006.

[8] I. Gurubhagavatula, "Consequences of obstructive sleep apnoea," *Indian Journal of Medical Research*, vol. 131, no. 2, pp. 188–195, 2010.

[9] J. Kokkarinen, "Obstructive sleep apnea-hypopnea and incident stroke: the sleep heart health study," *American Journal of Respiratory and Critical Care Medicine*, vol. 183, no. 7, p. 950, 2011.

[10] P. Lavie, P. Herer, and V. Hoffstein, "Obstructive sleep apnoea syndrome as a risk factor for hypertension: population study," *British Medical Journal*, vol. 320, no. 7233, pp. 479–482, 2000.

[11] M. H. Sanders, "Article reviewed: association of sleep-disordered breathing, sleep apnea, and hypertension in a large community-based study," *Sleep Medicine*, vol. 1, no. 4, pp. 327–328, 2000.

[12] C. F. Emery, M. R. Green, and S. Suh, "Neuropsychiatric function in chronic lung disease: the role of pulmonary rehabilitation," *Respiratory Care*, vol. 53, no. 9, pp. 1208–1216, 2008.

[13] D. I. Loube, P. C. Gay, K. P. Strohl, A. I. Pack, D. P. White, and N. A. Collop, "Indications for positive airway pressure treatment of adult obstructive sleep apnea patients: a consensus statement," *Chest*, vol. 115, no. 3, pp. 863–866, 1999.

[14] H. M. Engleman, S. E. Martin, I. J. Deary, and N. J. Douglas, "Effect of continuous positive airway pressure treatment on daytime function in sleep apnoea/hypopnoea syndrome," *The Lancet*, vol. 343, no. 8897, pp. 572–575, 1994.

[15] L. J. Epstein, D. Kristo, P. J. Strollo Jr. et al., "Clinical guideline for the evaluation, management and long-term care of obstructive sleep apnea in adults," *Journal of Clinical Sleep Medicine*, vol. 5, no. 3, pp. 263–276, 2009.

[16] M. Marklund, J. Verbraecken, and W. Randerath, "Non-CPAP therapies in obstructive sleep apnea: mandibular advancement device therapy," *European Respiratory Journal*, vol. 39, no. 5, pp. 1241–1247, 2012.

[17] W. J. Randerath, J. Verbraecken, S. Andreas et al., "Non-CPAP therapies in obstructive sleep apnoea," *European Respiratory Journal*, vol. 37, no. 5, pp. 1000–1028, 2011.

[18] S. Palmer, S. Selvaraj, C. Dunn et al., "Annual review of patients with sleep apnea/hypopnea syndrome—a pragmatic randomised trial of nurse home visit versus consultant clinic review," *Sleep Medicine*, vol. 5, no. 1, pp. 61–65, 2004.

[19] J. Pancer, S. Al-Faifi, M. Al-Faifi, and V. Hoffstein, "Evaluation of variable mandibular advancement appliance for treatment of snoring and sleep apnea," *Chest*, vol. 116, no. 6, pp. 1511–1518, 1999.

[20] Z. T. Lv, W. Song, J. Wu et al., "Efficacy of acupuncture in children with nocturnal enuresis: a systematic review and meta-analysis of randomized controlled trials," *Evidence-Based Complementary and Alternative Medicine*, vol. 2015, Article ID 320701, 12 pages, 2015.

[21] D. Moher, A. Liberati, J. Tetzlaff, D. G. Altman, and P. Group, "Preferred reporting items for systematic reviews and meta-analyses: the PRISMA statement," *PLoS Medicine*, vol. 6, no. 7, Article ID e1000097, 2009.

[22] A. O. Freire, G. C. M. Sugai, F. S. Chrispin et al., "Treatment of moderate obstructive sleep apnea syndrome with acupuncture: a randomised, placebo-controlled pilot trial," *Sleep Medicine*, vol. 8, no. 1, pp. 43–50, 2007.

[23] B. Chen, X. S. Zhang, H. Huang, Y. Jia, and X. M. Xie, "A study on differences of curative effects of acupuncture and nCPAP for treatment of OSAHS," *Chinese Acupuncture and Moxibustion*, vol. 28, no. 2, pp. 79–83, 2008.

[24] A. O. Freire, G. C. M. Sugai, S. Maria Togeiro, L. Eugênio Mello, and S. Tufik, "Immediate effect of acupuncture on the sleep pattern of patients with obstructive sleep apnoea," *Acupuncture in Medicine*, vol. 28, no. 3, pp. 115–119, 2010.

[25] P. Zhang, "Treating 30 patients with obstructive sleep apnea hypopnea syndrome by laryngeal three acupoints," *Western Journal of Traditional Chinese Medicine*, vol. 27, no. 10, pp. 129–130, 2014.

[26] L. Zhang, L. Shi, H. Zhou et al., "Clinical observation on the effect of acupuncturein the treatment of 90 cases with obstructive sleep apnea," *China Health Industry*, no. 20, pp. 192–193.

[27] Y. Song, W. Yu, T. Xu, and X. Gu, "Curative observation of the electro-acupuncture and nasal continuous positive airway pressure on patients with obstructive sleep apnea hypoventilation syndrome," *Journal of Emergency in Traditional Chinese Medicine*, vol. 24, no. 8, pp. 1352–1356, 2015.

[28] J. P. T. Higgins and S. Green, *Cochrane Handbook for Systematic Reviews of Interventions*, Version 5.1.0, The Cochrane Collaboration, 2011.

[29] E. Ernst and K. L. Resch, "Concept of true and perceived placebo effects," *British Medical Journal*, vol. 311, no. 7004, pp. 551–553, 1995.

[30] T. J. Kaptchuk, "The placebo effect in alternative medicine: can the performance of a healing ritual have clinical significance?" *Annals of Internal Medicine*, vol. 136, no. 11, pp. 817–825, 2002.

[31] H. A. Taub, J. N. Mitchell, F. E. Stuber, L. Eisenberg, M. C. Beard, and R. K. McCormack, "Analgesia for operative dentistry: a comparison of acupuncture and placebo," *Oral Surgery, Oral Medicine, Oral Pathology*, vol. 48, no. 3, pp. 205–210, 1979.

[32] H.-F. Guo, J. Tian, X. Wang, Y. Fang, Y. Hou, and J. Han, "Brain substrates activated by electroacupuncture (EA) of different frequencies (II): role of Fos/Jun proteins in EA-induced transcription of preproenkephalin and preprodynorphin genes," *Molecular Brain Research*, vol. 43, no. 1-2, pp. 167–173, 1996.

[33] G. C. M. Sugai, O. Freire Ade, A. Tabosa, Y. Yamamura, S. Tufik, and L. E. Mello, "Serotonin involvement in the electroacupuncture- and moxibustion-induced gastric emptying in rats," *Physiology and Behavior*, vol. 82, no. 5, pp. 855–861, 2004.

[34] K. K. Sun, H. P. Jung, J. B. Sang et al., "Effects of electroacupuncture on cold allodynia in a rat model of neuropathic pain: mediation by spinal adrenergic and serotonergic receptors," *Experimental Neurology*, vol. 195, no. 2, pp. 430–436, 2005.

[35] S. P. Zhang, J. S. Zhang, K. K. L. Yung, and H. Q. Zhang, "Non-opioid-dependent anti-inflammatory effects of low frequency electroacupuncture," *Brain Research Bulletin*, vol. 62, no. 4, pp. 327–334, 2004.

PERMISSIONS

LIST OF CONTRIBUTORS

Jin Bae Weon, Min Rye Eom and Youn Sik Jung
Department of Medical Biomaterials Engineering, College of Biomedical Science, Kangwon National University, Chuncheon 200-701, Republic of Korea

Eun-Hye Hong and Hyun-Jeong Ko
Laboratory of Microbiology and Immunology, College of Pharmacy, Kangwon National University, Chuncheon 200–701, Republic of Korea

Hyeon Yong Lee
Department of Food Science and Engineering, Seowon University, Cheongju 361-742, Republic of Korea

Dong-Sik Park
Functional Food & Nutrition Division, Department of Agro-Food Resources, Suwon 441-853, Republic of Korea

Choong JeMa
Department of Medical Biomaterials Engineering, College of Biomedical Science, Kangwon National UniversVity, Chuncheon 200-701, Republic of Korea
Institute of Bioscience and Biotechnology, Kangwon National University, Chuncheon 200-701, Republic of Korea

Maxi Meissner
Department of Organizational Psychology, Faculty of Behavioural and Social Sciences, University of Groningen, Netherlands

Marja H. Cantell
Centre for Special Educational Needs and Youth Care, Faculty of Behavioural and Social Sciences, University of Groningen, Netherlands

Ronald Steiner
Sport- und Rehamedizin Universitätsklinikum Ulm, Germany

Xavier Sanchez
Department of Medical and Sport Sciences, University of Cumbria, Lancaster, UK

Yanfei He, Siyu Chen, Hai Yu, Long Zhu, Yayun Liu, Chunyang Han and Cuiyan Liu
College of Animal Science and Technology, Anhui Agricultural University, 130 ChangjiangWest Road, Hefei, Anhui 230036, China

Fernando Almeida-Souza
Laboratório de Imunomodulaçaõ e Protozoologia, Instituto Oswaldo Cruz, Fiocruz, 21040-900 Rio de JaneViro, RJ, Brazil
Departamento de Patologia, Universidade Estadual do Maranhão, 65055-310 São Luís, MA, Brazil

Noemi Nosomi Taniwaki
Unidade de Microscopia Eletrônica, Instituto Adolf Lutz, 01246-000 São Paulo, SP, Brazil

Ana Cláudia Fernandes Amaral
Unidade de Microscopia Eletrônica, Instituto Adolf Lutz, 01246-000 São Paulo, SP, Brazil

Celeste da Silva Freitas de Souza and Kátia da Silva Calabrese
Laboratório de Imunomodulaçaõ e Protozoologia, Instituto Oswaldo Cruz, Fiocruz, 21040-900 Rio de Janeiro, RJ, Brazil

Ana Lúcia Abreu-Silva
Departamento de Patologia, Universidade Estadual do Maranhão, 65055-310 São Luís, MA, Brazil

Reza Farzinebrahimi, RosnaMat Taha and Bakrudeen Ali Ahmed
Institute of Biological Sciences (IBS), Faculty of Science, University of Malaya, 50603 Kuala Lumpur, Malaysia

Kamaludin A. Rashid and Shahril Efzueni Rozali
Biology Division, Center for Foundation Studies in Science, University of Malaya, 50603 Kuala Lumpur, Malaysia

Mahmoud Danaee
Academic Development Centre (AdeC),Wisma R&D, University of Malaya, 59990 Kuala Lumpur, Malaysia

Woo-Sang Jung, Seungwon Kwon, Seung-Yeon Cho, Seong-Uk Park, Sang-Kwan Moon, Jung-Mi Park, Chang-Nam Ko and Ki-Ho Cho
Department of Cardiology and Neurology, College of Korean Medicine, Kyung Hee University, Seoul 02447, Republic of Korea

Yang Yang and Eun-Hee Hwang
Department of Food and Nutrition, School of Human Environmental Sciences,Wonkwang University, Iksan 570-749, Republic of Korea

Bok-Im Park and Yong-Ouk You
Department of Oral Biochemistry, School of Dentistry,Wonkwang University, Iksan 570-749, Republic of Korea

You Yeon Choi, Mi Hye Kim and Woong Mo Yang
Department of Convergence Korean Medical Science, College of Korean Medicine, Kyung Hee University, Seoul 02447, Republic of Korea

Jongki Hong
College of Pharmacy, Kyung Hee University, Seoul 02447, Republic of Korea

Kyuseok Kim
Department of Ophthalmology, Otorhinolaryngology and Dermatology of Korean Medicine, College of Korean Medicine, Kyung Hee University, Seoul 02447, Republic of Korea

Shintaro Ishikawa,Misako Tamaki, Yui Ogawa, Kiyomi Kaneki, Meng Zhang, Masataka Sunagawa and Tadashi Hisamitsu
Department of Physiology, School of Medicine, Showa University, 1-5-8 Hatanodai, Shinagawa-ku, Tokyo 142-8555, Japan

Sheng-feng Lu, Ning Wang, Wei-xing Shen, Shu-ping Fu, Qian Li, Mei-ling Yu, Xia Chen and Xin-yue Jing
Key Laboratory of Acupuncture and Medicine Research of Ministry of Education, Nanjing University of Chinese Medicine, Nanjing 210023, China

Yan Huang
Key Laboratory of Acupuncture and Medicine Research of Ministry of Education, Nanjing University of Chinese Medicine, Nanjing 210023, China
Key Laboratory of Acupuncture and Immunological Effects, Shanghai University of Traditional Chinese Medicine, Shanghai 200030, China

Wan-xin Liu
School of Veterinary Medicine, University of Pennsylvania, 3800 Spruce Street, Philadelphia, PA 19104, USA

Bing-mei Zhu
Key Laboratory of Acupuncture and Medicine Research of Ministry of Education, Nanjing University of Chinese Medicine, Nanjing 210023, China
Jiangxi University of Traditional Chinese Medicine, Nanchang 330004, China

Chalinee Ronpirin
Department of Preclinical Science, Faculty of Medicine, Thammasat University, Pathumthani 12120, Thailand

Nattaporn Pattarachotanant and Tewin Tencomnao
Department of Clinical Chemistry, Faculty of Allied Health Sciences, Chulalongkorn University, Bangkok 10330, Thailand

Tao Liu and Li Zhang
Institute of Digestive Diseases, Longhua Hospital, Shanghai University of Traditional Chinese Medicine, Shanghai 200032, China

Ning Wang
School of Chinese Medicine, Li Ka Shing Faculty of Medicine, University of Hong Kong, Pok Fu Lam, Hong Kong

Linda Zhong
School of Chinese Medicine, Hong Kong Chinese Medicine Study Centre, Hong Kong Baptist University, Kowloon Tong, Hong Kong

Juan Zhao, Tong-Tong Cao, Jing Tian, Hui-hua Chen, Chen Zhang, Hong-Chang Wei, Wei Guo and Rong Lu
Department of Pathology, Shanghai University of Traditional Chinese Medicine, 1200 Cailun Road, Shanghai 201203, China

Hen-Yu Liu
Stem Cell Research Center, Taipei Medical University, Taipei 110, Taiwan
School of Dentistry, College of Oral Medicine, Taipei Medical University, Taipei 110, Taiwan

Chiung-Fang Huang
Department of Dentistry, Taipei Medical University Hospital, Taipei 110, Taiwan

Chun-Hao Li, Ching-Yu Tsai, Wei-Hong Chen and Hong-Jian Wei
Stem Cell Research Center, Taipei Medical University, Taipei 110, Taiwan

Ming-Fu Wang
Department of Food and Nutrition, Providence University, Taichung 433, Taiwan

Yueh-Hsiung Kuo
Department of Chinese Pharmaceutical Sciences and Chinese Medicine Resources, China Medical University, Taichung 404, Taiwan
Department of Biotechnology, Asia University, Taichung 413, Taiwan

Mei-Leng Cheong
Department of Obstetrics and Gynecology, Cathay General Hospital, Taipei 106, Taiwan
College of Medicine, Taipei Medical University, Taipei 110, Taiwan

Win-Ping Deng
Stem Cell Research Center, Taipei Medical University, Taipei 110, Taiwan
Graduate Institute of Biomedical Materials and Tissue Engineering, Taipei Medical University, Taipei 110, Taiwan
Institute of Medicine, Fu Jen Catholic University, Taipei 242, Taiwan

Caragh Brosnan
School of Humanities and Social Science, Faculty of Education and Arts, University of Newcastle, University Drive, Callaghan, NSW 2308, Australia
Australian Research Centre in Complementary and Integrative Medicine, Faculty of Health, University of Technology Sydney, 15 Broadway, Ultimo, NSW 2007, Australia

Vincent C. H. Chung
Australian Research Centre in Complementary and Integrative Medicine, Faculty of Health, University of Technology Sydney, 15 Broadway, Ultimo, NSW 2007, VAustralia
The Jockey Club School of Public Health and Primary Care,The Chinese University of Hong Kong, Prince of Wales Hospital, Shatin, New Territories, Hong Kong

Anthony L. Zhang
Australian Research Centre in Complementary and Integrative Medicine, Faculty of Health, University of Technology Sydney, 15 Broadway, Ultimo, NSW 2007, Australia
Health Sciences, RMIT University, P.O. Box 71, Bundoora, VIC 3083, Australia

Jon Adams
Australian Research Centre in Complementary and Integrative Medicine, Faculty of Health, University of Technology Sydney, 15 Broadway, Ultimo, NSW 2007, Australia

Qianqian Yang
Zhejiang Hospital of Traditional Chinese Medicine, Zhejiang Chinese Medical University, 54 Youdian RoaVd, Hangzhou 310006, China
2College of Agronomy and Plant Protection, Qingdao Agricultural University, Qingdao 266109, China

Lei Gao
Shandong Provincial Research Center for Bioinformatic Engineering and Technique, School of Life Sciences, Shandong University of Technology, 266 West Cunxi Road, Zibo 255049, China

Maocan Tao, Zhe Chen, Xiaohong Yang and Yi Cao
ZhejiangHospital of Traditional Chinese Medicine, Zhejiang Chinese Medical University, 54 Youdian Road, Hangzhou 310006, China

Qiu-Ju Jiang, Weiwei Chen, Jinhua Shen, Yong-Bo Peng, Ping Zhao, Lu Xue, Meng-Fei Yu, Liqun Ma, Xiao-Tang Si, Li Tan, He Zhu and Qing-Hua Liu
Institute for Medical Biology & Hubei Provincial Key Laboratory for Protection and Application of Special Plants in Wuling Area of China, College of Life Sciences, South-Central University for Nationalities, Wuhan 430074, China

Hong Dan
Key Laboratory of Chinese Medicine Resource and Compound Prescription, Hubei University of Chinese Medicine, Wuhan 430065, China

Guangzhong Yang
College of Pharmacy, South-Central University for Nationalities, Wuhan 430074, China

Zhuo Wang and Jiapei Dai
Wuhan Institute for Neuroscience and Engineering, South-Central University for Nationalities, Wuhan 430074, China

Gangjian Qin
Department of Medicine-Cardiology, Feinberg Cardiovascular Research Institute, Northwestern University Feinberg School of Medicine, Chicago, IL 60611, USA

Chunbin Zou
Acute Lung Injury Center of Excellence, Division of Pulmonary, Allergy, and Critical Care Medicine, Department of Medicine, University of Pittsburgh School of Medicine, Pittsburgh, PA 15213, USA

Boyan Liu, Yanhui Du, Lixin Cong and Ge Yang
Department of Geriatrics, Affiliated Hospital, Changchun University of Traditional Chinese Medicine, Changchun 130000, China

Xiaoying Jia
Department of Neurology, Jilin Province People's Hospital, Changchun 130000, China

Jia Wang, Jiani Wu and Zhishun Liu
Department of Acupuncture, Guang'anmen Hospital, China Academy of Chinese Medical Sciences, No. 5 Beixiange Street, Xicheng District, Beijing 100053, China

Yanbing Zhai
Department of Acupuncture, Guang'anmen Hospital, China Academy of Chinese Medical Sciences, No. 5 Beixiange Street, Xicheng District, Beijing 100053, China

Shitong Zhao and Jing Zhou
Beijing University of Chinese Medicine, No. 11 North Third Ring Road, Chaoyang District, Beijing 100029, China

Jialing Zhang, Yong Huang, Shanshan Qu and Jiping Zhang
School of Traditional Chinese Medicine, Southern Medical University, Guangzhou, Guangdong 510515, China

Kangbai Huang, Guoxin Zhong and Suhe Li
Clinical Medical College of Acupuncture, Moxibustion and Rehabilitation, Guangzhou University of Chinese Medicine, Guangzhou, Guangdong 510006, China

Hongzhuan Xuan
Key Laboratory of Pollinating Insect Biology, Ministry of Agriculture, Beijing 100093, China
School of Life Science, Liaocheng University, Liaocheng 252059, China

Chongluo Fu, Yuanjun Wang and Yuehua Wang
School of Life Science, Liaocheng University, Liaocheng 252059, China

Aifeng Li
College of Chemistry and Chemical Engineering, Liaocheng University, Liaocheng 252059, China

Wenjun Peng
Key Laboratory of Pollinating Insect Biology, Ministry of Agriculture, Beijing 100093, China

Zheng-tao Lv, Jun-ming Huang, Jin-ming Zhang and An-min Chen
Department of Orthopedics, Tongji Hospital, Tongji Medical College, Huazhong University of Science and Technology, Wuhan, Hubei 430030, China

Wen-xiu Jiang
Department of Otolaryngology, Tongji Hospital, Tongji Medical College, Huazhong University of Science and Technology, Wuhan, Hubei 430030, China

Index

www.ingramcontent.com/pod-product-compliance
Lightning Source LLC
Chambersburg PA
CBHW082028190326
41458CB00010B/3304